Burn Care for General Surgeons and General Practitioners

David G. Greenhalgh
Editor

Burn Care for General Surgeons and General Practitioners

Springer

Editor
David G. Greenhalgh
Shriners Hospitals for Children Northern California
University of California, Davis Medical Center
Sacramento, California, USA

ISBN 978-3-319-29159-8 ISBN 978-3-319-29161-1 (eBook)
DOI 10.1007/978-3-319-29161-1

Library of Congress Control Number: 2016935289

Printed on acid-free paper

This Springer imprint is published by Springer Nature
The registered company is Springer International Publishing AG Switzerland

I would like to dedicate this book to my three mentors in burns—Richard Gamelli, David Heimbach, and Glenn Warden. I would also like to thank my wife, Kathy, for all of her patience with me while I was working on this textbook. Her support has been tremendous.

Foreword

Burn Care: Introduction

Understanding the critical needs of the burn patient is vital to the delivery of the necessary treatment if we are to limit impact of the burn injury and return the patient to their preinjury health and functional status. Burn Care for the surgeon is a ready resource for those caring for burn patients. Covered in a clear and well-organized approach are topics covering the physiologic response to the burn injury and what treatments are required during the early treatment phase and recovery.

Chicago, IL, USA Richard L. Gamelli

Preface

There have been tremendous advances in the management of burns. Within the past few decades, patients with massive burns, who in the past were not even resuscitated, are now surviving. It is now expected that children and young adults will survive and live productive lives. In the past it was expected that the elderly did not have a chance to survive sizeable burns but as the population ages, the number of elderly burn patients also increases. The care of the older patient has also become more aggressive and outcomes are surprisingly good. The focus of burn care is to optimize functional and cosmetic outcomes so that the survivor can return to a productive and enjoyable life.

Fortunately, most burns are relatively small so survival is not the issue but even small burns treated poorly can lead to life-long problems. If a small but deep hand burn is not treated optimally, then the resulting scar can limit function and lead to an unproductive life. While many caregivers feel that they know how to treat such small burns, it is surprising how little knowledge exists for the management of these problems. The American Board of Surgery no longer requires burn experience during the training of surgical residents. Plastic surgery training emphasizes a burn experience but the training of the acute management of burns is sketchy at best. Many non-surgeons manage small burns (pediatricians, family practitioners, emergency physicians) but their training is limited. The decision as to when a burn might need surgery is one of the most important considerations to optimize its outcome. Those physicians who train in the vicinity of a burn center may be exposed to burn care but as the number of burn centers decreases the availability to interact with a burn team decreases.

The purpose of this textbook is to provide the basic medical and surgical management of burns. The target audience is the non-surgeon, the trainee, residents, and those surgeons who want exposure to the basic principles of burn care. The book is also a reference for those surgeons who are training to become burn surgeons. Finally, the principles can be applied to anyone who manages burns in the third world. The book does not focus on highly advanced techniques but stresses burn care using simple, inexpensive and straightforward techniques that can be used by any caregiver.

Sacramento, CA, USA David G. Greenhalgh

Acknowledgements

I would like to acknowledge Matthew Harrison for his assistance with many of the photographs used in the publication. I would also like to acknowledge Wendy Vetter and the Springer illustrators for their skillful drawings. Finally, I would like to thank Lorraine Coffey for all of her assistance while serving as the textbook's developmental editor.

Sacramento, CA David G. Greenhalgh, M.D.

Contents

Contributors

Amy Acton, R.N., B.S.N. Phoenix Society for Burn Survivors, Grand Rapids, MI, USA

Gretchen J. Carrougher, R.N., M.N. Department of Surgery, University of Washington Regional Burn Center, Harborview Medical Center University of Washington, Seattle, WA, USA

Damien Wilson Carter, M.D. Department of Surgery, Maine Medical Center, Tuft's University, Portland, ME, USA

Robert Cartotto, M.D., F.R.C.S.C. Department of Surgery, Ross Tilley Burn Centre, Sunnybrook Health Sciences Centre, University of Toronto, Toronto, ON, Canada

Amalia Cochran, M.D., F.A.C.S. Department of Surgery, University of Utah Healthcare, Salt Lake City, UT, USA

Sharmila Dissanaike, M.D., F.A.C.S. Department of Surgery, Texas Tech University Health Sciences Center, Lubbock, TX, USA

Geneviève Ferland-Caron, M.D., F.R.C.S.C. Division of Plastic and Reconstructive Surgery, University of Alberta, Edmonton, AB, Canada

Kevin N. Foster, M.D., M.B.A., F.A.C.S. Department of Surgery, The Arizona Burn Center, Maricopa Integrated Health Systems, Phoenix, AZ, USA

Nicole Gibran, M.D., F.A.C.S. David & Nancy Auth - Washington Research Foundation Chair in Restorative Burn Surgery, Seattle, WA, USA

Daniel Goldberg, M.D. Rhode Island Burn Center at Rhode Island Hospital, Alpert Medical School of Brown University, Providence, RI, USA

Ernest J. Grant, Ph.D., R.N., F.A.A.N. North Carolina Jaycee Burn Center, UNC Hospitals, Chapel Hill, NC, USA

David G. Greenhalgh, M.D. Shriners Hospitals for Children Northern California and University of California, Davis Medical Center, Sacramento, CA, USA

David T. Harrington, M.D. Rhode Island Burn Center at Rhode Island Hospital, Alpert Medical School of Brown University, Providence, RI, USA

Radha K. Holavanahalli, Ph.D. Department of Physical Medicine and Rehabilitation, University of Texas Southwestern Medical Center, Dallas, TX, USA

Victor C. Joe, M.D., F.A.C.S. Department of Surgery, Burn Center, School of Medicine, Orange, CA, USA

University of California, Irvine Medical Center, Departmennt of Surgery, Orange, CA, USA

Peter Kwan, B.Sc., M.D., F.R.C.S.C. Department of Burn Surgery, University of California Davis Medical Center and Shriners Hospitals for Children Northern California, Sacramento, CA, USA

Department of Plastic and Reconstructive Surgery, University of Alberta, Edmonton, AB, Canada

Steven Maximus, M.D. Department of Surgery, Burn Center, School of Medicine, Orange, CA, USA

University of California, Irvine Medical Center, Departmennt of Surgery, Orange, CA, USA

Samantha A. Moore, M.D., Ph.D. Department of Surgery, Texas Tech University Health Sciences Center, Lubbock, TX, USA

Kevin Mowbrey, B.M.Sc., M.D. Division of Plastic and Reconstructive Surgery and Critical Care, Department of Surgery, University of Alberta, Edmonton, AB, Canada

Tina L. Palmieri, M.D., F.A.C.S., F.C.C.M. Firefighters Burn Institute Burn Center, University of California, Davis, Sacramento, CA, USA

Shriners Hospital for Children Northern California, Sacramento, CA, USA

Ingrid Parry, M.S., P.T. Department of Physical and Occupational Therapy, Shriners Hospital for Children, Sacramento, CA, USA

Tam N. Pham, M.D., F.A.C.S. Department of Surgery, University of Washington Regional Burn Center, Harborview Medical Center University of Washington, Seattle, WA, USA

Kathleen Romanowski, M.D. Division of Acute Care Surgery, Department of Surgery, University of Iowa Hospitals and Clinics, Iowa City, IA, USA

John A. Scavone, M.D. Department of Anesthesiology, Shriners Hospitals for Children Northern California, Sacramento, CA, USA

Soman Sen, M.D., F.A.C.S. Division of Burn Surgery, Department of Surgery, University of California, Davis, Sacramento, CA, USA

Robert L. Sheridan, M.D., F.A.A.P., F.A.C.S. Division of Burns, Massachusetts General Hospital, Department of Surgery, Harvard Medical School, Boston Shriners Hospital for Children, Boston, MA, USA

Edward E. Tredget, M.D., M.Sc., F.R.S.C. Division of Plastic and Reconstructive Surgery and Critical Care, Department of Surgery, University of Alberta, Edmonton, AB, Canada

Sundeep Tumber, D.O. Department of Anesthesiology, Shriners Hospitals for Children Northern California, Sacramento, CA, USA

Shelley Wiechman, Ph.D., A.B.P.P. Department of Rehabilitation Medicine, University of Washington School of Medicine, Seattle, WA, USA

Steven E. Wolf, M.D. Department of Surgery, University of Texas – Southwestern Medical Center, Dallas, TX, USA

Derek Yang, B.S. Department of Surgery, Texas Tech University Health Sciences Center, Lubbock, TX, USA

Epidemiology of Burn Injuries and Burn Care

1

Steven Maximus and Victor C. Joe

Introduction

It is estimated by the American Burn Association that approximately 486,000 patients suffered burn injuries that required medical treatment in 2013 [1]. A total of 3240 deaths were attributed to burn and inhalation injuries during this time period, including 2855 deaths from residential fires, 300 from vehicle fires, and 85 from other sources. The odds of a US resident dying from exposure to fire, flames, or smoke is 1 in 1141. For comparison, the odds of dying in a motor vehicle accident are 1 in 112. Data from the Centers for Disease Control's (CDC) Web-based Injury Statistics Query and Reporting System (WISQARS™) showed that in 2013 there were 3220 fatal and 405,327 nonfatal burn-related injuries [2]. Over the past five years there has not been a significant change in the number of burn injuries. The average number of fatal burn injuries was 3122, while the mean number of nonfatal burn injuries was 412,597. Tables 1.1 and 1.2 show the breakdown of fatal and nonfatal burn injuries according to age for 2013.

In 2013, there were 1,240,000 fires reported in the United States [3]. These fires caused 3240 deaths and 15,925 injuries. Of these fires, 487,500 were structure fires, which caused 2855 deaths and 14,075 injuries; 369,500 were residential fires, which accounted for 2755 deaths and 12,200 injuries; and 188,000 were vehicle fires, which caused 320 deaths and 1050 injuries. A fire department responded to a fire every 25 s, and a structure fire was reported every 65 s. One fire injury was reported every 33 min, and a fatality occurred every 2 h and 42 min. Residential fires accounted for approximately 4 % of burn admissions. However these patients had a 12 % mortality rate compared to a 3 % mortality rate for patients burned in other types of fires [4]. This difference in mortality is attributed to the prevalence of inhalation injury in residential fires [5].

Prediction of Mortality

Prediction of mortality is critical to evaluating the process of care and providing triage criteria, in addition to analyzing and standardizing populations for research purposes [6]. There are several formulas used specifically for predicting mortality in burn. Formulas commonly used to predict

S. Maximus, M.D. • V.C. Joe, M.D., FA.C.S. (✉)
Department of Surgery, Burn Center,
School of Medicine, Orange, CA, USA

University of California, Irvine Medical Center,
Department of Surgery, 333 City Blvd West,
Suite 1600, Orange, CA 92868, USA
e-mail: vcjoe@uci.edu

D.G. Greenhalgh (ed.), *Burn Care for General Surgeons and General Practitioners*,
DOI 10.1007/978-3-319-29161-1_1

Table 1.1 Fatal burn injuries by age group (2013)

Age	Burns	Age adjusted rate
Fatal burn injuries—2013		
0–4	165	0.83
5–9	101	0.49
10–14	51	0.25
15–19	62	0.29
20–24	100	0.44
25–29	103	0.48
30–34	102	0.48
35–39	118	0.60
40–44	141	0.68
45–49	209	0.99
50–54	257	1.14
55–59	329	1.55
60–64	312	1.72
65–69	242	1.66
70–74	219	2.06
75–79	234	3.05
80–84	230	3.99
85+	241	3.99
Total	3220	0.95

Table 1.2 Nonfatal burn injuries by age group (2013)

Age	Burns	Age adjusted rate
Nonfatal burn injuries 2013		
0–4	63,297	318.59
5–9	21,706	105.52
10–14	15,654	75.81
15–19	28,107	132.84
20–24	45,134	197.99
25–29	37,379	173.21
30–34	33,640	158.20
35–39	25,318	129.15
40–44	26,510	127.15
45–49	26,421	124.58
50–54	24,034	106.54
55–59	21,091	99.51
60–64	11,539	63.67
65–69	9653	66.08
70–74	4740	44.68
75–79	4589	59.76
80–84	2732	47.35
85+	3736	61.84
Total	405,327	131.28

mortality include the Ryan Score, Baux Scores, and the Abbreviated Burn Severity Index (ABSI). The Ryan Score is based on a study that included adult and pediatric patients admitted between 1990 and 1994 and identified three variables as major risk factors for mortality: burn size greater than 40 % total burn surface area (TBSA), age greater than 60, and the presence of inhalation injury [6, 7]. Mortality was found to be a function of the number of the risk factors present, and this study showed that inhalation injury significantly contributed to mortality [7]. The classic Baux Score was introduced in 1961 in order to predict mortality after burn injuries. It was defined as: *age+percent body burned=Baux Score* [8–10]. Traditionally, a Baux Score of 100 is associated with a mortality of 50 %. This method of scoring has been criticized for overestimating mortality risk since so many advances have been made in antibiotic therapy, surgical therapy, and critical care. In 2010, Osler et al. modified it to account for the presence of inhalation injury [10]. The revised score, R-Baux, is defined as: *age+percent burn+17 (if inhalation injury is present)=R-Baux Score*, which is then converted into a percent mortality. The advantage of the Baux score is that it is simple to perform quickly. However, more accurate predictions can be made using more complex statistical analysis [10, 11].

The Abbreviated Burn Severity Index (ABSI) was formulated in 1982 by Tobiasen et al., and it was derived from multivariate logistic regression [12]. The ABSI score is based upon five variables—sex, age, presence of inhalation injury, presence of full-thickness burn, and TBSA. It provides a probability of survival as a percentage based on the aforementioned variables. These formulas all were developed using nonhomogenous populations with TBSA ranging from 0–10 % to 90–100 %, and they have been validated in other studies [13–17]. Although simple to use and shown in studies to have predictive value, none of them has been externally validated in a population consisting only of extensively burned adults and children (TBSA >20 %) [7].

Causes of Burn Injuries

Cooking is the leading cause of residential fires and residential fire injuries [18]. From 2007 to 2011, there was an average of 156,600 residential fires per year in which cooking equipment was deemed to be the cause of the fire. These fires caused an average of 400 deaths per year and 5080 injuries. Ranges with or without ovens caused the majority of fires started with cooking equipment (57 %), and unattended equipment was the leading cause of cooking fires. Overall, 43 % of residential fires were thought to cooking related, and they accounted for 38 % of home fire injuries and 16 % of home fire deaths.

In 2011, heating equipment was reported to be the cause of 53,600 residential fires. This accounted for 14 % of all home fires, which was the second highest single cause, after cooking. 16 % of home fire deaths involved heating equipment, which was third highest after cooking and smoking. Overall, heating equipment was involved in 400 deaths and 1520 injuries. Stationary and portable heaters were the most common equipment involved [19]. Defective heating devices and the improper use of heating devices accounted for a higher proportion of deaths in low-income areas [20].

In 2011, 90,000 smoking-related fires occurred in the United States, being one of the leading causes of domestic fatal burn injuries. Fires started by smoking materials were associated with an estimated 540 deaths, 1640 injuries, and $621 million in property damage. One out of four of those fatalities was suffered by someone other than the cigarette smoker. Most of the deaths resulted from fires that started in bedrooms, living rooms, family rooms, or dens. Smoking-related fires accounted for 8 % of all fires, 20 % of associated deaths, and 9 % of injuries [21].

Nevertheless, the long-term trend in fires caused by smoking materials has decreased by 73 % from 1980 to 2011. This decline is attributed to the decline in smoking, standards, and regulations requiring mattresses and upholstered furniture to resist cigarette ignition and a recent adoption of fire-safety regulations among cigarette makers. Canada and the United States have passed laws that require all cigarettes sold to have reduced ignition strength by ASTM Standard E2187-04. Fire-safe cigarettes are made with two or three thin bands of less-porous paper that act to slow down a burning cigarette. If a fire-safe cigarette is left unattended, the burning tobacco will reach this paper and self-extinguish. New York was the first state to adopt the fire-safe cigarette requirements in 2003. In 2000–2003, smoking material fire deaths averaged 43 per year. After implementation of the bill, smoking material fire deaths averaged 25 per year in 2006–2008, a 42 % drop [22].

Sleeping while smoking was the primary factor contributing to 31 % of all home smoking material fire deaths, while alcohol or drug impairment and physical disability both accounted for 18 % of deaths. Age was a factor in 10 % of those deaths. Up to 50 % of burn patient fatalities have a history of alcohol use, and alcohol intoxication has been shown to increase the risk of infection and mortality in burn patients [23]. Forty percent of home fire deaths involving smoking were started in the bedroom, and 35 % were started in the living room, family room, or den. Not surprisingly, smoking-related home fire deaths peaked during winter months, with the highest rate of deaths in December through March.

There is an increasing association between cannabis and burn patients. Several states have legalized the use of cannabis for medicinal purposes, while others also have legalized it for recreational use. The use of cannabis in the US population has increased from 6.2 % in 2002 to 7.0 % in 2014, [24] but this rate has increased more quickly in burn patients. A recent study from the University of Kansas using data from the National Burn Repository 2002–2011 showed 6.0 % of burn unit patients testing positive for cannabis in 2002. This number increased to 27 % in 2011 ($P=0.0022$). That study showed that flame injuries, which accounted for more than 60 % of injuries, were the most common type of injury caused by cannabis. They were followed by scald injuries, which accounted for approximately 15 % of injuries. This study also found that patients who tested positive for cannabis had larger burns (TBSA 12.94 % vs. 10 %, $P<0.001$), longer length of stay (13.31 vs. 12.6 days, $P=0.16$), longer ICU length of stay (7.84 vs. 6.39, $P=0.0006$), and more operations (2.78 vs. 2.05, $P<0.001$). These patients tended to be male (80 %), were less likely to be insured (25.2 % vs. 17.26 % $P<0.0001$), and were younger, on average (35 years old vs. 42, $P<0.0001$) [25]. The increased association between burn patients and cannabis use may be due to the physiologic and psychological effects of cannabis on the patient, as these effects may lead to increased accidents. As more states legalize cannabis, it is safe to assume that there may be a correlating increase in these types of burns [26].

Playing with fire caused an average of 49,300 fires between 2007 and 2011, and it resulted in an average of 80 deaths. A child under six started 43 % of these fires, and the majority of these fires were caused by males (83 %). Sixty-four percent of these fires began at home, and the remainder began outdoors or at educational properties. For outdoors fires, 24 % were started during the month of July and were thought to be influenced by Independence Day-related festivities [27].

Burn injuries due to recreational activities are an ongoing problem for many communities [28, 29]. A total of 9600 firework-related injuries were treated in US emergency rooms, 26 % of those patients were under the age of 15, and 68 % were male. Sixty-one percent of these injuries were to the extremities, and the hand or finger was the most commonly injured extremity at 46 %; followed by the leg at 11 %, and the arm, shoulder, or wrist accounting for 4 %. Most of the remainder of the injuries were to the head (34 %), and eye injuries accounted for 17 % of the total. 89 % of firework-related injuries involved fireworks that were approved for consumer use by Federal regulations [30].

Outdoor campfires are another frequent cause of burn injury. A retrospective study done by UC San Diego that examined data from 1999 to 2007 found 241 patients admitted to their burn center during that time period. Each year, 12–39 patients were injured by these types of fires, and 84 % were men. Patients fell into two age groups: 2–9 years old and 18–64 years old. The beach was the most common location for recreational fire injuries. Alcohol was a contributing factor in 60.6 % of adult burns, and 80.7 % of patients sustained partial-thickness and full-thickness burns. 36.6 % of these patients required skin grafts, and the mean length of staying was 8.6 days [28].

In order to prevent injuries from recreational fires, New Mexico implemented a ban on them from June to August 2011, due to the prevalence of drought, high winds, and uncontrolled wildfires. The New Mexico Burn Center then looked at the results of the ban on recreational fires and charts from burn patients admitted from May 27 through September 6, 2010 were compared to burn patients admitted from May 28 through September 5, 2011 [31]. There were a total of 14 burn injuries in 2010, compared with 4 in 2011, which represents a statistically significant decrease in admissions ($P=0.02$). There was a total decrease of campfire-related injuries from 91 in 2010 to 25 in 2011 [31]. Legislation aimed at limiting recreational fires during summer months seems to be effective in preventing injury.

Arson is another leading cause of fires which accounted for 420 annual deaths, 1360 civilian injuries, and $1.3 billion dollars in property damages. The majority of these fires (75 %) were outdoors, while 18 % involved structures, and 7 % were vehicle fires. Structure fires accounted for 92 % of deaths due to arson, despite accounting for only 18 % of the total. A majority (51 %) of arson fires occur between 3 p.m. and midnight, and according to FBI statistics, two out of five individuals arrested for arson are under 18 years of age [32].

Electrical fires, which are defined as a fire involving electrical failure or malfunction, accounted for 47,700 home fires in 2011. They resulted in 418 deaths and 1570 injuries. 16,400 nonresidential electrical fires were reported to the US fire departments, and these resulted in 13 deaths and 243 injuries [33]. High voltage (>1000 V) electrical burns can result in severe injuries, and they account for an estimated 1000 fatalities annually in the United States. Electrical injuries represent 3–5 % of burn unit admission annually [34, 35]. Electrical burn injuries resulting from attempted theft of copper have become more frequent as the value of this metal rises

[36]. The commercial price of copper tripled in 2006 [37], and since then, this has been reported as a risk factor for electrical burn injuries [38–40].

Although it has been estimated that 486,000 burn injuries occurred in the USA in 2013, the exact number of burn injuries that occur in the USA is not known. Only 21 states require reporting of burn injuries, two states only require reporting of burns resulting from assault or arson, and seven others only require burns >15 % TBSA be reported [41]. Therefore, the total number of annual burn injuries in the USA is estimated by extrapolating data collected in these states [42].

Not all patients with burn injuries require care at a burn center. Approximately 25,000 patients met criteria for burn center care (Table 1.3). There are 128 self-identified burn care facilities in the USA, and only 62 are verified by the American Burn Association. Geographic access to verified burn centers and self-identified burn facilities varies greatly across states and regions in the United States. Eighty percent of the population lives within two hours of some type of burn center via ground or air travel. However, one-third of the US population must be transported by air in order to reach an ABA-verified burn care center within 2 h [43].

Table 1.3 Mortality rate based on total burn surface area (2013)

%TBSA	Lived Cases	Died Cases	Mortality rate
0.1–9.9	133,242	864	0.6
10–19.9	25,660	699	2.7
20–29.9	7156	659	8.4
30–39.9	3082	621	16.8
40–49.9	1532	561	26.8
50–59.9	798	463	36.7
60–69.9	515	417	44.7
70–79.9	284	347	55.0
80–89.9	185	461	71.4
>90	96	544	85.0
Subtotal	172,550	5636	3.2
Missing or 0 %	24,369	867	3.4
Total	196,919	6503	3.2

TBSA total burn surface area

Patients and Complications

The American Burn Association maintains the National Burn Repository (NBR) database that contains data sets of acute burn admissions beginning in 1947. A total of 203,422 records of patients from 99 hospitals in 36 states and the District of Columbia have been contributed to the database. The NBR releases an annual report detailing patients that are treated at burn centers in the USA [44]. The 2015 NBR reports reflect data from 2014.

Some key findings from the 2015 NBR report include:

- Over 68 % of burn patients were men.
- The mean age of all reported cases was 32 years old. Children under the age of five accounted for 19 % of the cases, while patients age 60 and older represented 13 % of cases.
- The mortality rate for all cases was 3.2 %, and it was 5.7 % for injuries from fire and flame. Mortality increased with an increase in TBSA, and patients with TBSA > 90 % had a mortality rate of 85 %. More than 75 % of reported burns were less than 10 % TBSA, but these cases had a mortality rate of 0.6 %.
- The most common etiologies of burn injuries were fire/flame and scalding, which accounted for almost eight of every ten reported injuries. Scald injuries were most prevalent in children under five, while fire/flame injuries were the most common in all other age categories. Nine percent of burn injuries were of unknown etiology.
- Seventy-three percent of burn injuries with known occurrence locations happened at home. 72 % of cases were identified as non-work-related accidents, and 13.7 % of burn injuries were work-related accidents.
- Child abuse was suspected in 1.1 % of patients, and 1.1 % of burn injuries were self-inflicted.

The 2015 NBR Report further noted that the average length of stay (LOS) for patients with burn injuries declined from 9.3 days to 8.6 days from 2005 to 2014. During that same period, the mortality rate slightly increased from 3.1 to 3.2 %

for males, while it decreased from 4.9 to 3.6 % for females. Advanced age, burn size, and inhalation injury were all related to an increased risk of death, which has also been validated in other database studies [45]. For patients under the age of 60, with a TBSA between 0.1 and 19.9, the presence of inhalation injury increased the likelihood of death by almost 24 times. Other studies have also shown significant increases in mortality with the presence of inhalation injury [46].

A correlation exists between complications and number of days on the ventilator. In total, 7.6 % of patients experienced complications including arrhythmia, bacteremia, cellulitis, blood/systemic infection, pneumonia, respiratory failure, septicemia, urinary tract infections, and wound infections. Patients with zero ventilator days had a 7.1 % complication rate, patients with 1–3 ventilator days had a 22.3 % complication rate, and patients with >4 ventilator days had a 59.5 % complication rate. Pneumonia was the most frequent clinical complication, occurring in 5 % of fire/flame-injured patients and over 40 % of patients with 4+ ventilator days. Pneumonia, alone, has been shown to increase burn mortality by 40 %, while the combination of inhalation injury and pneumonia leads to a 60 % increase in death. Children and the elderly are especially prone to pneumonia after burn injuries, due to limited physiological reserve [47, 48]. Duration of ventilation may actually be a cause of some complications (pneumonia). However, it is more likely a marker of severity of illness, and it correlates with other complications that occur in critically ill patients [42].

Infection is a common problem in burn units, and it is thought that up to 75 % of deaths occurring after the initial resuscitation period are attributable to infectious complications [5]. Burn injuries cause significant immunological stress, and wounds are at risk of bacterial infection due to breakdown of the skin barrier as well as to alterations to innate and acquired immunity [5, 49]. Methicillin-resistant *Staphylococcus aureus* (MRSA) is a frequent cause of nosocomial infection in burn injuries, and their prevalence is increasing due to extended hospitalization and antibiotic therapy [43]. A 2014 retrospective study by DiMuzio et al. reviewed data from acute burn patients in a pediatric burn hospital from 2004 to 2011 [50]. They found that the incidence of MRSA increased from 20 % in 2004 to 45 % in 2009 to 2011. The most common infectious organisms were *Staphylococcus aureus* (25 %), *Pseudomonas aeruginosa* (13 %), and *E. coli* (6 %). The Infectious Disease Society has published guidelines on the use of broad spectrum antibiotics for serious bacterial infections, and they recommend a susceptibility of greater than 80 % based on the institution's antibiogram [51, 52]. With the increasing use of antibiotics, emerging multidrug-resistant bacteria outbreaks (MDRB) in burn units have become problematic. A systematic review by Genessay et al. in 2015 analyzed 29 peer-reviewed articles on such outbreaks [53]. They found that the most common organisms in MDRB outbreaks were MRSA and *Acinetobacter baumannii*, with mortality rates among infected patients ranging from 0 to 33 %. Sixteen screening studies of staff showed carrier rates of 0–20 %. There was a lack of consensus on how to manage such outbreaks, because implementation of isolation precautions does not always suffice, and unit closure was necessary in five of the outbreaks. MDRB infections are responsible for increased morbidity and mortality in burn patients, and management is difficult due to multifactorial transmission and limited therapeutic possibilities [51].

Diabetics are at particular risk for multisystem complications, given their alterations in vascular supply. McCampbell et al. reviewed data from the New York Presbyterian-Weill Cornell Medical Center from 1996 to 2000. They found that 167 diabetics from 18 to 65 years old had a higher rate of full-thickness burns (51 vs. 31 %; $P=0.025$), skin grafts (50 vs. 28 %; $P=0.01$), burn-related procedures (57 vs. 32 %; $P=0.001$), and infections (65 vs. 51 %; $P=0.05$), in addition to longer LOS (23 vs. 12 days; $P=0.0001$). Although there was no statistically significant difference in incidence of specific infections, the rates of cellulitis, wound infection, urinary tract infection, line infection, and osteomyelitis were consistently higher in the diabetic population. Scald burns were the most common etiology, while flame burns were the second most common [54]. Another study done by Kimball et al. who collected data on 43 diabetic patients with isolated leg or foot burns from 1999 to 2009 showed that diabetic patients had significantly higher burn ICU admission rates compared to nondiabetics with similar injuries (16.3 % of vs. 8.5 % of patients, $P<0.001$), total length of hospital stay (14.1 vs. 9.8 days, $P<0.01$), and renal failure (4.7 % vs. 0.6 %, $P<0.05$) [55]. A study in 2013 from the University of California, Davis Burn Center, found 68 adult diabetic patients with lower extremity burns. It also showed that the most common etiology was scald burns, and the patients had increased complication rates. They found that the majority of lower extremity burns resulted from intentional exposure to heat sources. These patients also showed increased morbidity and mortality [56]. The presence of diabetes and peripheral neuropathy is thought to hamper these patients' ability to detect injuries, and they can lead to a more complicated hospital course.

Patients with perineal and buttock burns are another group of patients with high infection risk, as these wounds have a contamination risk as well as shear stress that is always present [57]. Although these wounds occur infrequently (incidence as low as 1.2 % in the United States population), they are quite difficult to manage, and these patients often experience systemic infections and complications. Several studies have shown that one-third of patients with perineal injuries die within 48 h of injury, and their overall mortality ranges from 25 to 50 % [51–54]. For these patients, data supports the use of prophylactic ostomy, especially if the burn directly involves the anus. However, its use does not seem to affect mortality [57]. Most published studies recommend reserving the use of diverting ostomies for complicated patients, but there are no large volume, randomized clinical trials [58, 59].

Breakdown in terms of race showed that 113,407 (58.6 %) of patients were white, 38,226 (19.8 %) were black, 26,926 (13.9 %) were Hispanic, 8622 (4.5 %) identified as other, 4743 (2.5 %) were Asian, 1550 (0.8 %) were Native American, and 9.948 were identified as unknown. Of note, nonwhite burn patients outnumbered white patients in ages 0–5, while white patients outnumbered nonwhite patients in all other age groups.

In the end, 86.7 % of patients who suffered perineal burn injuries were discharged to home, while 5.7 % of these patients required home health services. Another 2.7 % were discharged to a rehabilitation facility, and 2.2 % were discharged to a skilled nursing facility. Finally, 2.5 % of patients were transferred to another hospital, extended care facility, another service, or to another acute burn facility. Only 0.4 % of these patients were discharged to inpatient psychiatry.

Burn Geography

The South and the Midwest had the highest overall fire rate for the 5-year period from 2007 to 2011, with 5.4 fires per 1000. The South had 12.8 average fire deaths per 1 million people, while the Midwest experienced an average of 13.0 deaths per one million people during that period. The Midwest also had an average injury rate of 71.8 for the five-year period, which was 27 % higher than the national rate. The South had the highest death rates for most community sizes under 100,999. Mississippi had the highest average fire death rate at 27.5, and it was one of the top ten states in poverty, level of education, rural factors, and composite race index. When 5-year averages of fire-related deaths are compared by state, correlations in states with higher death rates include poverty, race, smoking, rural settings, and education [60]. Colder weather during the winter, substandard housing, and a lack of adequate smoke detectors are all thought to be risk factors for home fires [3]. Racial differences in house fire death rates have been shown to decrease as income increases, which implies that the death rate from fires is an effect of economic status [61].

Mobile homes have been found to carry twice the death rate compared to other types of housing. 65 burn patients were admitted from 2002 to 2004. The average age of these patients was 39; 77 % were male, 67 % were white, and 79 % were residents of Georgia, South Carolina, North Carolina, and Florida. The patients had an average TBSA of 21 %, 64 % had an associated inhalation injury, and 69 % of those patients required ventilator support. The average LOS per TBSA percentage was 1.01 days. 88 % of these patients had preexisting medical comorbidities. 74 % were smokers, 64 % were alcoholics, and 28 % were uninsured. In 40 % of the cases, the cause of the fire was unknown. In 31 %, the cause was accidental explosion, and 29 % were due to other causes. 40 % of the burns occurred between December and February [27].

An estimated 25,000 vacant residential building fires were reported annually in the USA from 2010 to 2012. These accounted for 7 % of all residential building fires, which resulted in 60 deaths, 225 injuries, and $777 million in property loss each year [62]. Vacant residential buildings are rarely maintained, and they often serve as sites for illegal activities. The homeless population often uses these properties as shelter, although there is little known about the buildings' overall condition. Only 12.6 % of these structures had working smoke alarms, while only 1 % had automatic extinguishing systems present. By comparison, only 3 % of US households lack functional smoke alarms according to the US Consumer Product Safety Commission [63]. 37 % of vacant residential fires are intentionally set (37 %), while other causes include the presence of open flame (13 %), carelessness (11 %), other heat sources (8 %), and electrical malfunction (7 %).

Types of Burns

Flame Burns

Flame and fire burns are typically associated with the highest risk of death and complications, when compared to other etiologies [44]. They result in the most common admission to burn centers, with 42.6 % of admissions in the NBR. Table 1.4 shows common burn injuries as well as considerations with these injuries. The most common cause is non-work-related accidents (72.6 %),

Table 1.4 Types of burns—complications, treatments, considerations, and referral criteria

Type of burn	Common complications	Treatments	Considerations	Referral to burn center
Flame	Inhalation injury, pneumonia	Partial thickness—daily antibiotic dressing changes or occlusive dressings (Biobrane) Surgery for full-thickness burns and partial-thickness burns unlikely to heal within 3 weeks	Assess for inhalation injury, consider early intubation if signs of respiratory distress	Partial thickness burns with TBSA > 10 %, burns, Third degree burns, burns involving face hands, feet, genitalia, perineum or major joints
Scald/contact burns	Cellulitis	Partial thickness—small blisters can be left intact Wound care with daily antibiotic dressing changes or occlusive dressings (Biobrane) Up to 40 % of grease burns may require excision and grafting	Children at higher risk of full-thickness injury	
Electrical burns	Pneumonia, wound infection, cellulitis	Aggressive wound exploration, early debridement	Can have very deep burns with muscle necrosis, joint destruction, and vascular thrombosis	All patients with electrical injuries should be referred to burn centers
Chemical Burns	Cellulitis	Removal of offending agent, dilution with high-density shower for 20–30 min—no immersion	Systemic toxicity can occur Injuries often deeper than initially thought	All patients with chemical burns should be referred to burn centers

TBSA total burn surface area

while 72.8 % occurred in the home. Work-related injuries accounted for 12.7 % of flame and fire burns, and recreational fires cause 6.6 % of these injuries. These types of burns are associated with the highest rate of complication, and the rate increases with age. The overall complication rate was found to be 16.4 %. Infants had complication rate of 12.8 % of complications, patients under 20 had a 6.6–10.8 % complication rate, and those over 80 had a 27.8 % rate. Pneumonia was the most common infection, as it accounted for 11.9 % of all complications, and it occurred in 5.0 % of all patients. The next most common complications were urinary tract infections (3.3 %) and cellulitis (2.3 %). In all, 17.6 % of these patients had excisions, and 12.4 % underwent grafting.

Health care providers should be particularly vigilant for inhalation injury in patients injured by flame burns, particularly when fires occur in closed spaces. Smoke inhalation has a significant effect on morbidity and mortality of flame burns, as inhalation injury is reported in 14.9 % of these patients. Smoke inhalation is associated with a 22 % mortality rate, while patients without smoke inhalation have a 2.8 % mortality rate. Patients with flame burns should be assessed for signs of inhalation injury upon initial assessment. Dyspnea, burns involving the oropharynx, singed hairs, and cough are risk factors for inhalation injury. If any of these signs is present, humidified oxygen with a non-rebreathing reservoir mask at a rate of 10–12 L/min should be administered. Patients with respiratory compromise or distress should be intubated and ventilated with 100 % oxygen. Since edema in the upper airways typically develops 12–24 h after the injury [64], intubation should be used liberally in patients with any sign of upper airway injury. Patients who are not intubated should be monitored closely with continuous checking of pulse oximetry and arterial blood gasses to assess both oxygenation and ventilation.

Surgery is reserved for full-thickness burns or partial-thickness burns that are unlikely to heal within 3 weeks. As previously mentioned, patients with partial-thickness burns greater than 10 % TBSA should be referred to a burn center for further management [65].

Scald Burns and Contact Burns

Scald injury is the second most common mechanism of injury reported to the NBR over the last 10 years. Eighty percent of these injuries occurred in the home and 94 % were classified as accidental. Intentional injuries accounted for 3.9 % of scald injuries. Unlike flame burns, scald injuries are associated with an overall low rate of complications, and complications are mostly infectious in nature. Cellulitis was the most common complication, occurring in 2.2 % of patients and accounting for 17.7 % of total complications. Urinary tract infection (1.4 %), pneumonia (0.8 %), and wound infection (08 %) were the next most common complications, and they accounted for 11.2 %, 6.6 %, and 6.4 % of complications, respectively. The most common procedure these patients undergo is excisional debridement (18.9 %), while 12.6 % require skin grafts. Mortality from scald injuries correlates with TBSA, and the overall mortality is less than 1 % for these types of injuries. However, mortality exceeds over 40 % in burns with TBSA >70 %.

A 10-year retrospective study of hot oil scalds from the Yorkshire Regional Burn Center showed an increase in the number of admissions from 1995 to 2004, with a peak occurrence in ages 1–5 and 30–40 age groups. TBSA of adults and children were found to be similar (7.15 vs. 7.23 %, respectively), but the incidence of full-thickness injury in adults was twice that of children (67 % vs. 26 %). In the 1–6 year age group, 92 % of the injuries were due to pulling a handle or cord of a container of hot liquid [66].

Contact burns make up 8.4 % of NBR entries in the last decade, with 75 % of these injuries occurring in the home. 80 % are non-work related, and less than 3 % are suspected to be intentional injuries. This group was reported to have a 7.2 % complication rate, with complications rising with age. Patients age 20–29 have a complication rate of 7.6 %, while those between 70 and 79 have a 21.2 % complication rate. The most common complications were cellulitis (2.2 % of patients), UTI (1.2 %), and wound infection (0.8 %). Pneumonia and respiratory failure only occurred in 0.8 and 0.7 % of patients, respectively.

Contact burns had an overall mortality of 0.7 %. Only 10 cases with TBSA over 40 % were reported to the NBR in the last decade. Overall, 19.5 % of these patients underwent excisional debridement, and 12.5 % required skin grafts.

Scald burns secondary to grease are particularly damaging, with 40 % of patients requiring at least one excision and grafting procedure [67]. Patients with partial-thickness scald burns that are not caused by grease can be managed conservatively. Multiple studies show that conservative treatment with wound care is superior to early excision [68, 69]. Occlusive dressings such as Biobrane and amnion have been shown to have superior results in terms of LOS and pain for treatment of partial-thickness burns, and they also can be used in these types of burns successfully [69–71].

Electrical Burns

Electrical admissions comprise only 3.6 % of all reported admissions in the 2015 NBR report. However, these patients tend to have some of the most devastating and debilitating injuries. The majority of electrical burns occurred in the workplace (60.8 %), while 30.8 % occurred in the home. Case reports of electrical injury also have been reported secondary to cardioversion [72, 73]. Unlike flame, scald, and contact burns, there is not a linear correlation between age and risk of complications. Patients aged 1–2 have a 1.7 % complication rate, while patients 2–5 had a 1.3 % complication rate. Patients aged 20–29 had a complication rate of 13 %, which was second only to patients over 60 (13.5 % complication rate). The overall complication rate was 10.5 %, which is second only to flame burns (16.4 %). Pneumonia is the most common complication rate reported, at a rate of 2.1 % and accounting for 10 % of all complications. Wound infection (1.4 % of patients), cellulitis (1.4 %), septicemia (1.2 %), respiratory failure (1.1 %), and urinary tract infection (0.9 %) were the next most common complications. Of note, renal failure occurred in 0.8 % of these patients, and compartment syndrome occurred in 0.7 %. The main mechanism of electrical burn damage is thought to be the abnormal flow of electrons flowing throughout the body, which causes heating and poration of the cellular membranes. Damage is secondary to increased transmembrane potentials induced by strong electric fields [74]. Injury is also produced by depolarization of muscles and nerves, which initiates abnormal electrical rhythms in the heart and brain, resulting in both internal and external electrical burns [40]. These types of burns are difficult to manage, because quantification of burn extension and localization of the point of entry are difficult to ascertain [75]. These patients typically have very deep burns with muscle necrosis, joint destruction, and vascular thrombosis. The upper and lower limbs are the main parts of the body affected by electrical injuries, and there is a high rate of hand and digit involvement [75]. The protocol for treatment during initial resuscitation of these patients should follow general burn management principles. The optimal management of these patients includes aggressive wound exploration and early debridement [76]. It is recommended that these patients be referred to burn centers for further management [65].

Chemical Burns

Chemical injuries accounted for 3.4 % of the data reported to the NBR, and they occurred most commonly in the home (42.9 %). 45.9 % of these injuries were work-related. Cellulitis was the most common complication, and it occurred in 2 % of this group of patients. Wound infection (0.9 %), pneumonia (0.9 %), and urinary tract infection (0.9 %) were the next most common complications. Sepsis was rare after chemical burns, and it developed in only 0.6 % of patients. 17.8 % of patients underwent excisional debridement, and 12.8 % required skin grafting. Initial trauma primary and secondary assessment still applies to patients with chemical burns, and the offending agent should be removed immediately [77]. Copious, high-density shower should be done with tap water for up to 20–30 min to remove the chemical. Patients should not be immersed or placed in a tub, as this can cause spread of the chemical to unaffected areas. Dry chemicals should be brushed off before shower is initiated

[77]. Systemic toxicity is a concern with chemical burns. Hydrofluoric acid can cause hypocalcaemia and ventricular fibrillation [78], and formic acid exposure is associated with intravascular hemolysis, renal failure, and necrotizing pancreatitis [79]. Respiratory failure may also occur with inhalation of chemicals. It should be managed similarly to smoke inhalation injuries, with early intubation for those patients exhibiting signs of respiratory distress. The extent of chemical burn injuries is often deeper than it seems externally, as many agents cause unusual tanning and have local anesthetic properties. Due to the unique and difficult nature of these injuries, it is recommended that these patients be referred to burn centers for treatment as soon as possible [65, 80].

Intentional Burns

Intentional burns include both deliberately self-inflicted burns and assault burns. These patients represent a unique patient population in terms of clinical presentations and outcomes. A study from the University of Alabama at Birmingham by Reiland et al. compared 96 patients with intentional burns to all other burn injuries. The intentional burn patient group had a higher mean TSBA (26.1 % vs. 13.8 %), a higher percentage of men (85.7 % vs. 55.7 %), a longer mean LOS (19.9 days vs. 13.2 days), a higher incidence of inhalational injury (20.8 % vs. 8.7 %), a higher rate of mortality (20.0 % vs. 9.8 %), and a higher likelihood of elevated blood alcohol content (14.6 % vs. 7 %) and positive drug screen (11.4 % vs. 0 %). The most common location of intentional burns involved the arms and hands (76.0 %), the trunk (69.8 %), the head and neck (67.8 %), and the legs and feet (55.2 %). In all, 64.6 % of intentional burn patients were African-American, compared to 29.3 % in the other burn group ($P = < 0.0001$). 10.7 % of the intentional burn patients were discharged to a psychiatric facility (0 % in other group), while 7.1 % were discharged to jail (1.8 % in other group) [81].

Data is contradictory when analyzing patients with self-inflicted burn injuries. Single-institution studies have shown that intentionally injured burn patients have higher mortality rates—up to double the odds of death—than do those with unintentional mechanisms of injury [82]. Patients with intentional burns also have been shown to have larger TBSA, longer LOS, and higher morbidity and mortality [83]. A retrospective cohort study by Thombs et al. reviewed data from the NBR from 1995 to 2005 controlled for explicitly matched patients with self-inflicted injuries for the presence of psychiatric disorder. It did not find any statistical difference in terms of mortality, ICU LOS, or total hospitalization [84]. Patients with self-inflicted burns may be hesitant to report their injuries as self-inflicted. Studies have shown that up to 45 % of patients show a discrepancy between the reported etiology and appearance of the burn [85]. Patients with self-inflicted burns may benefit from psychological evaluation and treatment.

Conclusion

Fatalities from fires and burn injuries are not as prevalent as those occurring from other mechanisms of injury. Mortality from burn injuries has improved over the past 50 years due to advancements throughout the spectrum of care. Nevertheless, burn injuries remain a significant source of trauma that require general surgeons and general plastic surgeons, as well as burn surgeons and burn reconstructive surgeons. While there are commonalities in the pathophysiology of burn injuries regardless of the specific mechanism of injury, understanding the differences in terms of risk, natural history, and complications helps guide approaches to treatment, prevention, and triage to higher levels of care.

References

1. American Burn Association. http://www.ameriburn.org/resources_factsheet.php. Accessed 17 June 2015.
2. Centers for Disease Control and Prevention: Web-based Injury Statistics Query and Reporting System (WISQARS) [Online]. National Center for Injury Prevention and Control, Centers for Disease Control and Prevention (producer). http://www.cdc.gov/Injury. Accessed 17 June 2015.

3. National Fire Protection Association. http://www.nfpa.org/research/reports-and-statistics/fires-in-the-us. Accessed 17 June 2015.
4. Feck GA, Baptiste MS, Tate Jr CL. Burn injuries, epidemiology and prevention. Accid Anal Prev. 1979;11:129–36.
5. Mlcak RP, Suman OE, Herndon DN. Respiratory management of inhalation injury. Burns. 2007;33(1):2–13.
6. Tsurumi A, Que YA, Yan S, Tompkins RG, Rahme LG, Ryan CM. Do standard burn mortality formulae work on a population of severely burned children and adults? Burns. 2015;41(5):935–45.
7. Ryan CM, Schoenfeld DA, Thorpe WP, Sheridan RL, Cassem EH, Tompkins RG. Objective estimates of the probability of death from burn injuries. N Engl J Med. 1998;338(6):362–6.
8. Baux S. Contribution a l'Etude du traitement local des brulures thermigues etendues These, Paris, France. 1961.
9. Baux S, Mimoun M, Saade H, Lioret N, Esteve M, Nolland XB, et al. Burns in the elderly. Burns. 1989;15(4):239–40.
10. Osler T, Glance LG, Hosmer DW. Simplified estimates of the probability of death after burn injuries: extending and updating the Baux score. J Trauma. 2010;68(3):690–7.
11. Royston P, Sauerbrei W. Multivariable model-building: a pragmatic approach to regression analysis based on fractional polynomials for modeling continuous variables. Hoboken, NJ: Wiley; 2008. p. 115–83.
12. Tobiasen J, Hiebert JM, Edlich RF. The abbreviated burn severity index. Ann Emerg Med. 1982;11(5):260–2.
13. Forster NA, Zingg M, Haile SR, Künzi W, Giovanoli P, Guggenheim M. 30 years later – does the ABSI need revision? Burns. 2011;37(6):958–63.
14. Germann G, Barthold U, Lefering R, Raff T, Hartmann B. The impact of risk factors and preexisting conditions on the mortality of burn patients and the precision of predictive admission-scoring systems. Burns. 1997;23(3):195–203.
15. Gravante G, Delogu D, Esposito G, Monton A. Analysis of prognostic indexes and other parameters to predict the length of hospitalization in thermally burned patients. Burns. 2007;33(3):312–5.
16. Seo DK, Kym D, Yim H, Yang HT, Cho YS, Kim JH, et al. Epidemiological trends and risk factors in major burns patients in South Korea: a 10-year experience. Burns. 2015;41(1):181–7.
17. Hussain A, Dunn KW. Accuracy of commercial reporting systems to monitor quality of care in burns. Burns. 2014;40(2):251–6.
18. Ahrens M. Home Fires involving cooking equipment. National Fire Protection Association. November 2013. http://www.nfpa.org/research/reports-and-statistics/fire-causes/appliances-and-equipment/cooking-equipment. Accessed 17 June 2015.
19. Hall J. Home fires involving heating equipment. National Fire Protection Association. October 2013. http://www.nfpa.org/research/reports-and-statistics/fire-causes/appliances-and-equipment/heating-equipment. Accessed 17 June 2015.
20. National Fire Data Center: fire in the United States, 1983 to 1990. 8th ed. National Fire Data Center Emmitsburg October 1993.
21. Hall J. The smoking-material fire problem. National Fire Protection Association. July 2013. http://www.nfpa.org/research/reports-and-statistics/fire-causes/smoking-materials. Accessed 17 June 2015.
22. National Fire Protection Association. www.firesafe-cigarettes.org. Accessed 17 June 2015.
23. Holmes W, Hold P, James M. The increasing trend in alcohol-related burns: its impact on a tertiary burn centre. Burns. 2010;36:938–43.
24. United States Department of Health and Human Services. Results from the 2011 National Survey on Drug Use and Health: summary of National Findings (2012). Rockville, MD: Substance Abuse and Mental Health Services Administration, Department of Health and Human Services; 2012.
25. Jehle Jr CC, Nazir N, Bhavsar D. The rapidly increasing trend of cannabis use in burn injury. J Burn Care Res. 2015;36(1):e12–7.
26. Anderson DM, Hansen B, Rees DI. Medical marijuana laws, traffic fatalities, and alcohol consumption. J Law Econ. 2013;56:333–69.
27. Mierley MC, Baker SP. Fatal house fires in an urban population. JAMA. 1983;249:1466–8.
28. Fraga AM, Fraga GP, Noordenbos J, Tenenhaus M, Castle S, Bhavsar D, Lee JG, Coimbra R, Potenza BM. Beach and campfire burns: a site of pleasure and tragedy. J Burn Care Res. 2010;31(1):184–9.
29. Hultman CS, Tong WT, Surrusco M, Roden KS, Kiser M, Cairns BA. To everything there is a season: impact of seasonal change on admissions, acuity of injury, length of stay, throughput, and charges at an accredited, regional burn center. Ann Plast Surg. 2012;69(1):30–4.
30. National Fire Protection Association. http://www.nfpa.org/research/reports-and-statistics/fire-causes. Accessed 17 June 2015.
31. Hall J. Fireworks. National Fire Protection Association. April 2013. http://www.nfpa.org/research/reports-and-statistics/fire-causes/electrical. Accessed 17 June 2015.
32. Hoang DM, Reid D, Lentz CW. Statewide ban on recreational fires resulted in a significant decrease in campfire-related summer burn center admissions. J Burn Care Res. 2013;34(1):74–7.
33. Campbell, R. Intentional Fires. National Fire Protection Association. April 2014. http://www.nfpa.org/research/reports-and-statistics/fire-causes/arson-and-juvenile-firesetting/intentional-fires. Accessed 17 June 2015.
34. Hall, J. Electrical Fires. National Fire Protection Association. April 2013. http://www.nfpa.org/research/reports-and-statistics/fire-causes/electrical. Accessed 17 June 2015.
35. Spies C, Trohman RG. Narrative review: electrocution and life-threatening electrical injuries. Ann Intern Med. 2006;145:531–7.

36. Koumbourlis AC. Electrical injuries. Crit Care Med. 2002;30(Suppl):S424–30.
37. Curinga G, Pietramaggiori G, Scherer SS, Masellis A, Gherardini G, Brancato R, Conte F, Bistoni G. Electrical injuries due to theft of copper. J Burn Care Res. 2010;31(2):341–6
38. Report from the Italian Institute of Copper. http://www.ir.it/rame/statistiche/asp#Prezzi; http://www.iir.it/rame/caratteristiche_chimicofische. Accessed 17 June 2015.
39. Taylor AJ, McGwin Jr G, Brissie RM, Rue 3rd LW, Davis GG. Death during theft from electric utilities. Am J Forensic Med Pathol. 2003;24(2):173–6.
40. Adukauskiene D, Vizgirdaite V, Mazeikiene S. Electrical injuries. Medicina (Kaunas). 2007;43(3):259–66.
41. Francis EC, Shelley OP. Copper wire theft and high voltage electrical burns. Int J Burns Trauma. 2014;4(2):59–61.
42. Hammond J. The status of statewide burn prevention legislation. J Burn Care Rehabil. 1993;14:473–5.
43. Herndon D. Total burn care. Elsevier 2012.
44. Klein MB, Kramer CB, Nelson J, Rivara FP, Gibran NS, Concannon T. Geographic access to burn center hospitals. JAMA. 2009;302(16):1774–81.
45. 2015 NBR Report. http://www.ameriburn.org/2015NBRAnnualReport.pdf. Accessed 17 June 2015.
46. Burton KR, Sharma VK, Harrop R, Lindsay R. A population-based study of the epidemiology of acute adult burn injuries in the Calgary Health Region and factors associated with mortality and hospital length of stay from 1995 to 2004. Burns. 2009;35(4):572–9.
47. Santaniello JM, Luchette FA, Esposito TJ, Gunawan H, Reed RL, Davis KA, Gamelli RL. Ten year experience of burn, trauma, and combined burn/trauma injuries comparing outcomes. J Trauma. 2004;57(4):696–700.
48. Lionelli GT, Pickus EJ, Beckum OK, Decoursey RL, Korentager RA. A three decade analysis of factors affecting burn mortality in the elderly. Burns. 2005;31(8):958–63.
49. Murray CK. Burns. In: Mandell, Douglas, and Bennett's principles and practice of infectious diseases, vol. 2, Churchill Livingstone: Elsevier. p. 3905–9.
50. Cook N. Methicillin-resistant Staphylococcus aureus versus the burn patient. Burns. 1998;24:91–8.
51. DiMuzio EE, Healy DP, Durkee P, Neely AN, Kagan RJ. Trends in bacterial wound isolates and antimicrobial susceptibility in a Pediatric Burn Hospital. J Burn Care Res. 2014;35(5).
52. American Thoracic Society; Infectious Diseases Society of America. Guidelines on the management of adults with hospital-acquired, ventilator-associated, and healthcare-associated pneumonia. Am J Respir Crit Care Med. 2005;171:388–416. 10.1164/rccm.200405-644ST and http://www.atsjournals.org/doi/abs/10.1164/rccm.200405-644ST#.Vt0xW8ftVJo.
53. Boggan JC, Navar-Boggan AM, Jhaveri R. Pediatric-specific antimicrobial susceptibility data and empiric antibiotic selection. Pediatrics. 2012;130:e615–22.
54. Girerd-Genessay I, Bénet T, Vanhems P. Multidrug-resistant bacterial outbreaks in burn units: a synthesis of the literature according to the ORION statement. J Burn Care Res. 2015;28.
55. McCampbell B, Wasif N, Rabbitts A, Staiano-Coico L, Yurt RW, Schwartz S. Diabetes and burns: retrospective cohort study. J Burn Care Rehabil. 2002; 23(3):157–66.
56. Kimball Z, Patil S, Mansour H, Marano MA, Petrone SJ, Chamberlain RS. Clinical outcomes of isolated lower extremity or foot burns in diabetic versus non-diabetic patients: a 10-year retrospective analysis. Burns. 2013;39(2):279–84.
57. Barsun A, Sen S, Palmieri TL, Greenhalgh DG. A ten-year review of lower extremity burns in diabetics: small burns that lead to major problems. J Burn Care Res. 2013;34(2):255–60.
58. Merchant N, Boudana D, Willoughby L, Lin J, Rehou S, Shahrokhi S, Jeschke MG. Management of adult patients with buttock and perineal burns: The Ross Tilley Burn Centre experience. J Trauma Acute Care Surg. 2014;77(4):640–8.
59. Price CE, Cox S, Rode H. The use of diverting colostomies in paediatric peri-anal burns: experience in 45 patients. S Afr J Surg. 2013;51(3):102–5.
60. Kement M, Acar HA, Barlas IS, Aksakal N, Gezen C, Düzci U, Oncel M. Clinical evaluation of a temporary fecal containment device for non-surgical fecal diversion in perineal burns. Ulus Travma Acil Cerrahi Derg. 2011;17(2):123–7.
61. Pruitt BA Jr, Wolf SE, Mason AD Jr. Epidemiological, demographic, and outcome characteristics of burn injury. Chapter 3. In: Herndon DN, editor. Total burn care. 3rd ed. Philadelphia: Saunders Elsevier; 2007. p. 14–32.
62. Mullins RF, Alarm B, Huq Mian MA, Samples JM, Friedman BC, Shaver JR, Brandigi C, Hassan Z. Burns in mobile home fires – descriptive study at a regional burn center. J Burn Care Res. 2009;30(4):694–9.
63. FEMA. Vacant Residential Building Fires (2010-2012). Topical fire report series. 15(11). http://www.usfa.fema.gov/downloads/pdf/statistics/v15i11.pdf. Accessed 17 June 2015.
64. Greene, Michael and Craig Andres, "2004-2005 National Sample Survey of Unreported Residential Fires," Division of Hazard Analysis, Directorate for Epidemiology, U.S. Consumer Product Safety Commission, July 2009.
65. Harms BA, Bodai BI, Kramer GC. Microvascular fluid and protein flux in pulmonary and systemic circulations after thermal injury. Microvasc Res. 1982;23(1):77–86.
66. Harms BA, Bodai BI, Kramer GC. Microvascular fluid and protein flux in pulmonary and systemic circulations after thermal injury. Microvasc Res. 1982;23(1):77–86. http://www.ameriburn.org/BurnCenterReferralCriteria.pdf. Accessed 17 June 2015.
67. Hankins CL, Tang XQ, Phipps A. Hot oil burns – a study of predisposing factors, clinical course and prevention strategies. Burns. 2006;32(1):92–6. Epub 2005 Dec.
68. Klein MB, Gibran NS, Emerson D, Sullivan SR, Honari S, Engrav LH, Heimbach DM. Patterns of

grease burn injury: development of a classification system. Burns. 2005;31(6):765–7.
69. Desai MH, Rutan RL, Herndon DN. Conservative treatment of scald burns is superior to early excision. J Burn Care Rehabil. 1991;12(5):482–4.
70. Vloemans AF, Hermans MH, Van der Wal MB, Leibregts J, Middlekoop E. Optimal treatment of partial-thickness burns in children: a systematic review. Burns. 2014;40(2):177–90.
71. Thomson PD, Parks DH. Monitoring, banking and clinical use of amnion as a burn wound dressing. Ann Plast Srug. 1981;7(5):354–6.
72. Wood F, Martin L, Lewis D, Rawlins J, McWilliams T, Burrows S, et al. A prospective randomised clinical pilot study to compare the effectiveness of Biobrane(®) synthetic wound dressing, with or without autologous cell suspension, to the local standard treatment regimen in paediatric scald injuries. Burns. 2012;38:830–9.
73. Kennedy JM, Goldie C, Nickerson D. Burn progression secondary to cardioversion. J Burn Care Res. 2011;32(4):e143–5.
74. Alconero Camarero AR, Casaus Pérez M, Gutiérrez Caloca N. Incidents of cutaneous alteration secondary to external electrical cardioversion. Enferm Intensiva. 2006;17(4):163–72.
75. Luce EA. Electrical burns. Clin Plast Surg. 2000;27:133–43.
76. Curinga G, Pietramaggiori G, Scherer SS, Masellis A, Gherardini G, Brancato R, Conte F, Bistoni G. Electrical injuries due to theft of copper. J Burn Care Res. 2010;31(2):341–6.
77. Luz DP, Millan LS, Alessi MS, Uguetto WF, Paggairo A, Gomez DS, Ferreira MC. Electrical burns: a retrospective analysis across a 5 year period. Burns. 2009;35(7):1015–9.
78. Carlotto RC, Peters WJ, Neligan PC, Douglas LG, Beeston J. Chemical burns. Can J Surg. 1996;39:2.
79. Sheridan RL, Ryan CM, Quinby Jr WC, Blair J, Tompkins RG, Burke JF. Emergency management of major hydrofluoric acid exposures. Burns. 1995;21:62–3.
80. Pruitt BA. Chemical injuries: epidemiology, classification and pathophysiology. Presented at the annual meeting of the American Burns Association, Las Vegas, 1990.
81. Palao R, Monge I, Ruiz M, Barret JP. Chemical burns: pathophysiology and treatment. Burns. 2010;36(3):295–304.
82. Reiland A, Hovater M, McGwin Jr G, Rue 3rd LW, Cross JM. The epidemiology of intentional burns. J Burn Care Res. 2006;27(3):276–80.
83. Varley J, Pilcher D, Butt W, Cameron P. Self harm is an independent predictor of mortality in trauma and burns patients admitted to ICU. Injury. 2012;43(9):1562–5.
84. Modjarrad K, McGwin Jr G, Cross JM, Rue 3rd LW. The descriptive epidemiology of intentional burns in the United States: an analysis of the National Burn Repository. Burns. 2007;33(7):828–32. Epub 2007 May 24.
85. Thombs BD, Bresnick MG. Mortality risk and length of stay associated with self-inflicted burn injury: evidence from a national sample of 30,382 adult patients. Crit Care Med. 2008;36(1):118–25.
86. Friedman T, Shalom A, Westreich M. Self-inflicted burns. Ann Plast Surg. 2007;58(6):622–4.

Burn Pathophysiology

2

Kathleen Romanowski

Introduction

The physiologic changes that occur following a burn injury are both local and systemic. In the early decades of the 1900s, burn shock was the greatest threat to the survival of a burn patient; however, through the advancements in burn resuscitation, our management of shock has improved to the point that the management of the burn itself is now critical to the patients' outcomes. From the perspective of looking at the systemic effects of burn, one of the first advancements occurred due to the work of Frank Underhill. By studying the victims of the Rialto Theater fire in 1921, he demonstrated that burn shock which was not properly resuscitated was associated with increases in hematocrit. It was felt that this increase occurred due to fluid and electrolyte loss from the burn injury and was indicative of a plasma volume deficit [1]. The idea that burn shock was secondary to intravascular fluid loss was studied further by Cope and Moore following the Cocoanut Grove Nightclub fire in 1942. They introduced the concept of burn edema and the replacement of fluids using a body weight-based formula [2]. A number of other body weight-based formulas have been developed and are utilized in current practice and will be discussed further in a later chapter.

An understanding of both the burn and its systemic effects is critical to the care of the burn-injured patient. The etiology of the burn can play an important role in determining the treatment and the extent and type of underlying physiologic derangements. Additionally, the physiology of the skin itself plays a role in determining the severity of injury, the systemic manifestations, and how the burn progresses. Despite technologic advances in many areas of burn care, clinical assessment of the wound remains the standard technique for determining burn wound size and depth. Ideally, someone with experience caring for burn wounds will perform this assessment. Assessment of the wound, its depth, and its etiology are critical, as these determine not only the type of treatment needed (surgery versus topical wound care) for the wound but also its healing potential. Typically it is accepted that burns that are going to heal within 2–3 weeks do so without hypertrophic scarring or severe functional impairment. However, there have been many studies that promote early surgical excision and split-thickness skin grafting as a method for improving survival and other outcomes from major burns [3–6]. The challenge now is determining which wounds

K. Romanowski, M.D. (✉)
Division of Acute Care Surgery,
Department of Surgery, University of Iowa
Hospitals and Clinics, 200 Hawkins Drive,
Iowa City, IA 52242, USA
e-mail: kathleen-romanowski@uiowa.edu

D.G. Greenhalgh (ed.), *Burn Care for General Surgeons and General Practitioners*,
DOI 10.1007/978-3-319-29161-1_2

will heal within 2–3 weeks (and thus have minimal scarring) and which wounds require skin grafting. To do this, one must have the clinical acumen to predict which wounds will take longer than 2–3 weeks to heal.

Beyond the local tissue injury, extensive thermal injury results in derangements of the cardiovascular, respiratory, renal, and integumentary systems that interact to create the recognized entity of burn shock. These physiologic changes lead to hypovolemia through the loss of fluid and protein in both the burned and non-burned tissue. A severe burn injury can result in significant hypovolemic shock. This inflammatory response, when paired with the tissue trauma, leads to the formation of local and systemic edema as well as the expression of mediators associated with inflammation and trauma [7–9]. Even when the initial hypovolemia is corrected, there remains a significant systemic inflammatory state. The increases in pulmonary and systemic vascular resistance and decrease in myocardial contractility remain even after the hypovolemia has been corrected and the preload is adequate [10–13]. This dysregulation of the cardiovascular system can exacerbate the systemic inflammatory response and lead to accelerated organ dysfunction [8, 9, 14].

Types of Burns

Flame and Flash Burns

Flame and flash burns are the most prevalent burns admitted to burn centers in the USA representing almost half of admissions. Flash burns generally occur due to the ignition of flammable gases such as natural gas, butane, propane, or gasoline. The vapors of these gases are significantly denser than air (3–4 times heavier for gasoline, 2 times for butane, and 1.5 times for propane) and therefore can accumulate in enclosed spaces. When these gases are used inappropriately as a fire accelerant or in the production of butane hash oil, there can be an explosion [15]. The explosion of the highly flammable vapors leads to intense heat for a very short period of time. Accordingly flash burns tend to affect exposed skin that is not protected by clothing (unless the clothing itself ignites shifting a flash burn to a flame burn). Because of the quick exposure times, flash burns are often partial thickness and frequently do not require skin grafting, but can have high percentage total body surface area (%TBSA) affected (Fig. 2.1). Many flash burns, however, end up needing grafting. Additionally, they can cause upper airway burns, edema, and inhalation injury.

While flash and flame burns are often combined for reporting purposes, they tend to have very different effects. Flame burns tend to be deep partial thickness or full thickness because the duration of exposure to intense heat tends to be longer than that experienced during flash injuries (Fig. 2.2). They tend to require surgical excision and grafting as treatment due to their depth. Traditionally many flame burns have been the result of house fires; however primary prevention efforts aimed at the proper use of smoke detec-

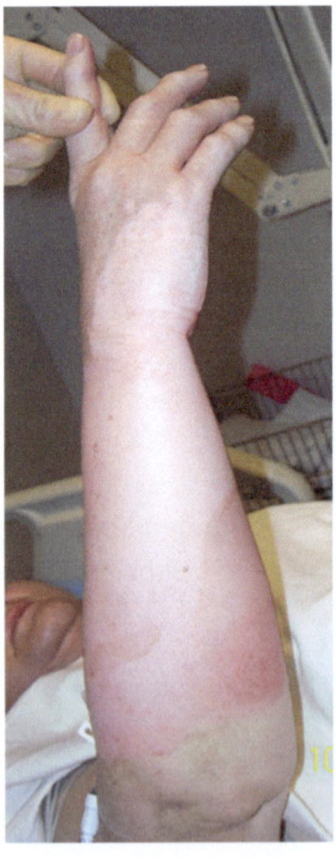

Fig. 2.1 This is a typical flash burn that led to well-demarcated burns to the forearm. The forearm was exposed, while the upper arm was covered with the sleeve of the shirt. The burn is of indeterminate depth

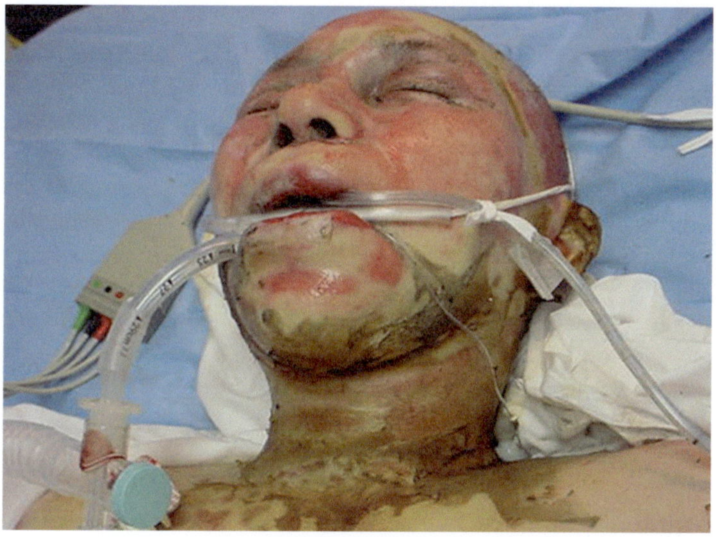

Fig. 2.2 This is a typical deep flame that was the result of a self-immolation with gasoline

tors have been successful in reducing the number of these incidents. Currently the more common causes of flame burns include careless smoking, automobile accidents, and the ignition of clothing. Frequently a flammable liquid is involved (66 % of the time) and gasoline is the most common liquid (63 % of cases) in these burns as well [16]. Gasoline-related burns occur during the summer months and reflect the increased use of gasoline for farming or recreation purposes (bonfires, burning leaves, boating, yard work) during this season. The highest incidence of flame burns occurs in those aged 15–29 years, and like all burns, they tend to occur more commonly in men. The most common contributing factor in flame burn injuries is a high blood ethanol level (28 %) leading to 51 % of those on fire using inappropriate attempts to escape the flames which leads to deeper burns [17].

Scald

Scald burn injuries are the second most common cause of burns in adults in the USA and the most common cause of burns in children under the age of 4 years [18]. While burn prevention has been very successful for other types of burns, the incidence of scalds has changed very little despite multiple educational programs. Liquids, grease, or steam can cause scald burns. Scalds caused by liquids or grease can be further divided into spill and immersion scalds. Most scalds are first- or second-degree burns, but third-degree burns can result, especially with prolonged contact (Fig. 2.3). The depth of the scald burn depends on the temperature of the liquid or steam, the thickness of the skin, and the duration of contact (which is somewhat determined by the viscosity of the liquid). The hotter the liquid, the shorter the contact time is needed to cause the same depth burn. For example, at 140 °F (60 °C), water causes a third-degree burn in 5 s, but when the temperature is increased 156 °F (69 °C), a similar burn will occur in 1 s. At 120 °F (49 °C), it would

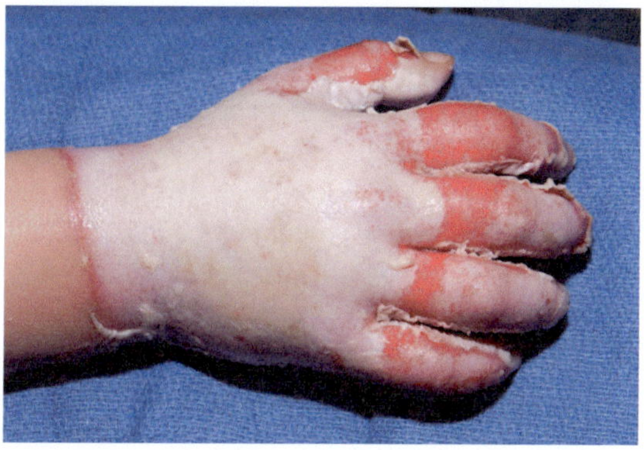

Fig. 2.3 This is a deep scald burn to a hand that was dipped into hot water

take 10 min of exposure to liquid to create a third-degree burn. Liquids that are thicker in consistency, such as soups or sauces, and therefore stay in contact with the skin longer, cause deeper burns. As opposed to flash and flame burns, areas exposed to hot liquids tend to sustain more shallow burns than clothed areas. Clothing holds the heat and keeps it in contact with the skin longer. As length of contact is critical in determining the depth of burn in scald injuries, immersion scalds are more often deeper than a spill scald with liquid at the same temperature [19, 20].

The treatment of scald burns also depends on the type of liquid that scalds the patient. Burns that are caused by grease and hot oil are generally deeper and are often full thickness. The most common scenario for sustaining grease burns is when a patient attempts to carry a burning pan of oil out of the house rather than putting a lid on the pan to extinguish the fire. This leads to a recognizable injury pattern where patients present with burns to either a single hand or the wrist (which is actually a flame burn) or more diffusely if the pan is dropped or the patient slips on the oil and falls [21]. Grease or oil burns require excision and grafting in 30–40 % of patients [22]. Tar and asphalt burns are another special type of scald injury. These burns are often deep, but the depth of the burn cannot be fully assessed until the tar is removed. Unfortunately tar is not easily removed from the patient and special consideration must be given to its removal. Tar can be removed by application of a petroleum-based ointment (such as bacitracin). This ointment is placed under a dressing and is changed every 2–4 h until the tar has dissolved.

The most significant scald injuries tend to occur in patients who cannot feel or perceive the discomfort of prolonged immersion (diabetics soaking their feet in hot water) or in patients who are not capable of escaping the hot water (young children, the elderly, or people with cognitive or physical disabilities that limit their ability to function independently). Because this latter group is an extremely vulnerable group, there is always a concern for non-accidental injury when they sustain scald injuries [23]. One must be cognizant of the risk for non-accidental burn and consider whether the story matches the pattern of injuries and look for patterns of burns that are suggestive of abuse even if the story of burn is plausible. These include circumferential extremity injuries and symmetrical burns to the buttocks and perineum (see Chap. 23). It is best to involve a burn surgeon if abuse is suspected given their experience with burn distribution and etiologies.

Scald burns are often partial thickness and can be managed nonoperatively if it is thought that they will heal within 10–14 days. Deep burns should be treated with excision and autografting early. Burns that are intermediate between superficial and deep should be excised and grafted whenever it becomes clear that they will not heal with local wound therapy in 2–3 weeks. This strategy was confirmed by Desai et al. [24] who compared children with large scald burns (greater than 25 % TBSA) that were either excised early (within 72 h) or after 2 weeks post injury. The children in the latter group were found to require excision of significantly smaller areas, and half of these delayed patients achieved reepithelialization without surgery. The ultimate decision depends on the likelihood of scarring. Small grafts in the middle of large healed areas are often more unsightly than healed burns with small scars.

Contact

Contact burns are the result of physical contact with a hot object. Common objects that cause contact burns are cigarettes, heaters, fireplaces, stoves, ovens, irons, exhaust pipes, soldering equipment, industrial equipment, and hot coals. These burns are generally small in size, but can be full thickness (Fig. 2.4). As with scald burns, the depth of contact burns can be predicted based on the temperature of the object that is contacted and the duration of the contact. Additionally, the situation surrounding the contact burn must be considered because there can be associated injuries which influence both the depth of the burn wound and concomitant resuscitation.

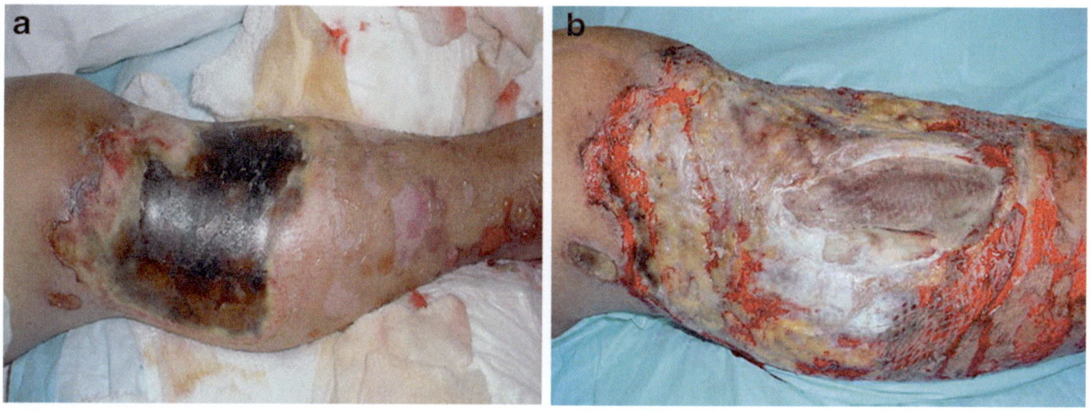

Fig. 2.4 (**a**) This is a typical contact burn of a leg being held against a hot engine block after a car crash. (**b**) With excision, it can be seen that this burn was a combination of crush and contact with the hot metal. These burns are often very severe

For example, a contact burn sustained in an industrial setting might involve contact with hot, heavy objects leading to deep full-thickness burns and crush injury. In these patients, the physician must anticipate the possibility of myonecrosis and myoglobinuria and alter their resuscitative efforts to account for this by increasing the amount of fluid given and targeting a higher urine output. Similarly burns sustained from contact with engine blocks after car crashes tend to be deeper than perceived and require significant excision and often require flaps for coverage [25]. Contact burns in children most often involve the palm and fingers. These tend to occur when toddlers put their hands on a hot object such as a woodstove, fireplace door, iron, or oven door [26]. Young children tend to freeze when in contact with a hot surface so the duration of contact is longer than for adults whose normal reflex is to immediately pull away. These wounds are often of intermediate depth and heal within 2–3 weeks, and while they require wound care and hand therapy, they do not require surgery if they heal in 2–3 weeks. Burns to palms that are deeper, especially in toddlers, are at risk of developing contractures and therefore require excision and grafting. Small hand burns are often treated with full-thickness skin grafts, but larger burns can be treated with split-thickness skin grafts with good cosmetic and functional outcomes [27, 28].

Electrical

An electrical burn results from the passage of electricity through the body with high-intensity heat generated as the patient becomes an inadvertent resistor. Electrical burns comprise only a small percentage of admissions to major burn centers (5–7 %) [29–31], but they may be the most devastating of all thermal injuries on a size-for-size basis as they involve both the skin and deeper tissues (Fig. 2.5). These injuries cause approximately 1,000 deaths per year in the USA. This results in a mortality rate of 3–5 % [32]. Burn injury due to electrical sources has three potential components. The first is a true electrical injury caused by current flow. Injuries can occur due to contact with either high- or low-voltage energy sources. Secondly injuries can result from the electrical flash (arc), which is generated as superheated ionized air flashes from the source to an object. These brief exposures to heat often result in burns that behave and are treated in much the same way as other flash burns. Finally, a flame injury can result from the ignition of clothes or the surrounding structures. These injuries are generally treated as any other flame burn would be treated. Electrical burns of all varieties have preponderance for affecting young working men employed as power company linemen, electricians, construction workers, laborers, and crane operators [33].

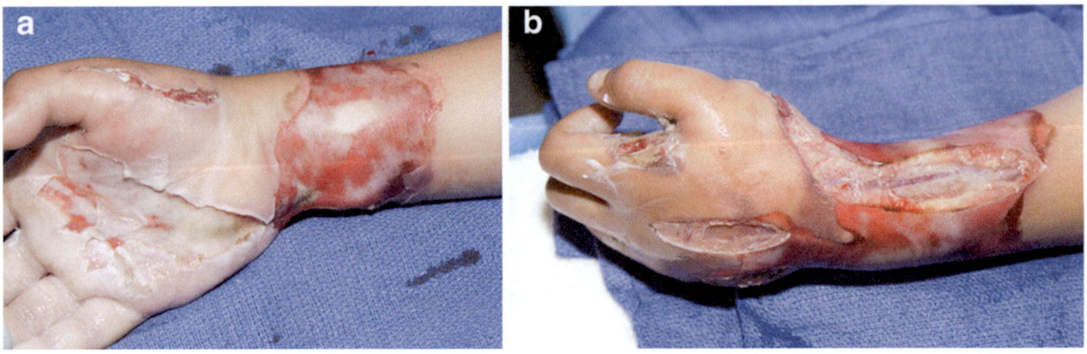

Fig. 2.5 There are two views of a classic high-voltage electrical burn to a hand. In (**a**), the contact with the wire on the palm can be seen. The current also affected the forearm. The hand is in the classic fixed and flexed position (**b**). The hand was ultimately amputated

The severity of electrical burns is dependent upon the voltage, current, type of current (alternating or direct), duration of contact, and resistance at the point of contact. Injuries caused by <1000 V are considered low voltage, while those caused by sources that are 1000 V or higher are considered high voltage. In general low-voltage injuries are localized and more superficial, while high-voltage injuries are associated with greater deep tissue injury [34]. In the USA, indoor wiring operates on an alternating current at 120 V, and as such most injuries are low voltage except in specialized industrial settings or incidents involving high-voltage electrical lines. Low-voltage injuries rarely cause significant tissue damage. They often present with small deep thermal burns at the contact points. The one special situation in which a low-voltage injury can cause significant injury is when a child chews on an active electrical connection [35]. The moisture in the child's mouth completes the circuit and causes severe burns inside the mouth and on the lips. If these burns involve the oral commissure, they are at high risk for late contracture and need to be followed closely with aggressive OT, splinting, and stretching regimen (Fig. 2.6) [36, 37]. High-voltage injuries tend to cause more deep tissue injury. These injuries often hide extensive deep tissue destruction underneath external wounds that are relatively small. Most high-voltage electrical burns are work related involving construction workers, linemen, utility, and electrical workers.

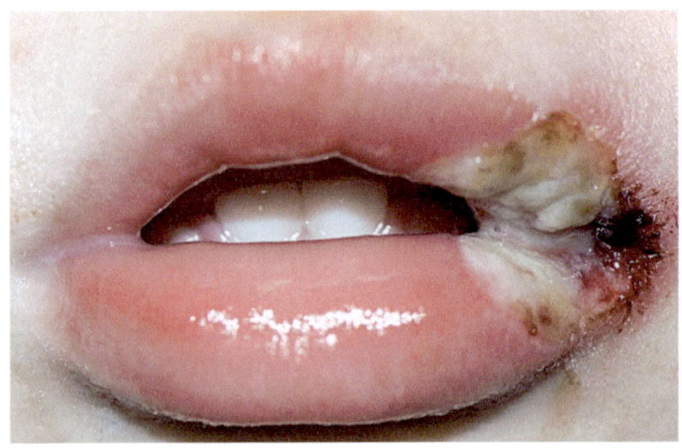

Fig. 2.6 This child sustained a typical commissure burn that resulted from chewing an electric cord. This small burn is quite disfiguring

With respect to current, the vast majority (~99 %) in the USA is alternating current, which reverses its polarity 120 times per second. Due to this fact, half of the time is spent positive with respect to ground and one-half is spent negative so one does not know whether a given point on the body contacted the wire or the ground making the terms "entrance" and "exit" wounds no longer appropriate. "Entrance" and "exit" have now been replaced by the term "contact points." Additionally alternating current causes tetanic muscle contractions. This can result in either throwing the patient away from the contact or drawing them into continued contact with the source of electricity. This inability to let go of the electricity source increases injury severity because of prolonged contact time [38].

Resistance is also critical to determining the extent of injury in electrical burns. At the level of the skin, high resistance is protective, but within the body, areas of increased resistance are at increased risk. Areas of dry calloused skin are partially protective as they have twice the resistance of normal skin and five times the resistance of wet skin. In the body the tissue resistance is lowest in the nerves and highest in the fat and bone. While in theory the current would be distributed in proportion to resistance throughout the body, this has not been seen to be the case in animal models. These models have shown that the body acts as a single uniform resistor rather than a collection of separate resistors [39]. However, as electricity travels through the body, the electrical injury is converted to heat. This results in deep muscle necrosis adjacent to the bone as these areas have the highest resistance and retain the most heat. This is especially true in the periosseous tissues between two bones such as the radius and ulna or the tibia and fibula [40, 41]. The increased retention of heat as well as the fact that there is less surface area for dissipation makes these areas particularly sensitive. In fact, the severity of injury is often inversely proportional to the cross-sectional area of the body part which is involved because of these factors. This leads to more destruction of the fingers, hands, forearms, ankles, and feet, while the damage has been traditionally thought to be less to the trunk and abdomen unless the injury is directly to those areas [42–44]. It has also been felt that the internal solid organs are generally preserved and protected from damage but recent animal studies suggest that this may not be the case. A recent study using a rabbit model of electrical injury found that there was severe injury to blood vessels and necrosis of vascular walls, which led to severe progressive muscular necrosis during the 72 h following injury. Additionally, they noted that there was evidence of injury to solid organs remote from the contact points such as the heart, lung, liver, and kidney [45]. This high-energy model does not reflect the clinical situation where major organs are rarely damaged.

When it comes to treating patients who have sustained electrical injuries, it is important to remember that they differ from other burn patients in likelihood of two important complications of burn injury: fluid resuscitation and need for fasciotomies. First, patients who sustain electrical injuries require increased amounts of fluid resuscitation per percent burn due to the myoglobinuria and acidosis secondary to the muscle destruction. If the increased fluid resuscitation fails, then fasciotomy, debridement, or amputation must be considered. Regardless of the development of myoglobinuria, these patients often require fasciotomies early in their hospitalizations due to tissue swelling and compartment syndrome. Due to the risk for compartment syndrome, affected extremities must be monitored closely. Fasciotomy is indicated for any sign of progressive peripheral neuropathy. If patients do not require immediate debridement, then a definitive operation can be postponed till post injury day 3–5. This allows debridement to take place before bacterial contamination but after the areas of deep necrosis are fully delineated [46, 47].

Chemical

Chemical burns are the result of chemicals contacting the skin. Many chemicals have the potential to cause damage to the skin and these injuries are relatively common. The American Association of Poison Control Centers (AAPCC) National Poison Data System (NPDS) 2013 annual report demonstrated 199,838 cases of exposure to cosmetic/personal care products; 196,183 household cleaning substances; 85,033 pesticides; and 33,081 hydrocarbons [48]. While these numbers have decreased somewhat over the last decade, there are still a significant number of exposures. Although chemical burns comprise only 3 % of all burns, they are responsible for almost 30 % of burn deaths. The majority of these deaths are the result of the ingestion of chemical substances [49]. In addition to ingestions, the most common sites of injury are the face, eyes, and extremities. Like electrical burns, chemical burns often occur on the job, especially in industrial settings; however they can result from contact with chemicals in the home as well. They often result from inadvertent contact with hazardous chemicals, cleaners, or solvents, but they can result from an assault. Usually these burns are caused by strong acids or alkalis. Unlike other burns where time of contact is usually limited, that is not always the case with chemical burns. The factors that contribute to the severity of a chemical burn are the concentration of the chemical, the quantity of chemical, the manner and duration of contact, mechanism of action of the chemical, and phase of the chemical agent (liquid, solid, or gas). The various mechanisms of action include reduction, oxidation, corrosion, protoplasmic poisoning, vesicants, and desiccants described in Chap. 16 [50]. Chemicals continue to cause damage to the skin until they are diluted by the flushing of the skin or inactivated by a reaction with the tissue. Burns that are caused by acid are generally less severe than those caused by an alkaline substance. Acids cause coagulation necrosis and precipitation of proteins that "tan" the skin which limit further penetration into the deeper tissues. Burns that are secondary to alkaline compounds lead to liquefactive necrosis of the cutaneous and subcutaneous lipids that leads to the destruction of deeper tissues [51]. Chemical burns can appear deceptively superficial as they may only be a brownish discoloration of the skin, but they are often deep dermal or full thickness. An example of this is burns caused by wet cement (calcium oxide [CaO]). These burns do not become symptomatic for hours after contact, and often by the time they seek medical attention, the wounds are so deep that they require skin grafting [52–54].

The initial management of all chemical burns is dilution of the chemical with copious water for 15–20 min. In the ideal situation, this would occur at the scene of the incident, prior to transport to the healthcare facility. In fact, almost all industrial and laboratory workplaces now have showers and areas for eye wash that facilitate the dilution of chemicals from the skin and eyes should an incident occur. The only exception to the use of irrigation as treatment is those chemicals, which are powders. Powdered chemicals, such as dry concrete, cement, and sodium hydroxide, should be brushed off of the skin prior to the utilization of irrigation. Although at first it might seem like a good idea to neutralize the alkali with acid or the other way around, but this is contraindicated. When you attempt to neutralize either an acid or an alkali, this can induce an exothermic reaction that can lead to a thermal injury on top of the chemical injury. While most chemical burns are treated with dilution followed by excision and skin grafting if necessary, some chemicals have specific treatment algorithms. The treatments of burns caused by specific chemicals are addressed in Chap. 16.

Frostbite

Frostbite (covered in detail in Chap. 17) is considered similar to a burn wound in terms of its inflammatory response [55]. In fact investigators hypothesize that frostbite follows Jackson's model for burn wounds which will be discussed later in this chapter [56]. Frostbite results when local tissue temperatures fall below freezing. There are two pathophysiologic mechanisms that lead to tissue damage in frostbite. First, there is direct cellular damage that occurs due to cold insult [57–60]. Pathologically it is noted by the formation of extracellular and intracellular ice crystals which lead to direct injury to the cell membrane. This results in water leaving the cell and cellular dehydration due to a change in the osmotic gradient [61]. This in turn results in a change to the lipid and protein conformations and alters the biochemical cellular processes that maintain homeostasis [61–65]. The rate of cooling influences the timing and the extent of the development of extracellular and intracellular ice crystals. Faster cooling leads to the development of intracellular ice crystals and more severe cell damage. When cooling occurs more slowly, there is an increase in extracellular ice crystal formation. Eventually, as the temperature drops, the intracellular crystals develop irrespective of the rate of cooling.

The second mechanism of injury in frostbite is progressive tissue ischemia. Tissue ischemia results from microvascular pathophysiology. A number of processes were identified that lead to these microcirculatory changes. There appears to be a transient vasoconstriction of arteriole and venules, which leads to concomitant microemboli [66]. The venules are more profoundly affected than the arterioles most likely due to low flow and the role of stasis in the pathophysiologic process of frostbite [67]. When thawing occurs the blood flow is restored to the capillaries, but then the blood flow subsequently diminishes within minutes. Within 20 min of rewarming, the blood flow completely stops. A similar process is observed in models of random skin flaps after reperfusion. It is believed that this occurs secondary to reactive oxygen species [68]. Seventy-two hours following restoration of blood flow, there is a significant loss of the endothelial lining and fibrin deposition in the capillary beds. Examination of the endothelium reveals swelling, fluid extravasation, and endothelial cell dilation [69].

Determinants of Burn Severity

Skin Biology

The skin is the largest organ of the human body comprising a surface area of almost 2 m^2. It is composed of three layers: the epidermis, the dermis, and the subcutaneous fat. The epidermis is the thin, tough, outer layer of the skin. It varies in thickness throughout different areas of the body. At its thinnest it is 0.05 mm on the eyelids and as thick as 1 mm on the soles of the feet [70]. The epidermis is derived from ectoderm. It is mainly composed of keratinocytes. Keratinocytes begin their life cycle at the basal layer of the epidermis and then migrate to the surface over 2–4 weeks [71]. The outer layers of the epidermis are divided into the stratum spinosum, the stratum granulosum, the stratum lucidum, and the stratum corneum (see Chap. 8). Keratinocytes lose their nuclei in the stratum lucidum and by the time they reach the stratum corneum they are flattened dead cells. The other two cell types in the epidermis are melanocytes, which produce melanin pigment that serves as a protection against ultraviolet radiation and Langerhans cells which are responsible for phagocytosis and antigen presentation. Burn wounds that are confined to the epidermis will heal without surgery or scarring. The keratinocytes that proliferate to heal an epidermal wound originate from the basal layer of the epidermis as well as from the dermal appendages (hair follicles and sweat glands). Even wounds that only involve the epidermis can have permanent pigment changes due to the depletion of melanocytes after injury which regenerated more slowly and less predictably than keratinocytes [72, 73]. Deeper burns tend to have more pigment problems than those that are more superficial.

The epidermis is connected to the dermis in the basement membrane zone through the epidermal projections called rete ridges that interdigitate with the dermal papillae. The dermal–epidermal junction is stabilized by the keratinocyte-derived collagen VII anchoring fibrils that extend into the dermis [74, 75]. When the skin is burned to the level of the dermal–epidermal junction or deeper, then the anchoring fibrils are damaged. These structures often take longer to regenerate and for the dermal–epidermal junction to fully mature (on the order of weeks to months) than the overlying keratinocytes. In addition, it takes time for the rete pegs to redevelop. Because of this, even seemingly minor insults to newly healed skin can lead to shearing, blistering, and epidermal loss.

The majority of the skin's thickness is made up of the dermis. Its thickness varies with age, gender, and body location. The dermis is a thick layer of fibrous and elastic tissue. The dermis is derived from mesoderm and is divided into the papillary dermis which is superficial and the reticular dermis which is the deeper layer. The principal cell of the dermis is the fibroblast which synthesizes both collagen and elastin. The majority of the structure of the dermis is provided by collagen fibers that are organized to provide stretching and tensile strength [76]. The elastin fibers provide the elastic recoil of the skin. The nonfibrous components of the dermis are called ground substance. Glycosaminoglycans are its main components, and it functions to maintain the semifluid matrix of the dermis and to regulate cellular cross talk [77]. Running through the matrix of the dermis are the dermal plexus of capillary vessels, sensory nerves, and adnexal structures of the skin. The adnexal structures include the sweat glands, sebaceous glands, and hair follicles which originate in the dermis and traverse the epidermis. These structures are lined with epidermal keratinocytes. Due to this lining of keratinocytes, the adnexal structures provide the epithelial cells necessary for reepithelialization after a partial dermal burn injury. The blood vessels of the dermal plexus aid in the healing of the wound by delivering the necessary nutrients to the cellular structures of the dermis and epidermis. Finally, the sensory nerves are also affected when the dermis is injured. During the healing process, they serve to mediate pain and itching and modulate inflammation and contribute to the remodeling phase of wound healing [78, 79]. Unfortunately, burn wounds that involve the entire dermis heal through fibrosis rather than regeneration. This fibrosis, in turn, leads to scarring.

The third layer of the skin is the subcutaneous fat layer that lies below the dermis. It serves to insulate the body and provide protective padding, and it serves as an energy storage area. This layer also varies in thickness between individuals and between different areas of the body, e.g., fat on the eyelids is extremely thin, while it is thicker on the abdomen and buttocks. The functions of the skin are protection from the external environment, thermal regulation, sensation, and endocrine functions.

Zones of Burn Injury

When the skin is injured by a thermal injury, there is damage at the cellular level that leads to denaturation of proteins, loss of the integrity of the plasma membrane, and necrosis. This necrosis is the worst at the center of the wound and becomes less severe at the periphery of the wound. It was this observation that led to Jackson's description of the three zones of injury in 1953 which remains the conceptual model of burn injury even today [56]. The three zones of the burn wound are *coagulation*, *stasis*, and *hyperemia* (Fig. 2.7).

The *zone of coagulation* is the area of the most severe cellular damage at the center of the wound. This is the region where there are no viable cells

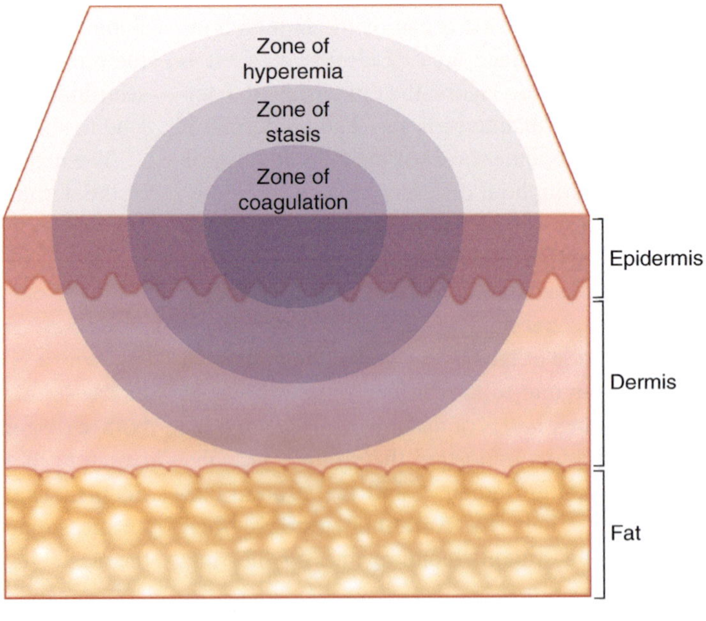

Fig. 2.7 This is a cartoon of the classic zones of a burn. The *zone of coagulation* contains the dead "eschar" that results from the heat of the injury. The *zone of stasis* contains capillaries that are jammed with leukocytes trying to enter the wound. This zone is at risk for necrosis with poor perfusion. The outer zone, the *zone of hyperemia*, is hyperemic because of vasodilation

remaining. As there are no remaining viable cells in this zone, its outcome is not affected by resuscitation or local wound care. The *zone of stasis* surrounds the *zone of coagulation*. The *zone of stasis* is composed of both viable and nonviable cells. The nonviable cells in this zone are either apoptotic or necrotic as a result of oxidative stress, inflammation, and decreased blood flow due to microthrombus formation [80]. This is the area that is vulnerable to low flow states and its outcome depends on proper medical care. The capillaries "clog" with leukocytes and debris to create a "traffic jam" that slows blood flow. Persistent stasis will lead to an increased risk of thrombosis. With inadequate wound care and resuscitation, this area will be exposed to hypoperfusion, edema, or infection and will progress to necrosis. Healthcare providers need to ensure the patient is properly resuscitated and avoid vasoconstrictors when possible to minimize burn depth progression [81, 82]. Wound care should consist of topical antibiotics and non-desiccating dressings to prevent further damage to the zone of stasis [83–85]. Additionally, patient factors such as advanced age, diabetes, or other chronic illnesses may contribute to worse outcomes for the zone of stasis. However, with proper care, the damage to this area is reversible as it is repopulated with viable cells. The outermost zone of a burn wound is the *zone of hyperemia*. This zone contains viable cells and is hyperemic due to local inflammatory-mediated vasodilation. This tissue will recover completely unless it is compromised by infection or hypoperfusion.

Determination of Burn Depth

Clinical Observation

Determination of burn wound depth is critical to determining the treatment approach for each patient. Burn wounds are classified as first degree (superficial burns), second degree (superficial dermal burns and deep dermal burns), third degree (full-thickness burns), and fourth degree (involving underlying structures such as the muscle or bone) (see Chap. 8). The traditional manner of determining burn depth is through clinical observation. Burn injury can involve the epidermis, the epidermis and the dermis, or may even affect the underlying subcutaneous fat, muscles, and bones [86]. First-degree burns (or superficial burns) only affect the epidermis. They are erythematous and extremely painful. As they only affect the epidermis and the keratinocyte-derived collagen VII anchoring fibrils between the dermis and the epidermis remain intact, there is no blister formation. Sunburns are a classic example of a first-degree, superficial burn affecting only the epidermis. These burns heal over the course of 3–5 days as the dead dermis sloughs and is replaced by new keratinocytes.

Second-degree burns extend into the dermis and are classified as either superficial dermal burns or deep dermal burns. Superficial dermal burns involve the epidermis and the papillary dermis. They are characterized by blister formation. Blisters may not form immediately following the injury and burns that are initially thought to be superficial may actually be superficial dermal injuries [4]. When the blister is debrided from a superficial dermal burn, the underlying wound is pink, but blanch to touch and also moist. It is also hypersensitive to touch making exposure to air and wound care extremely painful. The dermis in these injuries has increased blood flow due to vasodilation. Generally if treated appropriately, superficial dermal burns do not require an operation and heal on their own in 2–3 weeks with minimal risk of scarring. Deep dermal burns extend beyond the papillary dermis to the reticular dermis. These burns also develop blisters, but when the blisters are removed, the underlying wound surface appears mottled, pink, and white. This appearance occurs immediately following an injury. When pressure is applied to these wounds, the capillaries refill slowly. Deep partial-thickness wounds are characterized by discomfort rather than pain and have decreased sensation compared to the surrounding tissue. The management decisions for these wounds can be difficult because they are on the cusp of being full-thickness wounds. These wounds may or may not heal within 3 weeks and the differential between healing and not may only be a few tenths of a millimeter. These burns require serial assessment over the course of days. Even in the hands of an experienced surgeon, decisions about indeterminate deep dermal burns are only accurate 50–70 % of the time [87–89]. Those that do not heal in 3 weeks should be excised and skin grafted.

Third-degree burns are full-thickness injuries. They involve the epidermis and dermis and extend into the subcutaneous tissue. These wounds are firm and leathery. Some appear charred as well. The wounds that are not charred can be deceptive in appearance because they may also appear pink and mottled. However, unlike deep dermal wounds, full-thickness wounds do not blanch on pressure. They have decreased sensation to light touch and pain. In order to speed recovery and prevent infection and hypertrophic scarring, these wounds need to be excised and skin grafted early in their hospital course.

Adjuncts to Clinical Evaluation

Clinical determination of burn wound depth is not precise. In fact, clinical assessment of wound depth for all burn depths is 50–70 % accurate in the hands of senior burn surgeons [90]. This has led, over the last 80 years, to an intense search for a more precise method for determining burn wound depth, especially since it has been shown that patients benefit from early excision [90–92]. The ability to determine earlier which patients require excision would allow more patients to undergo early excision and skin grafting. Multiple modalities have been developed with this aim including thermography, photometry, nuclear imaging, pulse-echo ultrasound, and serial tissue biopsy. Each of these techniques attempts to take advantage of a different aspect of the changes in the burn wound. Serial biopsy, ultrasound, and vital dyes attempt to detect dead cells or denatured collagen [56, 93–96], while fluorescein, laser Doppler imaging, and thermography detect the altered blood flow of the wound to determine burn wound depth [97–99]. MRI attempts to detect physical changes such as edema [100]. One of the more recent techniques to show promise is noncontact laser Doppler imaging for burns that are of indeterminate thickness [90, 101, 102]. Noncontact laser Doppler has the advantage over some other adjunct methods for burn wound depth determination in that it is well tolerated by patients because it is held at a distance from the wound and does not exert pressure on the wound and can be used for serial measurements so that dynamic changes to the wound bed perfusion can be seen. To date none of these techniques has supplanted serial clinical assessment by an experienced clinician as the standard of care.

Systemic Responses to Burn Injury

Edema Formation in Acute Burn Injury

When a burn injury occurs, there is extravasation of the plasma into the burn wound. The movement of fluid to the extracellular space leads to hypovolemia and the consequent hemodynamic changes including decreases in plasma volume, cardiac output, and urine output with concomitant increase in systemic vascular resistance [7, 9, 103–105]. The primary goal in these situations is to restore intravascular volume and maintain tissue perfusion. This is not an easy task in the burn patient as there is the formation of extensive burn wound edema but also the extravasation and sequestration of fluid and protein in non-burned organs and soft tissues. Burn patients require large volumes of fluid resuscitation to maintain vascular volume during the initial hours following injury and it often takes 24–36 h before the goal of returning to a normal blood volume can be achieved [106]. Resuscitation is covered in Chap. 5.

Edema develops when the vascular fluid extravasates out of the microvessels at a rate that is faster than can be resorbed by the lymphatics draining the tissues. In extensive burns, edema follows a biphasic pattern where there is an immediate increase in the water content of the burn tissue within the first hour following injury [104, 107]. This initial edema formation within the burned tissue is extremely rapid in onset. In fact the tissue water content can double within the first hour after the injury [104, 108]. Leape found a 70–80 % increase in the water content of a full-thickness burn wound within the first 30 min after burn injury, with 90 % of this change occurring in the first 5 min [105, 109, 110]. Without resuscitation there was only a modest increase in burn wound water content. However, in resuscitated animals, adequate tissue perfusion continues to "feed" the edema for several hours. This extraneous fluid leads to the second phase of burn tissue edema which is a more gradual increase in fluid into the burn tissue and the non-burned soft tissue during the first 12–24 h following injury [8, 107]. The quantity of edema that forms is related to type and extent of injury, and on whether fluid resuscitation is provided, as well as the type and volume of fluid administered [104, 111, 112]. If vascular losses are not replaced, then the edema is self-limited as the tissue blood flow and capillary pressure decrease; however this causes other systemic issues.

Edema in Non-burned Tissue

In addition to the edema that develops within the burn injury, there is generalized edema that develops in the non-burned soft tissues when a patient sustains a burn injury. It has been reported that there is increased water content in non-burned skin even after as small as a 10 % burn with the peak of this edema occurring in the 12 h post injury [113]. Arturson reported an increased transcapillary lymph flow from non-burned tissue and a transient increase in permeability of vessels in these, as measured by an increase in the lymph concentration of the plasma [104, 108, 114]. Harms et al. [115] measured changes in lymph flow and protein transport in non-injured soft tissue for 3 days following injury and found that skin and muscle permeability were elevated for up to 12 h post burn for molecules the size of albumin and immunoglobulin G, but the microvascular permeability of the lung showed no increase. Severe hypoproteinemia correlates with increased lymph flow and tissue water content during the early resuscitation period and is also likely related to the sustained increase in water content and elevated lymph flow after the return of normal vascular permeability [9, 107–109, 115, 116]. Non-burn soft tissue edema can be ameliorated by the infusion of nonprotein colloids or the protein albumin, but it is unclear if either of these leads to an improvement in clinical outcomes [9, 117, 118]. In an effort to prevent edema, the use of hypertonic saline formulations as initial fluid therapies for burn shock has been studied. It has been shown that hypertonic saline can greatly reduce initial volume requirements [119, 120]. Unfortunately this is accompanied by a rebound increase in fluid requirements [116, 119]. Retrospective studies looking at correcting hypoproteinemia with early albumin use showed significant volume sparing during the first postburn day, but after 48 h, the effect is less apparent [121].

Edema in Muscle and the Nervous System

In addition to the changes seen in the burn and the surrounding soft tissues, there are changes following a thermal injury to the cellular membrane. Directly injured cells have a damaged cell membrane, which leads to increasing sodium and potassium fluxes and consequently cell swelling. In addition, this process also occurs in cells that are not directly injured by the burn. In skeletal muscle, the cellular transmembrane potentials are decreased even away from the site of injury [11]. The alterations in skeletal membrane functions and cellular edema following burn injury are similar to those seen in hemorrhagic shock [122, 123]. Following the burn injury, action potentials in general become dampened or nonexistent. Delays in signal propagation in the nerves, brain, skeletal muscle, heart, diaphragm, and gastrointestinal organs associated with major burn injury lead to encephalopathy, muscle weakness, impaired cardiac contractility, and gut dysfunction. It was initially thought that this delay in signal propagation was due to a decrease in adenosine triphosphate (ATP) levels or ATPase activity. More recent research suggests that increased sodium conductance in membranes, or an increase in sodium–hydrogen antiport activity, is the primary mechanism of delayed conduction [124]. Resuscitation of burn injury only partially restores the membrane potential and intracellular sodium concentrations to normal levels.

This demonstrates that hypovolemia alone is not completely responsible for the cellular swelling seen in burn shock [125]. Little is known about the time course of these changes in membrane potential in clinical burns, and it is not known to what extent the altered membrane potentials affect total volume requirements and organ function in burn.

Lungs

Pulmonary edema is common following a major burn injury and occurs more often following the initial fluid resuscitation phase than after the resuscitation. The pulmonary wedge pressure in the lung is increased secondary to the increased pulmonary vascular resistance that occurs with pre- and postcapillary vasoconstriction following burn injury. It is thought that this contributes to the formation of pulmonary edema [126, 127]. While there is likely some amount of left heart failure associated with burn injury that leads to the increased wedge pressure, the hypoproteinemia that was previously discussed is likely the greatest contributing fact to postburn pulmonary edema [127]. Animal models of burn injury revealed that there was not any evidence of increased capillary permeability in the lung, although they do suggest that albumin sequestration in the lung does increase following burn injury [128]. Clinical studies suggest that the burn-injured patients who have not sustained inhalation injury do not develop severe edema [129, 130]. This finding is consistent with the fact that there is virtually no change in the microvascular permeability of the lung and the fact that the lung lymph drainage rate may increase to prevent the accumulation of interstitial fluid.

Abdominal Compartment Syndrome

Abdominal compartment syndrome (ACS) is a life-threatening complication of edema [131, 132]. Intra-abdominal hypertension (IAH) is defined as an intra-abdominal pressure (IAP) >30 cm H_2O. ACS is a syndrome defined by sustained IAH in combination with a clinically tense abdomen, ventilation aberrations due to elevated pulmonary inspiratory pressures, and decreased urine output despite aggressive fluid resuscitation. Due to the large volumes of IV fluid resuscitation, decreased abdominal wall compliance (due to burn eschar), increased capillary permeability with leakage of large plasma volumes, and massive edema formation, severely burn-injured patients are especially at risk for ACS. In the critically ill burn-injured patient, ACS is often but not always fatal. It typically leads to multiple organ dysfunctions including impaired renal and hepatic blood flow, bowel ischemia, pulmonary dysfunction, depressed cardiac function, and increased intracranial pressures [133].

Hemodynamic Consequences of Acute Burn Injury

Myocardial Dysfunction

During the resuscitative phase of burn injury, the cardiac output (CO) is reduced, but the cause of this effect is the subject of much debate. Following burn injury there is an immediate depression of the cardiac output. This occurs even before there is any detectable reduction in plasma volume. The rapidity of this increase is thought to result from impaired electrical activity of the cardiac muscles and nerves and also due to an increase in afterload due to vasoconstriction. As more time passes following the burn injury, hypovolemia develops and leads to decreased venous return. This in turn contributes to reduced cardiac output. The cardiac output remains reduced even after adequate fluid therapy and restoration of a normal arterial blood pressure. This decrease has been attributed to circulating myocardial depressant factors, which possibly originate from the burn wound [12, 13]. In one study in sheep, a 15 % reduction in CO was found despite an aggressive volume repletion protocol [117]. Michie et al. found, upon looking at the CO and SVR in anesthetized dogs resuscitated after burn injury, that CO fell after the injury and over time returned to normal [134]. They also found that the reduced CO did not parallel the blood volume loss associated with the burn. They determined that the depression of CO is multifactorial and results from decreased blood volume, decreased venous return, and increased SVR and from a presumed circulating myocardial depressant substance. Following resuscitation and resolution of burn shock, patients develop a supranormal CO that is associated with the hypermetabolic state of burn.

In burn injury, myocardial function is compromised. The primary mechanism by which a burn injury alters myocardial cell membrane integrity and impairs myocardial function remains unclear. On a cellular level, it is thought that oxygen-derived free radicals may play a key causative role. Horton et al. found that a combination therapy of free radical scavengers and catalase significantly improved burn-mediated defects in left ventricular contractility and relaxation when administered with adequate fluid resuscitation, but antioxidant therapy did not alter the volume of fluid resuscitation required [135]. On a structural level, the decrease in myocardial function is thought to be due to the right heart overload and a direct depression in contractility [136, 137]. The decreased myocardial contractility is more pronounced following a burn injury because there are increases in the afterload of the right and the left heart due to increases in systemic vascular resistance (SVR) and peripheral vascular resistance (PVR). Unfortunately the right ventricle has very little ability to compensate for the increased afterload. The adrenergic stimulation associated with a burn injury helps maintain stroke volume (SV) and CO despite the myocardial depression. This comes at the cost of increased myocardial oxygen demands. It has been demonstrated that burn injury leads to contractile defects and both systolic and diastolic dysfunction which is present for the first few weeks following injury and is not corrected with early and aggressive fluid resuscitation [138–142]. This proves that hypovolemia is not the sole mechanism underlying the myocardial defects seen with burn shock. Additionally, researchers have found that serum from patients that fail to sustain a normal CO after a burn injury exhibits markedly negative inotropic effect on an in vitro heart preparation, while the serum of patients who had normal cardiac indices had no depressant activity [107, 135]. In addition to their work on antioxidants, Horton et al. demonstrated that there is decreased left ventricular contractility following burn injury, and that this is worse in the hearts of the aged [140]. They found that this was not reversed by resuscitation with isotonic fluid, but was reversed with early (first 4–6 h) resuscitation with 4 ml/kg of hypertonic saline dextran [141, 142]. In opposition to what was found in most other studies, Cioffi and colleagues found that persistent myocardial depression only occurred when animals in their model received no resuscitation. They found that immediate and full resuscitation completely reversed the alterations to myocardial function [143]. All of these studies emphasize the importance of early and adequate fluid therapy and suggest that functional myocardial depression may not occur in patients who receive prompt and adequate volume therapy.

Effects of Burns on Other Organ Systems

Several organ systems are particularly susceptible to ischemia and organ failure when burn resuscitation is delayed or not adequate. The kidney and the gastrointestinal tract are especially sensitive to ischemia. Hypovolemia, increased sympathetic tone, myocardial depression, inflammatory mediators (cytokines, eicosanoids, and platelet-aggregating factor), nephrotoxic agents, and pigmenturia can contribute to renal ischemia and injury [144–146]. Renal failure rates have improved dramatically over the last several decades owing to standardized adequate fluid resuscitation. However, when therapy is delayed or the patient develops hypotension, acute renal failure can occur. The gastrointestinal tract is extremely sensitive to ischemia as well. Occult ischemia and hypoxia can occur following burn due to vasoconstriction that occurs secondary to inflammatory mediators and increased sympathetic tone. This can occur even in the face of seemingly adequate resuscitation [147]. The ischemia of the bowel leads to a reduction in mucosal pH, degradation of the mucus layer, bacterial overgrowth, and bacterial translocation that can lead to the development of sepsis, Curling's ulcers, and irreversible bowel ischemia. Fortunately, the gut is remarkably tolerant of the insults of a major burn.

Cellular Mediators of Inflammation in Burn Injury

Following burn injury there are many inflammatory mediators which act both locally and systemically to cause burn shock. These mediators play complex roles in the pathogenesis of edema and the cardiovascular abnormalities of burn injury and burn shock. These mediators act in a myriad of ways including altering vascular permeability and transcapillary fluid flux, increasing the microvascular hydrostatic pressure, causing vasodilation, and altering membrane permeability. The mediators most often associated with burn shock include histamine, serotonin, bradykinin, oxygen-free radicals, prostaglandin, thromboxane, epinephrine, norepinephrine, vasopressin, angiotensin II, and interleukins. For a summary of the cellular mediators that play a role in burn shock, refer to Table 2.1 [128, 148–166].

Table 2.1 Cellular mediators of burn wound injury

Cellular mediator	Effect in the setting of a burn injury
Histamine	• Responsible for increased microvascular permeability immediately after burn injury • Causes large endothelial gaps to form due to the contraction of venular endothelial cells • Released from mast cells • Causes a rise in capillary pressure through arteriolar dilation and venular contraction • In animals, histamine blockers reduce localized edema, but the same benefit has not been demonstrated in humans [148]
Prostaglandins	• Synthesized from the arachidonic acid that is released from burned tissue and inflammatory cells • Contributes to inflammatory response of burn injury [149, 150] • Released from activated macrophages and neutrophils • Have local and systemic effects • Prostaglandin E2 (PGE2) and leukotrienes LB4 and LD4 increase microvascular permeability [151] • Prostacyclin (PGI2) is a vasodilator produced in burn injury and increases capillary permeability • PGE2 causes vasodilation, increased microvascular surface area, and increased microvascular permeability amplifying edema formation [152, 153]
Thromboxane	• Produced locally by platelets in the burn wounds [148] • Less important in edema formation • Can contribute to a growing zone of ischemia and can convert a partial-thickness wound to a deeper, full-thickness wound • Thromboxane inhibitors prevent progressive dermal ischemia [154, 155]
Bradykinin	• Local mediator of inflammation that increases venular permeability • Increased after burn injury • Generalized inflammatory response after burn injury favors the release of bradykinin [156]
Serotonin	• Released early after burn injury [157] • Smooth muscle constrictor of large blood vessels • Anti-serotonin agents reduce peripheral vascular resistance after burn injury, but not to reduce edema
Epinephrine and norepinephrine	• Released in massive amounts after burn injury [158, 159] • Cause arteriolar vasoconstriction via α1-receptor activation [148] • Lead to reduced capillary pressure that may limit edema and induce autoresuscitation of protein-poor interstitial fluid • Inhibit increased capillary permeability via β-agonist activity [148] • Potentially beneficial effects may not be fully functional in injured tissue and may be offset by vasoconstriction and ischemia in uninjured tissue

(continued)

Table 2.1 (continued)

Oxygen radicals	• Highly unstable reactive metabolites of oxygen • Strong oxidizing agents • Superoxide anion (O^{2-}), hydrogen peroxide (H_2O_2), and hydroxyl ion (OH^-) are produced and released by activated neutrophils after any inflammatory reaction or reperfusion of ischemic tissue • Hydroxyl ion (OH^-) is most potent and damaging • Evidence of oxygen radical formation after burn injury is the increased lipid peroxidation found in circulating red blood cells and biopsied tissue [128, 160, 161]
Platelet aggregation factor	• Increase capillary permeability and released after burn injury [162, 163] • A PAF antagonist blocked edema formation in a burn wound and inhibited PAF increase in the damaged tissue in a dose-dependent manner when given following burn injury and subsequently decreased the degree of burn shock [163]
Angiotensin II and vasopressin	• Participate in the normal regulation of extracellular fluid volume by controlling sodium balance and osmolality through renal function and thirst [148] • During burn shock both hormones are at supranormal levels in the blood due to increased sympathetic tone • Potent vasoconstrictors of terminal arterioles • Angiotensin II may be responsible for the selective gut and mucosal ischemia [164] • In severely burn-injured patients, angiotensin II levels were elevated two to eight times normal in the first 1–5 days after injury, with peak levels occurring on day 3 [165] • Vasopressin had peak levels of 50 times normal upon admission and declined toward normal over the first 5 days after burn injury • Vasopressin may be responsible for increased system vascular resistance and the left heart afterload
Corticotropin-releasing factor	• Reduce the extravasation of protein and therefore reduce the incidence of edema in a rat burn model [166] • May be a powerful natural inhibitory mediator of the acute inflammatory response of the skin in response to a burn injury

Summary

There are many pathophysiologic changes that occur after a burn injury. There are major local effects that affect how well a burn will heal. To make matters worse, large burns lead to profound systemic changes that influence not only healing of the burn wound but also the survival of the burn patient.

References

1. Underhill FP, Carrington GL, Kapsinow R, Pack GT. Blood concentration changes in extensive superficial burns, and their significance for systemic treatment. Arch Intern Med. 1923;32:31–9.
2. Moore FD. The body-weight burn budget. Basic fluid therapy for the early burn. Surg Clin North Am. 1970;50:1249–65.
3. Burke JF, Bondoc CC, Quinby WC. Primary burn excision and immediate grafting: a method shortening illness. J Trauma. 1974;14(5):389–95.
4. Engrav LH, Heimbach DM, Reus JL, Harnar TJ, Marvin JA. Early excision and grafting vs. nonoperative treatment of burns of indeterminate depth: a randomized prospective study. J Trauma. 1983; 23(11):1001–4.
5. Thompson P, Herndon DN, Abston S, Rutan T. Effect of early excision on patients with major thermal injury. J Trauma. 1987;27(2):205–7.
6. Gray DT, Pine RW, Harnar TJ, Marvin JA, Engrav LH, Heimbach DM. Early surgical excision versus conventional therapy in patients with 20 to 40 percent burns. A comparative study. Am J Surg. 1982;144(1):76–80.
7. Aulick LH, Wilmore DW, Mason Jr AD, Pruitt Jr BA. Influence of the burn wound on peripheral circulation in thermally injured patients. Am J Physiol. 1977;233:H520–6.
8. Settle JAD. Fluid therapy in burns. J Roy Soc Med. 1982;1(75):7–11.
9. Demling RH. Fluid replacement in burned patients. Surg Clin North Am. 1987;67:15–30.
10. Demling RH, Will JA, Belzer FO. Effect of major thermal injury on the pulmonary microcirculation. Surgery. 1978;83(6):746–51.
11. Baxter CR. Fluid volume and electrolyte changes of the early postburn period. Clin Plast Surg. 1974;1(4):693–709.

12. Baxter CR, Cook WA, Shires GT. Serum myocardial depressant factor of burn shock. Surg Forum. 1966;17:1–3.
13. Hilton JG, Marullo DS. Effects of thermal trauma on cardiac force of contraction. Burns Incl Therm Inj. 1986;12:167–71.
14. Clark WR. Death due to thermal trauma. In: Dolecek R, Brizio-Molteni L, Molteni A, et al., editors. Endocrinology of thermal trauma. Philadelphia, PA: Lea & Febiger; 1990. p. 6–27.
15. Jensen G, Bertelotti R, Greenhalgh D, Palmieri T, Maguina P. Honey oil burns: a growing problem. J Burn Care Res. 2015;36(2):e34–7.
16. Williams 2d JB, Ahrenholz DH, Solem LD, Warren W. Gasoline burns: the preventable cause of thermal injury. J Burn Care Rehabil. 1990;11(5):446–50.
17. Byrom RR, Word EL, Tewksbury CG, Edlich RF. Epidemiology of flame burn injuries. Burns Incl Therm Inj. 1984;11(1):1–10.
18. Shriners Hospitals for Children. Burn awareness week [internet]. 2015. http://www.shrinershospitalsforchildren.org/education/burn-awareness.
19. Ding YL, Pu SS, Pan ZL, Lu X, Miao SG, Han CM, et al. Extensive scalds following accidental immersion in hot water pools. Burns Incl Therm Inj. 1987;13(4):305–8.
20. Walker AR. Fatal tap water scald burns in the USA, 1979–1986. Burns. 1990;16(1):49–52.
21. Klein MB, Gibran NS, Emerson D, Sullivan SR, Honari S, Engrav LH, et al. Patterns of grease burn injury: development of a classification system. Burns. 2005;31(6):765–7.
22. Murphy JT, Purdue GF, Hunt JL. Pediatric grease burn injury. Arch Surg. 1995;130(5):478–82.
23. Bird PE, Harrington DT, Barillo DJ, McSweeney A, Shirani KZ, Goodwin CW. Elder abuse: a call to action. J Burn Care Rehab. 1998;19(6):522–7.
24. Desai MH, Rutan RL, Herndon DN. Conservative treatment of scald burns is superior to early excision. J Burn Care Rehab. 1991;12(5):482–4.
25. Gibran NS, Engrav LH, Heimbach DM, Swiontkowski MF, Foy HM. Engine block burns: Dupuytren's fourth-, fifth-, and sixth-degree burns. J Trauma. 1994;37(2):176–81.
26. Yanofsky NN, Morain WD. Upper extremity burns from woodstoves. Pediatrics. 1984;73(5):722–6.
27. Pensler JM, Steward R, Lewis SR, Herndon DN. Reconstruction of the burned palm: full-thickness versus split-thickness skin grafts – long-term follow-up. Plast Reconstr Surg. 1988;81(1):46–9.
28. Merrell SW, Saffle JR, Schnebly A, Kravitz M, Warden GD. Full-thickness skin grafting for contact burns of the palm in children. J Burn Care Rehab. 1986;7(6):501–7.
29. Esselman P, Thombs B, Magyar-Russell G, Fauerbach JA. Burn rehabilitation: state of the science. Am J Phys Med Rehabil. 2006;85:383–418.
30. Hussmann J, Kucan J, Russell R, Bradley T, Zamboni WA. Electrical injuries – morbidity, outcomes, and treatment rationale. Burns. 1995;21:530–5.
31. Lee R. Injury by electrical forces: pathophysiology, manifestations and therapy. Curr probl Surg. 1997;34:738–40.
32. Electrical Injuries in Emergency Medicine. Medscape reference. n.p. n.d. Web. Accessed 29 Sept 2011. http://emedicine.medscape.com/article/770179-overview.
33. Arnoldo B, Purdue G, Kowalske K, Helm PA, Burris A, Hunt JL. Electrical injuries: a 20 year review. J Burn Care Rehab. 2004;25:479–84.
34. Artz C. Electrical injury simulates crush injury. Surg Gynecol Obstet. 1967;125:1316–7.
35. Rai J, Jeschke MG, Barrow RE, Herndon DN. Electrical injuries: a 30-year review. J Trauma. 1999;46(5):933–6.
36. Holt GR, Parel S, Richardson DS, Kittle PE. The prosthetic management of oral commissure burns. Laryngoscope. 1982;92(4):407–11.
37. al-Qattan MM, Gillett D, Thomson HG. Electrical burns to the oral commissure: does splinting obviate the need for commissuroplasty? Burns. 1996;22(7):555–6.
38. Grube B, Heimbach D, Engrav L, Copass MK. Neurologic consequences of electrical burns. J Trauma. 1990;30:254–8.
39. Hunt J, Mason A, Masterson T, Pruitt Jr BA. The pathophysiology of acute electric burns. J Trauma. 1976;16:335–40.
40. Chilbert M, Maiman D, Sances A, Myklebust J, Prieto TE, Swiontek T, et al. Measure of tissue resistivity in experimental electrical burns. J Trauma. 1985;25(3):209–15.
41. Lee RC, Kolodney MS. Electrical injury mechanisms: dynamics of the thermal response. Plast Reconstr Surg. 1987;80(5):663–71.
42. Yang JY, Tsai YC, Noordhoff MS. Electrical burn with visceral injury. Burns Incl Therm Inj. 1985;11(3):207–12.
43. Branday JM, DuQuesnay DR, Yeesing MT, Duncan ND. Visceral complications of electrical burn injury. A report of two cases and review of the literature. West Indian Med J. 1989;38(2):110–3.
44. Honda T, Yamamoto Y, Mizuno M, Mitsusada M, Nakazawa H, Sasaki K, et al. Successful treatment of a case of electrical burn with visceral injury and full-thickness loss of the abdominal wall. Burns. 2000;26(6):587–92.
45. Jia-ke C, Li-gen L, Quan-wen G, Xiao-peng S, Hai-jun Z, Zhi-yong S, et al. Establishment of soft-tissue-injury model of high-voltage electrical burn and observation of its pathological changes. Burns. 2009;5:1158–64.
46. Mann R, Gibran N, Engrave L, Heimbach D. Is immediate decompression of high voltage electrical injuries to the upper extremity always necessary? J Trauma. 1996;40(4):584–7. discussion 587–589.
47. Yowler CJ, Mozingo DW, Ryan JB, Pruitt Jr BA. Factors contributing to delayed extremity amputation in burn patients. J Trauma. 1998;45(3):522–6.

48. Mowry JB, Spyker DA, Cantilena Jr LR, McMillan N, Ford M. 2013 Annual Report of the American Association of Poison Control Centers' National Poison Data System (NPDS): 31st Annual Report. Clin Toxicol. 2014;52:1032–283.
49. Watson WA, Litovitz TL, Rodgers Jr GC, Klein-Schwartz W, Reid N, Youniss J, et al. 2004 Annual Report of the American Association of Poison Control Centers Toxic Exposure Surveillance System. Am J Emerg Med. 2005;23(5):589–666.
50. Jelenko 3rd C. Chemicals that burn. J Trauma. 1979;14(1):65–72.
51. Yano K, Hata Y, Matsuka K, Ito O, Matsuda H. Effects of washing with a neutralizing agent on alkaline skin injuries in an experimental model. Burns. 1994;20(1):36–9.
52. Lewis PM, Ennis O, Kashif A, Dickson WA. Wet cement remains a poorly recognized cause of full-thickness skin burns. Injury. 2004;35(10):982–5.
53. Fisher AA. Cement burns resulting in necrotic ulcers due to kneeling on wet cement. Cutis. 1979;23(3): 272–4.
54. Early SH, Simpson RL. Caustic burns from contact with wet cement. JAMA. 1985;254(4):528–9.
55. Robson MC, Heggers JP. Evaluation of hand frostbite blister fluid as a clue to pathogenesis. J Hand Surg Am. 1981;6(1):43–7.
56. Jackson DM. The diagnosis of the depth of burning. Br J Surg. 1953;40(164):588–96.
57. Eubanks RG. Heat and cold injuries. J Ark Med Soc. 1974;71(1):53–8.
58. Fuhrman FA, Crismon JM. Studies on gangrene following cold injury: general course of events in rabbit feet and ears following untreated cold injury. J Clin Invest. 1947;26(2):236–44.
59. Quintanilla R, Krusen FH, Essex HE. Studies on frost-bite with special reference to treatment and the effect on minute blood vessels. Am J Physiol. 1947;149(1):149–61.
60. Weatherley-White RC, Sjostrom B, Paton BC. Experimental studies in cold injury. II. The pathogenesis of frostbite. J Surg Res. 1964;4:17–22.
61. Lovelock JE. Physical instability and thermal shock in red cells. Nature. 1954;173(4406):659–61.
62. Lovelock JE. The denaturation of lipid-protein complexes as a cause of damage by freezing. Proc R Soc Lond B Biol Sci. 1957;147(929):427–33.
63. Markert CL. Lactate dehydrogenase isozymes: dissociation and recombination of subunits. Science. 1963;140(3573):1329–30.
64. Mazur P. Studies on rapidly frozen suspensions of yeast cells by differential thermal analysis and conductometry. Biophys J. 1963;3:323–53.
65. Mazur P. Causes of injury in frozen and thawed cells. Fed Proc. 1965;24:S175–82.
66. Zacarian SA. Cryogenics: the cryolesion and the pathogenesis of cryonecrosis. In: Zacarian S, editor. Cryosurgery for skin cancer and cutaneous disorders. St. Louis, MO: Mosby St. Louis; 1985.
67. Zacarian SA, Stone D, Clater M. Effects of cryogenic temperatures on microcirculation in the golden hamster cheek pouch. Cryobiology. 1970;7(1):27–39.
68. Bulkley GB. The role of oxygen free radicals in human disease processes. Surgery. 1983;94(3):407–11.
69. Rabb JM, Renaud ML, Brandt PA, Witt CW. Effect of freezing and thawing on the microcirculation and capillary endothelium of the hamster cheek pouch. Cryobiology. 1974;11(6):508–18.
70. Southwood WF. The thickness of the skin. Plast Reconstr Surg. 1955;15(5):423–9.
71. Rudolph R, Ballantyne Jr DL. Skin grafts. In: McCarthy J, editor. Plastic surgery. Philadelphia, PA: WB Saunders; 1990. p. 221–74.
72. Tyack ZF, Pegg S, Ziviani J. Post-burn dyspigmentation: its assessment, management, and relationship to scarring – a review of the literature. J Burn Care Rehab. 1997;18(5):435–40.
73. de Chalain TM, Tang C, Thomson HG. Burn area color changes after superficial burns in childhood: can they be predicted? J Burn Care Rehab. 1998;19(1 Pt 1):39–49.
74. Compton CC, Press W, Gill JM, Bantick G, Nadire KB, Warland G, et al. The generation of anchoring fibrils by epidermal keratinocytes: a quantitative long-term study. Epithelial Cell Biol. 1995;4(3):93–103.
75. Regauer S, Seiler GR, Barrandon Y, et al. Epithelial origin of cutaneous anchoring fibrils. J Cell Biol. 1990;111(5 Pt 1):2109–15.
76. Yannas IV, Burke JF. Design of an artificial skin. I. Basic design principles. J Biomed Mater Res. 1980;14(1):65–81.
77. Yannas IV, Burke JF, Gordon PL, Huang C, Rubenstein RH. Design of an artificial skin. II. Control of chemical composition. J Biomed Mater Res. 1980;14(2):107–32.
78. Crowe R, Parkhouse N, McGrouther D, Burnstock G. Neuropeptide-containing nerves in painful hypertrophic human scar tissue. Br J Dermatol. 1994;130(4):444–52.
79. Dunnick CA, Gibran NS, Heimbach DM. Substance P has a role in neurogenic mediation of human burn wound healing. J Burn Care Rehab. 1996;17(5): 390–6.
80. Shupp JW, Nasabzadeh TJ, Rosenthal DS, Jordan MH, Fidler P, Jeng JC. A review of the local pathophysiologic bases of burn wound progression. J Burn Care Res. 2010;31(6):1–25.
81. Rico RM, Ripamonti R, Burns AL, Gamelli RL, DiPietro LA. The effect of sepsis on wound healing. J Surg Res. 2002;102(2):193–7.
82. Knabl JS, Bauer W, Andel H, Schwendenwein I, Dado PF, Mittlböck M, et al. Progression of burn wound depth by systemical application of a vasoconstrictor: an experimental study with a new rabbit model. Burns. 1999;25(8):715–21.
83. Winter GD. Formation of the scab and the rate of epithelialization of superficial wounds in the skin of the young domestic pig. Nature. 1962;193:293–4.

84. Hinman CD, Maibach H. Effect of air exposure and occlusion on experimental human skin wounds. Nature. 1963;200:377–8.
85. Palmieri TL, Greenhalgh DG. Topical treatment of pediatric patients with burns: a practical guide. Am J Clin Dermatol. 2002;3(8):529–34.
86. Forage AV. The history of the classification of burns (diagnosis of depth). Br J Plast Surg. 1963;16: 239–42.
87. Hlava P, Moserova J, Konigova R. Validity of clinical assessment of the depth of a thermal injury. Acta Chir Plast. 1983;25(4):202–8.
88. Niazi ZB, Essex TJ, Papini R, Scott D, McLean NR, Black MJ. New laser Doppler scanner, a valuable adjunct in burn depth assessment. Burns. 1993;19(6):485–9.
89. Yeong EK, Mann R, Goldberg M, Engrav L, Heimbach D. Improved accuracy of burn wound assessment using laser Doppler. J Trauma. 1996;40(6):956–61. discussion 961–962.
90. Jaskille AD, Ramella-Roman JC, Shupp JW, Jordan MH, Jeng JC. Critical review of burn depth assessment techniques: part II. Review of laser Doppler technology. J Burn Care Res. 2010;31(1):151–7.
91. Jaskille AD, Shupp JW, Jordan MH, Jeng JC. Critical review of burn depth assessment techniques: part I historical review. J Burn Care Res. 2009;30(6): 937–47.
92. Hoeksema H, Van de Sijpe K, Tondu T, Hamdi M, Van Landuyt K, Blondeel P. Accuracy of early burn depth assessment by laser Doppler imaging on different days post burn. Burns. 2009;35(1):36–45.
93. Ho-Asjoe M, Chronnell CM, Frame JD, Leigh IM, Carver N. Immunohistochemical analysis of burn depth. J Burn Care Rehab. 1999;20(3):207–11.
94. Moserova J, Hlava P, Malinsky J. Scope for ultrasound diagnosis of the depth of thermal damage. Preliminary report. Acta Chir Plast. 1982;24(4): 235–42.
95. Cantrell Jr JH. Can ultrasound assist an experienced surgeon in estimating burn depth? J Trauma. 1984;24(9 Suppl):S64–70.
96. Kaufman T, Hurwitz DJ, Heggers JP. The India ink injection technique to assess the depth of experimental burn wounds. Burns Incl Therm Inj. 1984;10(6): 405–8.
97. Black KS, Hewitt CW, Miller DM, Ramos E, Halloran J, Bressler V, et al. Burn depth evaluation with fluorometry: is it really definitive? J Burn Care Rehab. 1986;7(4):313–7.
98. Pape SA, Skouras CA, Byrne PO. An audit of the use of laser Doppler imaging (LDI) in the assessment of burns of intermediate depth. Burns. 2001;27(3): 233–9.
99. Hackett ME. The use of thermography in the assessment of depth of burn and blood supply of flaps, with preliminary reports on its use in Dupuytren's contracture and treatment of varicose ulcers. Br J Plast Surg. 1974;27(4):311–7.
100. Koruda MJ, Zimbler A, Settle RG, Jacobs DO, Rolandelli RH, Wolf GL, et al. Assessing burn wound depth using in vitro nuclear magnetic resonance (NMR). J Surg Res. 1986;40(5):475–81.
101. Riordan CL, McDonough M, Davidson JM, Corley R, Perlov C, Barton R, et al. Noncontact laser Doppler imaging in burn depth analysis of the extremities. J Burn Care Rehab. 2003;24(4): 177–86.
102. Jeng JC, Bridgeman A, Shivnan L, Thorton PM, Alam H, Clark TJ, et al. Laser Doppler imaging determines need for excision and grafting in advance of clinical judgment: a prospective blinded trial. Burns. 2003;29(7):665–70.
103. Lund T, Reed RK. Acute hemodynamic effects of thermal skin injury in the rat. Circ Shock. 1986;20:105–14.
104. Arturson G. Pathophysiological aspects of the burn syndrome. Acta Chir Scand. 1961;274(Supp 1): 1–135.
105. Leape LL. Kinetics of burn edema formation in primates. Ann Surg. 1972;176:223–6.
106. Cioffi Jr WG, Vaughan GM, Heironimus JD, Jordan BS, Mason Jr AD, Pruitt Jr BA. Dissociation of blood volume and flow in regulation of salt and water balance in burn patients. Ann Surg. 1991;214(3):213–8. discussion 8–20.
107. Demling RH, Mazess RB, Witt RM, Wolberg WH. The study of burn wound edema using dichromatic absorptiometry. J Trauma. 1978;18:124–8.
108. Arturson G, Jakobsson OR. Oedema measurements in a standard burn model. Burns. 1985;1:1–7.
109. Leape LL. Early burn wound changes. J Pediatr Surg. 1968;3:292–9.
110. Leape LL. Initial changes in burns: tissue changes in burned and unburned skin of rhesus monkeys. J Trauma. 1970;10:488–92.
111. Lund T, Wiig H, Reed RK. Acute postburn edema: role of strongly negative interstitial fluid pressure. Am J Physiol. 1988;255:H1069.
112. Onarheim H, Lund T, Reed R. Thermal skin injury: II. Effects on edema formation and albumin extravasation of fluid resuscitation with lactated Ringer's, plasma, and hypertonic saline (2,400 mosmol/l) in the rat. Circ Shock. 1989;27(1):25–37.
113. Brouhard BH, Carvajal HF, Linares HA. Burn edema and protein leakage in the rat. I. Relationship to time of injury. Microvasc Res. 1978;15:221–8.
114. Arturson G. Microvascular permeability to macromolecules in thermal injury. Acta Physioi Scand. 1979;463(Suppl):111–222.
115. Harms BA, Bodai BI, Kramer GC, Demling RH. Microvascular fluid and protein flux in pulmonary and systemic circulations after thermal injury. Microvasc Res. 1982;23(1):77–86.
116. Kramer GC, Gunther RA, Nerlich ML, Zweifach SS, Demling RH. Effect of dextran 70 on increased microvascular fluid and protein flux after thermal injury. Circ Shock. 1982;9:529–43.

117. Zetterstrom H, Arturson G. Plasma oncotic pressure and plasma protein concentration in patients following thermal injury. Acta Anaesth Scand. 1980;24: 288–94.
118. Demling RH, Kramer GC, Harms B. Role of thermal injury–induced hypoproteinemia on edema formation in burned and nonburned tissue. Surgery. 1989;95:136–44.
119. Elgjo GI, Traber DL, Hawkins HK, Kramer GC. Burn resuscitation with two doses of 4ml/kg hypertonic saline dextran provides sustained fluid sparing: a 48-hour prospective study in conscious sheep. J Trauma Inj Infect Crit Care. 2000;49(2):251–63. discussion 263–265.
120. Elgjo GI, Poli de Figueiredo LF, Schenarts PJ, Traber DL, Traber LD, Kramer GC. Hypertonic saline dextran produces early (8-12h) fluid sparing in burn resuscitation: a 24 hour prospective double blind study in sheep. Crit Care Med. 2000;28(1):163–71.
121. Andritsos MJ, Kinsky MP, Herndon DN, Kramer GC. Albumin only transiently reduces fluid requirements following burn injury. Shock. 2001;12(1):6.
122. Shires GT, Cunninham Jr JN, Baker CR, Reeder SF, Illner H, Wagner IY, et al. Alterations in cellular membrane dysfunction during hemorrhagic shock in primates. Ann Surg. 1972;176(3):288–95.
123. Arango A, Illner H, Shires GT. Roles of ischemia in the induction of changes in cell membrane during hemorrhagic shock. J Surg Res. 1976;20(5):473–6.
124. Mazzoni MC, Borgstrom P, Intaglietta M, Arfors KE. Luminal narrowing and endothelial cell swelling in skeletal muscle capillaries during hemorrhagic shock. Circ Shock. 1989;29(1):27–39.
125. Button B, Baker RD, Vertrees RA, Allen SE, Brodwick MS, Kramer GC. Quantitative assessment of a circulating depolarizing factor in shock. Shock. 2001;15(3):239–44.
126. Demling RH, Wong C, Jin LJ, Hechtman H, Lalonde C, West K. Early lung dysfunction after major burns: role of edema and vasoactive mediators. J Trauma. 1985;25(10):959–66.
127. Demling RH, Niehaus G, Perea A, Will JA. Effect of burn-induced hypoproteinemia on pulmonary transvascular fluid filtration rate. Surgery. 1979;85:339–43.
128. Till GO, Guilds LS, Mahrougui M, Friedl HP, Trentz O, Ward PA. Role of xanthine oxidase in thermal injury of skin. Am J Pathol. 1989;135(1):195–202.
129. Tranbaugh RF, Lewis FR, Christensen IM, Elings VB. Lung water changes after thermal injury: the effects of crystalloid resuscitation and sepsis. Ann Surg. 1980;192:47–9.
130. Tranbaugh RF, Elings VB, Christensen JM, Lewis FR. Effect of inhalation injury on lung water accumulation. J Trauma. 1983;23:597–604.
131. Ivy ME, Atweh NA, Palmer J, Possenti PP, Pineau M, D'Aiuto M. Intra-abdominal hypertension and abdominal compartment syndrome in burn patients. [Comment]. J Trauma Inj Infect Crit Care. 2000; 49(3):387–91.
132. Oda J, Ueyama M, Yamashita K, Inoue T, Noborio M, Ode Y, et al. Hypertonic lactated saline resuscitation reduces the risk of abdominal compartment syndrome in severely burned patients. J Trauma Inj Infect Crit Care. 2006;60(1):64–71.
133. Bloomfield GL, Dalton JM, Sugerman HJ, Ridings PC, DeMaria EJ, Bullock R. Treatment of increasing intracranial pressure secondary to the acute abdominal compartment syndrome in a patient with combined abdominal and head trauma. J Trauma Inj Infect Crit Care. 1995;39(6):1168–70.
134. Michie DD, Goldsmith RS, Mason Jr AD. Effects of hydralazine and high molecular weight dextran upon the circulatory responses to severe thermal burns. Circ Res. 1963;13:46–8.
135. Horton JW, White J, Baxter CR. The role of oxygen derived free radicals in burn-induced myocardial contractile depression. J Burn Care Rehab. 1988; 9(6):589–98.
136. Martyn JAJ, Wilson RS, Burke JF. Right ventricular function and pulmonary hemodynamics during dopamine infusion in burned patients. Chest. 1986;89:357–60.
137. Adams HR, Baxter CR, Izenberg SD. Decreased contractility and compliance of the left ventricle as complications of thermal trauma. Am Heart J. 1984;108(6):1477–87.
138. Merriman Jr TW, Jackson R. Myocardial function following thermal injury. Circ Res. 1962;11:66–9.
139. Horton JW, White J, Baxter CR. Aging alters myocardial response during resuscitation in burn shock. Surg Forum. 1987;38:249–51.
140. Horton JW, Baxter CR, White J. Differences in cardiac responses to resuscitation from burn shock. Surg Gynecol Obstet. 1989;168(3):201–13.
141. Horton JW, White DJ, Baxter CR. Hypertonic saline dextran resuscitation of thermal injury. Ann Surg. 1990;211(3):301–11.
142. Horton JW, Shite J, Hunt JL. Delayed hypertonic saline dextran administration after burn injury. J Trauma Inj. 1995;38(2):281–6.
143. Cioffi WG, DeMeules JE, Gameili RL. The effects of burn injury and fluid resuscitation on cardiac function in vitro. J Trauma. 1986;26:638–43.
144. Emara SS, Alzaylai AA. Renal failure in burn patients: a review. Ann Burns Fire Disasters. 2013;26(1):12–5.
145. Holm C, Horbrand F, von Donnersmarck GH, Mühlbauer W. Acute renal failure in severely burned patients. Burns. 1999;25(2):171–8.
146. Chrysopoulo MT, Jeschke MG, Dziewulski P, Dziewulski P, Barrow RE, Herndon D. Acute renal dysfunction in severely burned adults. J Trauma. 1999;46(1):141–4.
147. Tokyay R, Zeigler ST, Traber DL, Stothert Jr JC, Loick HM, Heggers JP, et al. Postburn gastrointestinal vasoconstriction increases bacterial and endotoxin translocation. J Am Physiol. 1993;74(4): 1521–7.

148. Goodman-Gilman A, Rall TW, Nies AS, et al. The pharmacological basis of therapeutics. New York: Pergamon Press; 1990.
149. Anggard E, Jonsson CE. Efflux of prostaglandins in lymph from scalded tissue. Acta Physiol Scand. 1971;81:440–3.
150. Harms B, Bodai B, Demling R. Prostaglandin release and altered microvascular integrity after burn injury. J Surg Res. 1981;31:27–8.
151. Arturson G. Anti-inflammatory drugs and burn edema formation. In: May R, Dogo G, editors. Care of the burn wound. Basel: Karger; 1981. p. 21–4.
152. Arturson G, Hamberg M, Jonsson CE. Prostaglandins in human burn blister fluid. Acta Physiol Scand. 1973;87:27–36.
153. LaLonde C, Knox J, Daryani R. Topical flurbiprofen decreases burn wound-induced hypermetabolism and systemic lipid peroxidation. Surgery. 1991;109: 645–51.
154. Heggers JP, Loy GL, Robson MC, Del Beccaro EJ. Histological demonstration of prostaglandins and thromboxanes in burned tissue. J Surg Res. 1980;28:11–5.
155. Heggers JP, Robson MC, Zachary LS. Thromboxane inhibitors for the prevention of progressive dermal ischemia due to thermal injury. J Burn Care Rehab. 1985;6:46–8.
156. Jacobsen S, Waaler BG. The effect of scalding on the content of kininogen and kininase in limb lymph. Br J Pharmacol. 1966;27:222.
157. Carvajal H, Linares H, Brouhard B. Effect of antihistamine, antiserotonin, and ganglionic blocking agents upon increased capillary permeability following burn edema. J Trauma. 1975;15:969–75.
158. Wilmore DW, Long JM, Mason AD, Skreen RW, Pruitt Jr BA. Catecholamines: mediator of the hypermetabolic response to thermal injury. Ann Surg. 1974;80:653–9.
159. Hilton JG. Effects of sodium nitroprusside on thermal trauma depressed cardiac output in the anesthetized dog. Burns Incl Therm Inj. 1984;10:318–22.
160. McCord J, Fridovieh I. The biology and pathology of oxygen radicals. Ann lntern Med. 1978;89: 122–7.
161. Demling RH, LaLonde C. Early postburn lipid peroxidation: effect of ibuprofen and allopurinol. Surgery. 1990;107:85–93.
162. Ono I, Gunji H, Hasegawa T, Harada H, Kaneko F, Matsuzaki M. Effects of a platelet activating factor antagonist on edema formation following burns. Burns. 1993;3:202–7.
163. Hafner JA, Fritz H. Balance anti inflammation: the combined application of a PAF inhibitor and a cyclooxygenase inhibitor blocks the inflammatory takeoff after burns. Int J Tissue React. 1990;12:203.
164. Fink MP. Gastrointestinal mucosal injury in experimental models of shock, trauma, and sepsis. Crit Care Med. 1991;19(5):627–41.
165. Crum RL, Dominie W, Hansbrough JF. Cardiovascular and neurohumoral responses following burn injury. Arch Surg. 1990;125:1065–70.
166. Kiang JG, Wei ET. Corticotropin releasing factor inhibits thermal injury. J Pharmacol Exp Ther. 1987;2:517–20.

Airway Management

3

Sundeep Tumber and John A. Scavone

Introduction

Acute burn injuries are a special category of trauma, which impose the risk of potentially devastating airway loss. A patient with a major burn injury may present with a life-threatening difficult airway scenario which would challenge even the most experienced physician. The management of the airway is precarious and requires a multidisciplinary approach involving an experienced anesthesiologist playing a critical role. Burn injury induced airway edema, and outright airway obstruction from acute facial burns can result in the so-called "cannot intubate-cannot ventilate" situation; this is fatal unless the burn surgeon creates an emergency surgical airway. The establishment of a secure airway is an essential and often initial step in the management of acute burn patients.

After the acute phase of burn care, major burn survivors will present for postburn skin reconstruction. Orofacial-cervical postburn scar contractures can cause significant anatomical distortions, which may create a difficult airway if a general anesthetic is needed. Losing this airway during the course of an anesthetic could also produce a devastating airway crisis with dire consequences.

The management of the airway in both the acute burn phase and the postburn scar reconstruction involves different airway issues, evaluations, and approaches in order to safely establish a secure airway.

Acute Burn Injury

Thermal injury to the face, oral cavity, and airway causes soft tissue edema (see Fig. 3.1), and subsequent airway obstruction may result from swelling of either the supraglottic or infraglottic airway tissues [1]. Airway edema may often occur without burns to the face in patients with burns covering a large surface area. The mechanism of injury should be identified and an airway exam performed in any patient with burns greater than 30 % total body surface area (TBSA) with special attention being paid to burns to the face. Thermal injury of the upper airway (occurring above the glottis) spares the structures below the larynx due to the dissipation of heat energy. Thermal injury of the lower airway is very rare but may occur when there is closed space exposure to steam or prolonged exposure to products of combustion. Other less reliable predictors of smoke inhalation injury may include singing of facial or nasal hair, evidence of oropharyngeal carbonaceous deposits,

S. Tumber, D.O. (✉) • J.A. Scavone, M.D.
Department of Anesthesiology, Shriners Hospitals for Children Northern California, 2425 Stockton Boulevard, Sacramento, CA 95817, USA
e-mail: stumber@shrinenet.org; jscavone@shrinenet.org

D.G. Greenhalgh (ed.), *Burn Care for General Surgeons and General Practitioners*,
DOI 10.1007/978-3-319-29161-1_3

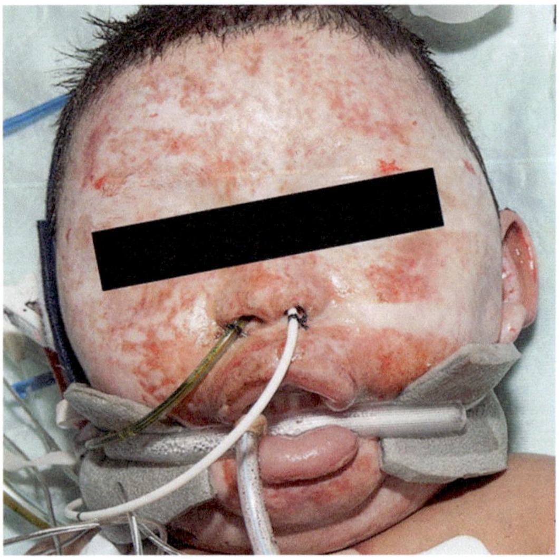

Fig. 3.1 Acute edema observed in a burn patient typifies the type of difficult airway that may be encountered in the burn center

or carboxyhemoglobin levels greater than ten percent [2]. Smoke inhalation injury is not truly a burn to the lower airway but, instead, is the result of smoke particles damaging the mucosa of the distal airways leading to sloughing, obstruction, and atelectasis. Observing soot or injury below the vocal cords while performing bronchoscopy makes the diagnosis. Epithelial damage in the airway is present in approximately one-third of patients with flame burns treated in burn centers. Patients with inhalation injury have increased fluid resuscitation requirements and have a higher likelihood of pulmonary complications and mortality, compared with those having an isolated burn injury [2–5]. Inhalation of products of combustion damages the epithelial lining of the larynx, trachea, and bronchi. Clinical signs include wheezing, dyspnea, coughing, and the presence of copious secretions. Beyond a direct insult to the tissue of the airway is an inflammatory response that occurs during the first 48 h following a major thermal injury. Inflammatory mediators such as IL-6, leukotrienes, and thromboxane increase capillary permeability leading to a loss of plasma proteins and electrolytes into the airway and alveolar tissue beds causing edema [6, 7]. Edema and obstruction of the airway following fluid resuscitation may not present until 8–36 h after the initial insult [1, 8, 9].

All burn patients suffering from flame burns should receive 100 % oxygen via a non-rebreather face mask on presentation. After a thorough airway assessment, early tracheal intubation should be considered before the development of clinically significant edema results in a compromised airway. Intubation should take place if any of the following are present: stridor, hypoxemia, hypercapnia, a Glasgow Coma Scale less than eight, deep facial burns, or oropharyngeal edema [10]. Because airway edema may not develop for many hours after the initial burn injury, frequent reevaluations of the airway and respiratory status are required. The consequences of upper airway edema will present sooner and be more severe in infants and small children. The epiglottis is of particular concern because it can be the focal point of airway obstruction [7].

Early intubation, *before* the development of edema, is the most conservative approach to take in the patient with a major burn who has significant facial involvement or an inhalational injury causing respiratory compromise. Intubation, while necessary to secure airway patency, carries the following significant risks to the patient: (1) esophageal intubation, (2) direct damage to laryngeal soft tissue or cartilages due to laryngoscopy or placement of the endotracheal tube, (3) pulmonary aspiration during intubation, and (4) failed intubation with loss of the airway. Intubation can subsequently lead to granuloma formation, tracheal stenosis, vocal cord paralysis, bleeding, or formation of a tracheoesophageal fistula [11–14]. The 2001 American Burn Association Practice Guidelines For Burn Care does not recommend intubation for inhalation injury alone, but "immediate intubation" for inhalation injury is recommended if "airway patency is threatened, gas exchange or compliance mandate mechanical ventilatory support, or mental status is inadequate for airway protection" [15]. The deeper and more extensive the burn, the more likely the patient will require intubation. Unless the burn is superficial, any patient with burns >40 % TBSA should be intubated due to the expected large volume of fluid resuscitation. Serial examinations of the upper airway with fiberoptic laryngoscopy may permit objective evaluation of supraglottic mucosal edema, secretions, and the mobility of the true vocal cords and has been described as one method to help guide the clinical decision to intubate [11]. Another reason to consider early intubation (in the intensive care unit or emergency department) is when the patient has a large burn injury and the burn team has decided to proceed with a major excision in the very near future. In this instance, securing the airway as soon as possible averts the complexities of intubating the patient later on in the operating room where laryngeal edema may have supervened.

Prior to securing an airway, the patient should be evaluated for clinical evidence suggesting difficulty with routine direct laryngoscopy. Preexisting airway abnormalities (e.g., retrognathia, maxillary protrusion) in a patient with major burns can confer additional complexity to direct laryngoscopy. Preoxygenation and mask ventilation can be suboptimal if not outright ineffective in a patient with facial burns. A two-provider approach to bag valve mask ventilation may be required. Excessive secretions, soot, and edema leading to distortion of the glottic and supraglottic tissue may make both direct and fiberoptic laryngoscopy quite difficult [15, 16]. Pulmonary aspiration during induction and intubation is more common in any emergency non-fasting patient, and this certainly applies to the burned trauma victim.

Early intubation in the acute burn patient who does not meet NPO criteria will require either an awake intubation or the use of a rapid sequence technique to avert aspiration. Depending on the mechanism of injury, cervical spine precautions during intubation may be necessary to prevent exacerbation of any spinal cord injury. If a cervical spine injury is suspected, an additional provider is necessary to provide manual in-line immobilization by grasping the mastoid process to maintain the cervical spine in a neutral position. If a rigid collar is in place, the front of the collar can be removed so it will not impede mouth opening. The circumstance of a severely burned patient with airway edema and an unstable C-spine may require up to four providers: one to give intravenous drugs, a second to provide in-line immobilization, a third to provide cricoid pressure, and a fourth to intubate.

Succinylcholine, a depolarizing muscle relaxant, may be used for an emergent rapid sequence intubation within the first 48 h after a burn injury provided that the patient is otherwise healthy. However, after 48 h following the burn injury, administration of succinylcholine can induce acute severe hyperkalemia resulting in a cardiac arrest. The etiology of this phenomenon has been elegantly elucidated by Martyn et al. who have demonstrated increased potassium release from upregulated immature extra junctional nicotinic acetylcholine receptor subunits [17, 18]. The upregulation is attributable to inflammation associated with the burn injury and local denervation of muscle [17–20]. This hyperkalemic response to succinylcholine can persist for up to 1 year postburn [10].

Non-depolarizing muscle relaxants have substantially altered pharmacokinetics in burn patients resulting in an increase in both dose requirements and time of onset to achieve effective paralysis. This occurs approximately 3–7 days after burn injury and may persist. This increase in dose requirement is due to the upregulation of acetylcholine receptors and to the increased binding of non-depolarizing muscle relaxants to plasma proteins such as alpha-1-acid glycoprotein, which increases twofold in burn patients [7, 20]. The dose of rocuronium required for muscle relaxation may be as high as 1.5 mg/kg for rapid sequence induction in patients with a major burn injury. The time to effective paralysis can be as long as 90 s, and this is a sharp comparison to the results in a healthy patient where the dose requirement is 0.9 mg/kg producing paralysis in 60 s [7, 21].

The induction dose of propofol will likely need to be reduced to avoid hypotension from a reduction in systemic vascular resistance and further cardiovascular depression in the setting of an acute burn injury with hypovolemic shock [2]. Etomidate generally preserves cardiovascular function on induction and is effective in preventing hypotension in moderate doses, but still carries the risk of cardiovascular instability in the hypovolemic patient. Nevertheless, its use in critically ill patients has fallen out of favor because of associated adrenal suppression. Stimulation of the sympathetic nervous system during a ketamine induction usually results in an increase in mean arterial pressure and heart rate. However, even with ketamine, caution must be used, as hypotension may occur if the burn patient has concurrent hypovolemic shock due to its mild direct myocardial depressant effects [2, 7]. The recommended doses of induction agents and neuromuscular blockers are summarized in Tables 3.1 and 3.2. Endotracheal tube sizes are summarized in Table 3.3.

Early intubation is the key to success in ensuring airway patency and stabilizing ventilation in acute burn patients. The caveat is that the loss of the ability to maintain spontaneous ventilation from pharmacologic interventions will be catastrophic in the event that the patient subsequently cannot be intubated or ventilated. If laryngeal edema is present or if there is a preexisting difficult airway, the use of any muscle relaxant or potent sedative to aid intubation can result in morbidity or mortality if the airway cannot be intubated. Mask ventilation or ventilation with a laryngeal airway may not be adequate in a patient with facial and airway edema. Direct laryngoscopy may result in an inadequate view for intubation because edematous tissue can lead to airway distortion, decreased neck and mandibular mobility, and suboptimal mouth opening [22–24]. Significant airway edema may thwart the use of newer airway video scopes and make intubation impossible even with these devices [25].

In a patient who has severe airway edema but who is conscious and spontaneously breathing, an awake fiberoptic intubation or a surgical airway under local anesthesia is the safest option in securing a definitive airway. Averting the loss of the airway rests on a judicious approach to

Table 3.1 Dosage of induction agents

Induction agent	IV dose (mg/kg)	Onset (seconds)	Duration (minutes)
Propofol	1–1.5	30	3–10
Ketamine	1–2	30–60	10–15
Etomidate	0.15–0.3	30–60	6–10
Midazolam	0.05–0.1	60–300	30

Table 3.2 Dosage of neuromuscular blocker agents

Neuromuscular blocker	Dose (mg/kg)	Onset (seconds)	Duration (minutes)
Succinylcholine[a]	1.5–2	30–60	6–12
Rocuronium	0.6–1.2 (high dose for RSI)	45–90	15–40

[a]Succinylcholine should be used within initial 48 h post-injury only

Table 3.3 Endotracheal tube sizing and laryngoscope blade selection

Uncuffed tube size ID (mm)	Cuffed tube size ID (mm)	Age/weight (years/kg)	Laryngoscope blade Miller	Laryngoscope blade Macintosh
3.0		<3 kg	0	–
3.0	3.0	Term >3 kg up to <8 months	0	–
3.5	3.5	8 months to <2 years	1	–
4.0	4.0	2 to <4 years	1.5	–
4.5	4.5	4 to <6 years	1.5	2
Use cuffed	5.0	6 to <8 years	2	2
Use cuffed	5.5	8 to <10 years	2	2
Use cuffed	6.0	10 to <12 years	2	3
Use cuffed	6.5	12 to <14 years	2	3
Use cuffed	7.0	14 to <16 years	2	3
Use cuffed	7.5–8.0	>16 years	2–3	3–4

sedation which has the following critical goals: (1) maintain spontaneous ventilation at all times—this is the most important goal, (2) maintain oxygenation, and (3) maintain the ability of the patient to follow commands. This construct ensures that even if a fiberoptic approach cannot be accomplished, there will not be loss of life. In a pediatric patient or an adult patient who cannot cooperate or tolerate an awake fiberoptic intubation, the goal becomes the preservation of spontaneous ventilation. Intubation can be accomplished after the induction of general anesthesia but the patient will no longer be able to follow commands. Drugs such as sevoflurane and ketamine are widely used for this purpose and the safest approach is to avoid neuromuscular blocking agents altogether. The use of a muscle relaxant is appropriate only after it can be demonstrated that the patient can be ventilated by bag valve mask or a laryngeal airway. Techniques for awake fiberoptic intubation and fiberoptic intubation after the induction of general anesthesia in a spontaneously ventilating patient will be discussed later in the chapter.

Postburn Contractures

Major burn survivors commonly present after their acute injury for reconstructive procedures including release of postburn contractures, placement of tissue expanders, scar excisions, and resurfacings. In addition, these survivors may undergo nonelective procedures such as an appendectomy, abscess drainage, central venous catheterization, or orthopedic interventions. The problem is that a major burn injury will often have a profound, long-term effect on the airway, and this alone will substantially increase the risk of anesthesia. Patients considered at risk are those with severe burn injuries to the head, face, neck, upper chest, or upper back. A significant decrease in the cervical range of motion may be highly problematic if it produces a fixed flexion deformity of the neck. In addition, facial and neck burn contractures may lead to microstomia from cicatrized angles of the mouth, obliterated nasal passages, reduced submandibular space compliance, and altered tracheal position (see Fig. 3.2) [26]. In children, these facial and neck contrac-

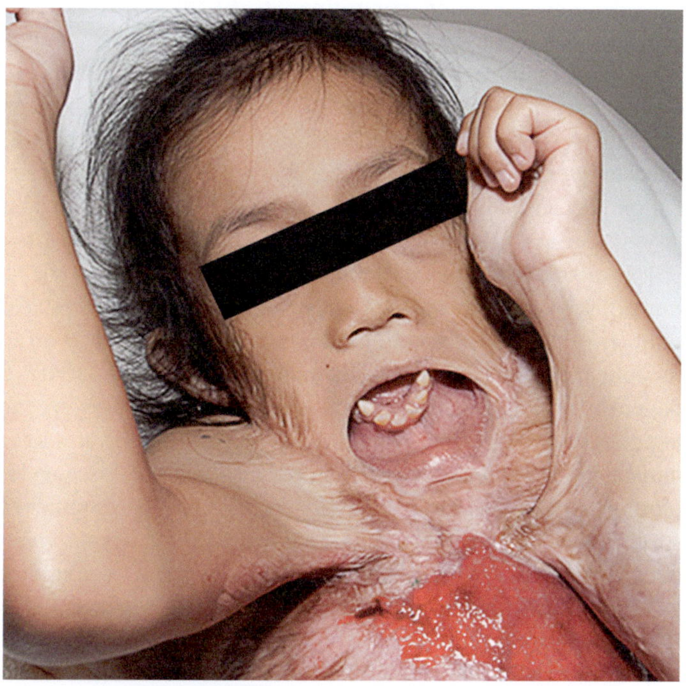

Fig. 3.2 This patient presented 16 months after her burn injury with a severe postburn scar contracture. It is obvious that obtaining her airway will be very difficult

tures can eventually result in oro-maxillofacial skeletal deformities, such as micrognathia, which further complicates airway management [27]. Any one of these aforementioned changes in normal anatomy can lead to difficulty with any technique of intubation, ventilation, or both. There is special importance surrounding the use of muscle relaxants, which can worsen the degree of scar retraction acutely due to the loss of muscle tone in the airway [28]. Burn contractures may also eliminate certain techniques that are otherwise feasible in the non-burned patient when the anesthesiologist needs to secure a difficult airway. An example of this issue is the difficulty in placing a video laryngoscope when circumoral scars limit mouth opening. Additional examples are obliterated or contracted nares that obviate a nasal fiberoptic intubation or thick neck scars that decrease the quality of transillumination necessary with the use of a light wand or make obtaining a surgical airway difficult.

Preoperative assessment of the patients must include a history, physical, and a thorough airway exam. Contractures of the face and neck can lead to obstructive sleep apnea, and a history of snoring may predict difficulty with mask ventilation during induction and necessitate vigilant postoperative ventilation monitoring [26, 29, 30]. Previous anesthetic records may be helpful, but airway contractures worsen over time and this is a variable dynamic in growing children. There is special relevance in a history of a previous tracheostomy, inhalation injury, or prolonged intubation because these events may result in laryngotracheal stenosis or tracheomalacia [26, 30]. Endotracheal tubes of smaller size must be immediately available when proceeding with intubation. Standard airway exams may not be reliable predictors of airway difficulty in burn patients, and a high index of suspicion signaling a potentially difficult airway may rest on the clinical judgment of the experienced anesthesiologist. Assessment of the airway in postburn scar contracture patients should include the evaluation of mouth opening, range of neck motion, sternomental distance with an emphasis on contractures and scarring, patency of the nasal passages, and the compliance of the submandibular space [26]. A noncompliant submandibular space results in difficult displacement of the tongue during laryngoscopy resulting in a poor view of the larynx. Scar formation around the neck may cause the epiglottis and vocal cords to be displaced anteriorly or retracted toward the side of the scar [26, 28]. Obtaining the so-called sniffing position, which is used to facilitate intubation, may be impossible in patients with postburn contractures of the neck. In the normal patient, this position involves the alignment of the oral-pharyngeal-laryngeal axes with the head by flexing the lower cervical spine and extending the upper cervical spine and atlanto-occipital joint to facilitate endotracheal tube insertion [31].

Psychological preparation of the patient is essential, particularly in older children who frequently have high levels of anxiety resulting from recalling pain or emotional trauma during the original injury or any prior procedures. The physician should take an unhurried, reassuring approach with the patient, and there should be an easy-to-understand emphasis that powerful sedatives will be administered to minimize or ablate discomfort.

Airway Management: Introduction

A multidisciplinary approach to the airway must be taken, with the anesthesiologist often assuming the lead role. For a difficult airway, a second anesthesia provider is vital in providing direct assistance to the primary anesthesiologist while a surgeon experienced with securing surgical airways and adept at burn contracture releases of the neck/face should be present. At least two contingency airway management plans should be formulated *before the procedure* and communicated to everyone. All equipment should be checked prior to commencement. Frequently, tube exchangers, laryngeal airways, and fiberoptic equipment are used during intubation, and it is imperative that all these devices are functional, compatible with one another, and physically present in the room.

There are a wide variety of successful techniques available to manage the difficult airway of a child or adult with acute burns or postburn contractures [26, 30]. To some extent, however, it would be misleading to think that all of the following techniques are feasible for every anesthesiologist. What assures safety and success is total familiarity with a given technique. This involves rehearsal, use, and repetition to attain expertise. It also means that every effort must be made *not* to lose the airway of a patient by prematurely disabling their ability to spontaneously ventilate before bag mask ventilation and/or tracheal intubation are known to be possible. The authors will present techniques which have been especially safe and consistently effective in the care of pediatric burn patients at our institution.

Airway Management: Awake Fiberoptic Intubation

The American Society of Anesthesiologists (ASA) Difficult Airway Algorithm (see Fig. 3.3) is a key resource as an important safety and decision-making tool when preparing for a difficult airway in an acute or postburn patient [32]. It is particularly important to assess the level of risk and the potential consequences associated with a particular airway management choice. Then one must determine the most prudent technique based on the merits and feasibility analysis of the patient's unique airway problem. Reference is made here to the top of algorithm. Due to contractures in postburn patients and severe edema in acute burn patients, there may be difficulty with mask ventilation, supraglottic airway device placement, direct laryngoscopy, fiberoptic intubation, and surgical airway access [32]. Anxiety and pain can lead to difficulty with cooperation and too often this prompts the wrong decision—inducing general anesthesia with or without the patient breathing spontaneously. If a "cannot intubate-cannot ventilate" scenario ensues, and an emergent surgical airway cannot be placed, catastrophe including death can result.

The gold standard and the safest approach for the management of the anticipated difficult airway in any patient is an awake fiberoptic intubation. This technique requires substantial skill and training, prudent choices and careful titration of drugs for sedation, and includes the necessity of adequate topical anesthesia of the structures of the airway. Poor topical anesthesia has a very significant downfall because it often leads to the administration of additional sedative drugs with the consequent inability to follow commands, loss of consciousness, and ultimately the loss of the airway. Ineffective sedation can lead to an uncooperative patient and suboptimal conditions including excess patient movement, agitation, undue discomfort, and adverse psychological or physiological responses to stress. The term "awake" means that the patient retains the ability to follow commands and clearly has spontaneous ventilation without assistive airway support. It is often best to have one anesthesiologist perform the fiberoptic intubation while an additional anesthesiologist titrates sedation, monitors the patient's vital signs, and ensures spontaneous ventilation with unequivocal responses to verbal stimulation. The two roles are divided, as they would be during a formal surgical procedure, to ensure adequate focus is maintained on the fiberoptic airway procedure and the patient's well-being. Supplemental oxygen is necessary throughout the intubation procedure and the second anesthesiologist also ensures this.

The utilization of a second anesthesiologist deserves special comment because it improves patient safety, which is achieved in the operating room whereby a surgeon performs a procedure but is *not* distracted from the surgical tasks by the anesthesia/analgesia needs of the patient. It is the author's opinion that the presence of two anesthesiologists during awake fiberoptic intubation creates the ideal safety environment and that, ultimately, this should become a standard of care in the USA. The difficult airway guidelines counsel us to call for help as soon as an airway becomes unmanageable; we think securing help *before* this possibility occurs is the most prudent approach.

Only minimal to moderate sedation should be used when performing an awake fiberoptic intubation. The ASA clearly defines minimal sedation as a drug-induced state during which patients respond normally to verbal commands.

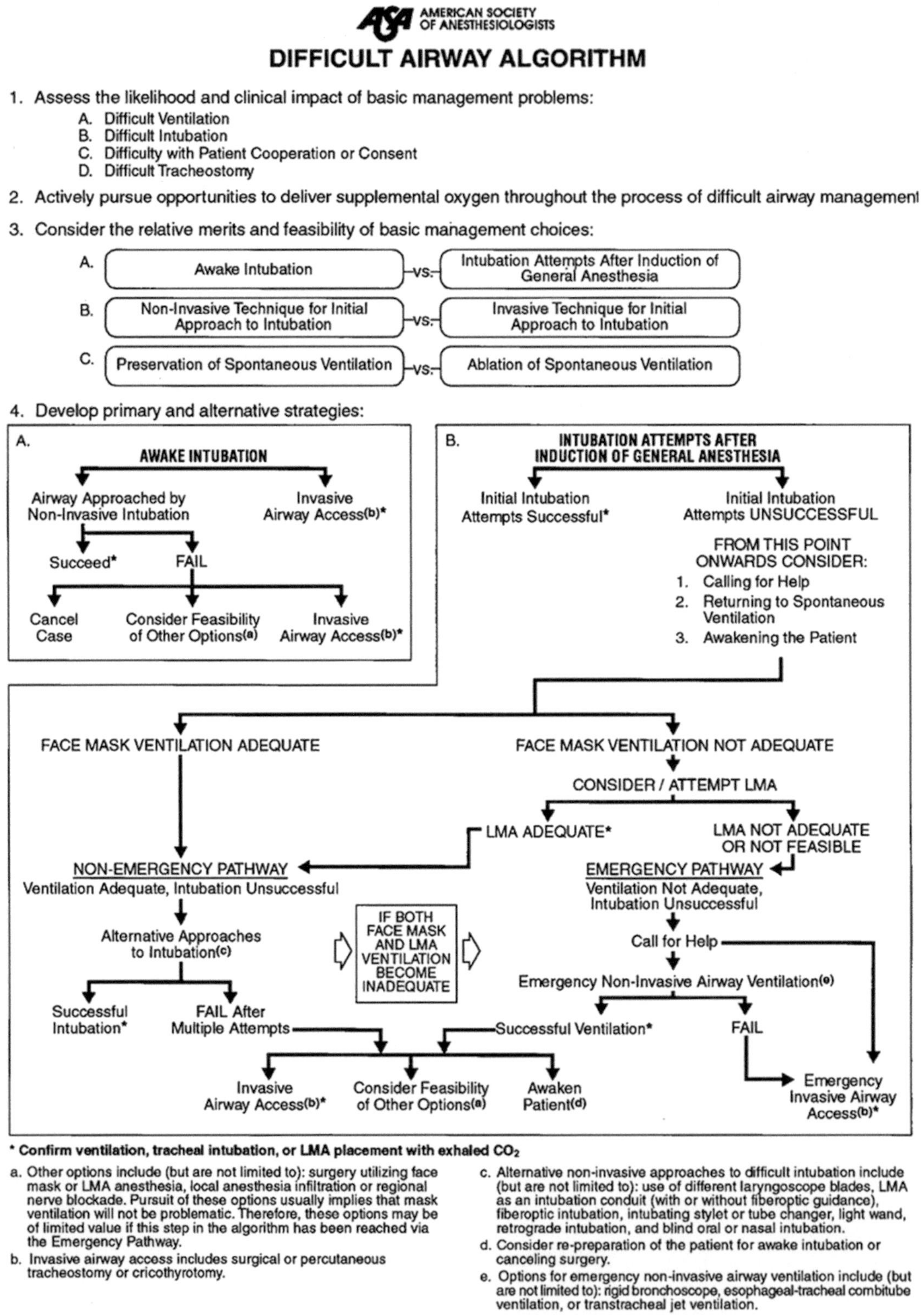

Fig. 3.3 The American Society of Anesthesiologists Difficult Airway Algorithm (Reprinted from: Apfelbaum JL, Hagberg CA, Caplan RA, et al. Practice guidelines for management of the difficult airway: an updated report by the American Society of Anesthesiologists Task Force on Management of the Difficult Airway. Anesthesiology. 2013;118(2):251–70 [32] with permission from Wolters Kluwer Health, Inc.)

Although cognitive function and coordination may be impaired, ventilatory and cardiovascular function is unaffected. Moderate sedation is a drug-induced depression of consciousness during which patients respond purposefully to verbal commands, either alone or accompanied by light tactile stimulation. No interventions are required to maintain a patent airway, and spontaneous ventilation is adequate while cardiovascular function is usually maintained. Importantly, reflex withdrawal from a painful stimulus is *not* considered a purposeful response [33]. Deep sedation defeats the entire purpose of an awake fiberoptic intubation. It lowers the safety of the procedure because deep sedation has the capacity to easily progress to general anesthesia with airway loss.

The ideal drugs for titration during an awake fiberoptic intubation are those drugs which provide sedation, analgesia, anxiolysis, amnesia, and suppression of both cough and gag reflexes. Drugs which have sedative properties but which can be quickly reversed offer an additional layer of safety because their effects can be immediately mitigated if there is oversedation. This is limited to opioids and benzodiazepines, which are rapidly and easily reversed by naloxone and flumazenil, respectively. The level of consciousness is assessed virtually continuously during the procedure, and a slow titration of drugs is accomplished by asking the patient to follow simple commands such as "inhale deeply" and "give a thumbs-up."

Dexmedetomidine has been described throughout the literature as a useful sedative for awake fiberoptic intubation in a variety of patients [34–36]. Dexmedetomidine, an alpha$_2$-agonist, acts centrally by stimulating receptors in the locus ceruleus. This results in a decreased sympathetic CNS outflow and consequent sedation. It has a shorter elimination half-life and an eightfold greater selectivity for the alpha$_2$ receptor than does clonidine, a drug in the same class. Dexmedetomidine can produce profound sedation without respiratory depression and can provide anterograde amnesia, anxiolysis, analgesia, and some antisialagogue effects [34]. Several different dose schedules of dexmedetomidine have been described for awake fiberoptic intubation, but typically is administered as an intravenous loading dose of 1 mcg/kg over 10 min, followed by a continuous infusion ranging between 0.1 and 0.7 mcg/kg/h. Intravenous glycopyrrolate is usually administered as a bolus dose of 5–10 mcg/kg specifically for its antisialagogue effects and for preventing bradycardia induced by the loading dose of dexmedetomidine [34].

Table 3.4 Ramsay scores

Score	Description
0	Awake, oriented
1	Agitated, anxious
2	Awake, cooperative
3	Sleeping, but cooperative
4	Deep sedation, quick reaction to pain
5	Deep sedation, slow reaction to pain
6	Deep sedation, no reaction to pain

If dexmedetomidine is not sufficient, midazolam, a short-acting, rapidly titratable benzodiazepine, can be added for additional sedation [37]. This dose can be repeated to achieve a Ramsay sedation score of 2 or more (see Table 3.4) but the maximum recommended dose in this setting is 0.05 mg/kg. Midazolam is an excellent anxiolytic and amnestic and confers a distinct safety advantage in that it can easily be reversed.

Remifentanil is a potent, ultrashort-acting opioid with a context-sensitive half time of 3 min and elimination half time of 6 min. It has been used as a sole agent or in combination with other drugs for awake fiberoptic intubation due to its short acting but intense level of analgesia. Additionally it suppresses airway reflexes and has only a minimal effect on cognitive function [34]. Similar to all narcotics, remifentanil exhibits a dose-dependent depression of respiratory rate and therefore can cause apnea. It is particularly advantageous due to its short half-life, ease of titratability, and its ability to be reversed with naloxone [38]. A bolus dose of 0.75 mcg/kg followed by an infusion of 0.075 mcg/kg/min, preceded by premedication with midazolam 0.05 mg/kg intravenously, has proved safe and effective in achieving sufficient patient comfort and adequate intubating conditions with stable hemodynamics during awake nasal fiberoptic intubation [39].

The combination of dexmedetomidine, midazolam, and remifentanil is the author's preference for sedation for awake fiberoptic intubation and is already a well-described technique for patients undergoing flexible bronchoscopy [40]. Intravenous midazolam and glycopyrrolate defined above are administered in the preoperative holding area. In the operating room, a loading dose of 1 mcg/kg of dexmedetomidine is given over 10 min. Concurrently, a remifentanil infusion is started at 0.075 mcg/kg/min. Additional boluses of remifentanil are given incrementally at the dose of 0.25 mcg/kg (maximum dose of 1 mcg/kg) to achieve adequate sedation and analgesia, but the objective is to maintain the patient's ability to fully follow commands. Additionally, intravenous midazolam can be administered incrementally at the dose of 0.02 mg/kg up to a maximum total dose of 0.05 mg/kg. A second provider must continually assess the patient's level of consciousness and be prepared to immediately reverse the sedation if necessary. During the 10 min required to load dexmedetomidine, nebulized lidocaine (4 %, 2–4 ml, maximum dose 3 mg/kg) via face mask is administered with oxygen at a flow of 8 l/min. Oxymetazoline spray is applied to the nares after which a small nasopharyngeal airway lubricated with 2 % lidocaine jelly is placed. Alternatively, pledgets soaked in 4 % cocaine inserted into the nares with bayonet forceps provide topical anesthesia and excellent hemostasis as well. The maximum dose of cocaine is 1–2 mg/kg with the total dose not to exceed 200 mg in any patient. Then, insertion of a nasopharyngeal airway with viscous lidocaine jelly is well tolerated and serves as a functional conduit permitting the nebulized lidocaine to reach the posterior pharynx and vocal cords. The total dose of local anesthetic should not exceed the calculated doses known to produce toxic levels by the agents selected (see Table 3.5).

If nasal intubation is planned, the nares are dilated with 2–3 progressively larger nasopharyngeal airways pre-lubricated with 2 % lidocaine jelly until the diameter of the last nasopharyngeal airway is slightly larger than the endotracheal tube that will be used. This facilitates a smoother passage of the fiberscope into the pharynx since it prevents collapse of the surrounding nasal tissues and eliminates contact with blood or secretions that can obscure the view. The largest nasal airway should be modified into a split nasopharyngeal airway, which is fashioned by making a lengthwise cut over its entire length [41]. The fiberscope is passed through this longitudinally split nasopharyngeal airway and aligned with a direct view of the vocal cords. Retraction of the tongue, jaw lift, or patient phonation assists in visualization of the vocal cords and epiglottis. A 20-gauge multiport epidural catheter is inserted through the vocal cords via the channel of the fiberscope. Then, as the epidural catheter is withdrawn and while the vocal cords remain under direct visualization via the fiberscope, 4 % lidocaine (2–3 ml) is sprayed first below and then above the vocal cords. The fiberoptic scope is removed, and oxygen via face mask is administered while the endotracheal tube is loaded onto the fiberscope and the lidocaine spray to the vocal cords achieves full effect. The fiberoptic scope is once again passed through the nares via the split nasopharyngeal airway, and this time it is advanced through the anesthetized vocal cords. The split nasopharyngeal airway allows for easy removal from the nares by peeling it off the fiberscope. The fiberscope is advanced into the right main stem bronchus and the endotracheal tube is then advanced over the fiberscope into the trachea. If the endotracheal tube does not pass easily, it is likely "hung up" at the level of the vocal cords and may need to be rotated 90° to facilitate its passage. Failing this, a change to a smaller endotracheal tube or to a flexible tube may be necessary for passage [42]. Once endotracheal tube placement is confirmed with end-tidal CO_2 and visualization of tracheal rings with the fiberscope, induction agents can be

Table 3.5 Topical local anesthetic toxic doses

Local anesthetic	Toxic dose (mg/kg)	Maximum dose (total mg)
Lidocaine	4.5	500
Cocaine	3	200

administered. The nasal route is preferred over the oral route due to the direct alignment with the vocal cords and a decreased gag reflex when a nasopharyngeal airway is used as a conduit for the fiberscope.

When the nasal route is unavailable due to structural obliteration or surgery is planned around the nares, the oral route can be used for an awake fiberoptic intubation. The patient is sedated using the same protocol as described above for the nasal route. If possible, it is useful to place a small nasopharyngeal airway, which efficiently permits nebulized lidocaine to reach the posterior pharynx and vocal cords. The nasal airway also allows for the spraying of the cords and posterior pharynx via the epidural catheter through the fiberscope. Then an oral atomizer is used to spray the base of the tongue and posterior pharynx with additional 4 % lidocaine. Several different methods have been described for oral intubation, but our clear preference is to use an intubating laryngeal airway such as the Air-Q (Mercury Medical, Clearwater, Florida). Following adequate topical anesthesia of the tongue and oral structures with nebulized lidocaine, the Air-Q laryngeal airway is lubricated with 2 % lidocaine jelly and inserted while the patient is awake. The fiberscope is advanced via the Air-Q to the glottic structures. The vocal cords are anesthetized with 4 % lidocaine delivered by an epidural catheter, which has been advanced through the fiberscope under direct vision. The objective is to inject lidocaine onto both the supra- and infraglottic areas with extension into the tracheobronchial tree. The fiberscope is removed; the endotracheal tube is loaded and then reinserted into the hypopharynx via the laryngeal airway. The fiberscope is gently advanced past the vocal cords and into the trachea. Then the endotracheal tube is "railroaded" over the fiberscope and into the trachea after which the fiberscope is removed while the endotracheal tube is manually held in place. An appropriately sized blue pushing device, which is available with the Air-Q laryngeal airway, is affixed to the endotracheal tube (the 15 mm airway connector must be removed to allow this) and this holds the tube in place while the laryngeal airway is extracted. The airway connector is then reattached, the breathing circuit is connected, and the patient is ventilated with confirmation of end-tidal CO_2. A quick reinsertion of the fiberscope confirms the proper depth of the ETT in the trachea. If prolonged intubation is *not* planned, our recommendation is to leave the Air-Q in place and to secure it along with the endotracheal tube, taped together to the patient's face. This reduces the risk of dislodgment of the newly placed endotracheal tube, which could occur during extraction of the laryngeal airway over the endotracheal tube. Induction agents can be administered after the proper placement of the endotracheal tube is confirmed.

Because the sedation techniques described above are also especially effective in children and adolescents, an awake fiberoptic intubation should be attempted first when a difficult airway is present. Preoperative anxiety can further be relieved by the administration of lorazepam or midazolam orally, if needed. Supplemental use of low-dose intravenous ketamine (0.1–0.2 mg/kg) effectively removes the impediment to use this technique for fear that the child/adolescent cannot cope.

Airway Management: "Asleep" Fiberoptic Intubation in a Spontaneously Ventilating Patient

If the patient is unable or too young to cooperate, then an "asleep" fiberoptic intubation can be performed. In this instance, the patient will require general anesthesia, and the primary goal is to maintain the patient's ability to spontaneously ventilate, followed by the anesthesiologist's confirmation of the ability to ventilate the patient with a face mask or a supraglottic airway. By far, the safest approach is to perform the fiberoptic intubation while maintaining the patient in a deep plane of anesthesia with the patient spontaneously ventilating the entire time. Sevoflurane and ketamine are two of the most commonly used drugs for this purpose, but sevoflurane is superior to ketamine in blunting the pharyngeal and laryngeal reflexes. Topical anesthesia of the airway is often required to prevent laryngospasm and coughing during airway manipulation even if the patient is in a deep plane of anesthesia. Nebulization of aerosolized lidocaine is omitted. Topical anesthesia of the airway is best accomplished by introducing a fiberscope through a laryngeal airway and using direct visualization of the vocal cords to position a multiport epidural catheter across the glottic opening via the working port of the fiberoptic scope. If the patient is not under a deep plane of anesthesia, application of topical agents can cause laryngospasm, coughing, or emesis, which can result in difficulty ventilating the patient and the possibility of losing the airway. Neuromuscular blocking agents are to be administered only after confirmation of the endotracheal tube in the trachea, which is done by end-tidal CO_2 measurement and direct visualization of the end of the endotracheal within the trachea via the fiberscope.

Intravenous access is an absolute safety requirement and must be established *before* proceeding with a mask induction with sevoflurane so that emergency medications can be administered if required. For example, an intravenous line allows for the administration of propofol to break laryngospasm and quickly deepen the anesthetic. The use of any neuromuscular blocking drug in this situation caries a certain peril and should be avoided unless there is no other way to restore the airway. Obtaining an intravenous line can be difficult and the use of an ultrasound is often needed. Premedication can be accomplished with the patient receiving preoperative oral midazolam or lorazepam prior to intravenous placement. Nitrous oxide in addition to preoperative benzodiazepines may help with sedation for placement of lines. If the above techniques fail to adequately sedate the patient, intramuscular ketamine (2–4 mg/kg) can be administered to provide sedation, while spontaneous ventilation is preserved during peripheral or central line placement. If intravenous access cannot be quickly established, there should be no hesitation in inserting an interosseous line; this immediately establishes intravenous access and has an excellent safety record.

Once intravenous access has been obtained, a mask induction with sevoflurane is initiated with the goal of maintaining spontaneous ventilation. After a deep plane of anesthesia is achieved, an Air-Q laryngeal airway can be placed to facilitate endotracheal intubation via the fiberscope. The cords should be treated with topical lidocaine to advancement of the endotracheal tube past the vocal cords. Alternatively, a nasal fiberoptic intubation using a split nasopharyngeal airway can be used to help facilitate intubation, and the airway should be anesthetized with lidocaine prior to advancement of the nasal endotracheal tube.

Airway Management: "Asleep" Fiberoptic Intubation Without Spontaneous Ventilation

The last approach to fiberoptic intubation that can be taken is the induction of anesthesia with fiberoptic intubation after potent induction agents have been administered. Spontaneous ventilation will be ablated, and this approach may be appropriate if the provider has had recent experience in managing the particular patient's airway during a recent anesthetic. The critical safety key is that the anesthesiologist learned that the patient was easily ventilated by mask. Usually intravenous propofol along with inhaled sevoflurane is administered on induction, and the ability to mask ventilate or ventilate via a supraglottic airway is demonstrated before additional drugs are administered. Neuromuscular blocking agents may be administered, but are not advised, until endotracheal intubation is confirmed by end-tidal CO_2 monitoring and direct visualization via the fiberscope. This method can be done via the oral route using an Air-Q laryngeal airway or via the nasal route.

Airway Management: Surgical Release of Postburn Neck Contracture Under Ketamine Prior to Securing the Airway

If an awake fiberoptic intubation is not successful, a surgical release of postburn neck contractures can be done under ketamine and tumescent local anesthesia prior to securing the airway. The release of the contracture allows for sufficient extension of the atlanto-occipital joint to make it possible to perform direct laryngoscopy, fiberoptic intubation, or a video laryngoscope intubation [43]. Once the trachea is intubated, surgery for grafting can proceed under general anesthesia. There are numerous reports in the literature of successful surgical release of neck contractures under local anesthesia and ketamine sedation and general anesthesia with inhalation agents while maintaining spontaneous ventilation prior to intubation [26, 30]. The risk of airway obstruction with a general anesthetic mask induction along with the difficulty of maintaining a good seal with a face mask could complicate airway management in a postburn contracture patient. Intravenous ketamine (0.5–1 mg/kg) sedation for neck release along with local tumescent anesthesia may be the best choice and has been well described in the literature for both adult and pediatric patients [44, 45].

Airway Management: Other Techniques

The difficult airway can be managed with several additional techniques including but not limited to video laryngoscopes, blind nasal intubation, alternative laryngoscope blades, awake look intubation via direct laryngoscopy, intubating optical stylets, several different types of laryngeal airways to aid in intubation, light wand, retrograde intubation, and invasive surgical access. Even the use of extracorporeal membrane oxygenation (ECMO) has been reported as a bridge to intubation [30, 46].

A variety of techniques and methods can be used in an effort to safely secure the airway in a patient with acute burns or postburn contractures. Difficulties with intubation should be anticipated and careful planning by the care team is essential. Contingency plans should be well developed, practiced, and communicated. Using the principles of difficult airway management for non-burn patients, an awake attempt at intubation should be considered first, followed by the consideration of intubation with general anesthesia in the spontaneously ventilating patient. These concepts and techniques allow for the safe care of patients with acute burns or severe postburn contractures. These patients have precarious airways and are therefore at risk of catastrophe leading to either a serious morbidity or death attributable to a loss of the airway.

Summary

Like any trauma patient, the airway is the first consideration in managing a burn patient. The main concern is for edema that leads to obstruction. Early intubation is always preferable to attempting to deal with an emergent airway. Dealing with the edematous airway requires expertise that includes a team approach with anesthesiologists and surgeons. Patients with scar contractures of the neck and mouth are even more difficult. These difficult patients must be approached with planning and skill.

References

1. Moylan JA, Chan CK. Inhalation injury – an increasing problem. Ann Surg. 1978;188(1):34–7.
2. Sharar SR, Olivar H. Anesthesia for burn patients. In: Post TW, editor. UpToDate, Waltham, MA. Accessed 23 Apr 2015.
3. Dai NT, Chen TM, Cheng TY, et al. The comparison of early fluid therapy in extensive flame burns between inhalation and noninhalation injuries. Burns. 1998;24(7):671–5.
4. Suzuki M, Aikawa N, Kobayashi K, Higuchi R. Prognostic implications of inhalation injury in burn patients in Tokyo. Burns. 2005;31(3):331–6.
5. Clark WR. Smoke inhalation: diagnosis and treatment. World J Surg. 1992;16(1):24–9.
6. Kumar P. Grading of severity of the condition in burn patients by serum protein and albumin/globulin studies. Ann Plast Surg. 2010;65(1):74–9.
7. Bittner EA, Shank E, Woodson L, Martyn JA. Acute and perioperative care of the burn-injured patient. Anesthesiology. 2015;122(2):448–64.
8. Tricklebank S. Modern trends in fluid therapy for burns. Burns. 2009;35(6):757–67.
9. Monafo WW. Initial management of burns. N Engl J Med. 1996;335(21):1581–6.
10. Bishop S, Maguire S. Anaesthesia and intensive care for major burns. Continuing Educ Anaesth Critic Care Pain Adv Access. Feb 23, 2012.

11. Muehlberger T, Kunar D, Munster A, Couch M. Efficacy of fiberoptic laryngoscopy in the diagnosis of inhalation injuries. Arch Otolaryngol Head Neck Surg. 1998;124(9):1003–7.
12. Reinhold H, Deloof T, Jortay A, Mathieu M, Vandesteene A. The risks of tracheal intubation. Acta Anaesthesiol Belg. 1978;29(1):69–84.
13. Peppard SB, Dickens JH. Laryngeal injury following short-term intubation. Ann Otol Rhinol Laryngol. 1983;92(4 Pt 1):327–30.
14. Colice GL, Munster AM, Haponik EF. Tracheal stenosis complicating cutaneous burns: an underestimated problem. Am Rev Respir Dis. 1986;134(6): 1315–8.
15. Ahrenholz DH, Cope N, Dimick A, Gamelli RL, Gillespie RW, Kagan RJ, et al. American burn association practice guidelines for burn care. J Burn Care Rehabil. 2001;22:S23–6.
16. Oscier C, Emerson B, Handy JM. New perspectives on airway management in acutely burned patients. Anaesthesia. 2014;69(2):105–10.
17. Martyn J, Goldhill DR, Goudsouzian NG. Clinical pharmacology of muscle relaxants in patients with burns. J Clin Pharmacol. 1986;26(8):680–5.
18. Martyn JA, Richtsfeld M. Succinylcholine-induced hyperkalemia in acquired pathologic states: etiologic factors and molecular mechanisms. Anesthesiology. 2006;104(1):158–69.
19. Osta WA, El-osta MA, Pezhman EA, et al. Nicotinic acetylcholine receptor gene expression is altered in burn patients. Anesth Analg. 2010;110(5):1355–9.
20. Martyn JA, Abernethy DR, Greenblatt DJ. Plasma protein binding of drugs after severe burn injury. Clin Pharmacol Ther. 1984;35(4):535–9.
21. Han TH, Martyn JA. Onset and effectiveness of rocuronium for rapid onset of paralysis in patients with major burns: priming or large bolus. Br J Anaesth. 2009;102(1):55–60.
22. Maclennan N, Heimbach DM, Cullen BF. Anesthesia for major thermal injury. Anesthesiology. 1998;89(3):749–70.
23. Woodson LC. Anesthesia for acute burn injuries, Principles and practice of burn surgery. New York, NY: Marcel Dekker; 2005. p. 103–33.
24. Fuzaylov G, Fidkowski CW. Anesthetic considerations for major burn injury in pediatric patients. Paediatr Anaesth. 2009;19(3):202–11.
25. Greathouse JS, Stuart JL, White WA. Difficult airway management following severe gasoline burn injury: a case report. AANA J. 2012;80(4):268–72.
26. Prakash S, Mullick P. Airway management in patients with burn contractures of the neck. Burns. 2015;41(8): 1627–35.
27. Nahlieli O, Kelly JP, Baruchin AM, Ben-meir P, Shapira Y. Oro-maxillofacial skeletal deformities resulting from burn scar contractures of the face and neck. Burns. 1995;21(1):65–9.
28. Han TH, Teissler H, Han RJ, Gaines JD, Nguyen TQ. Managing difficult airway in patients with post-burn mentosternal and circumoral scar contractures. Int J Burns Trauma. 2012;2(2):80–5.
29. Robertson CF, Zuker R, Dabrowski B, Levison H. Obstructive sleep apnea: a complication of burns to the head and neck in children. J Burn Care Rehabil. 1985;6(4):353–7.
30. Caruso TJ, Janik LS, Fuzaylov G. Airway management of recovered pediatric patients with severe head and neck burns: a review. Paediatr Anaesth. 2012;22(5):462–8.
31. El-orbany MI, Getachew YB, Joseph NJ, Salem MR, Friedman M. Head elevation improves laryngeal exposure with direct laryngoscopy. J Clin Anesth. 2015;27(2):153–8.
32. Apfelbaum JL, Hagberg CA, Caplan RA, et al. Practice guidelines for management of the difficult airway: an updated report by the American Society of Anesthesiologists Task Force on Management of the Difficult Airway. Anesthesiology. 2013;118(2): 251–70.
33. Practice guidelines for sedation and analgesia by non-anesthesiologists. Anesthesiology. 2002;96(4):1004–17.
34. Johnston KD, Rai MR. Conscious sedation for awake fibreoptic intubation: a review of the literature. Can J Anaesth. 2013;60(6):584–99.
35. He XY, Cao JP, He Q, Shi XY. Dexmedetomidine for the management of awake fibreoptic intubation. Cochrane Database Syst Rev. 2014;1:CD009798.
36. Gaszynski T, Gaszynska E, Szewczyk T. Dexmedetomidine for awake intubation and an opioid-free general anesthesia in a superobese patient with suspected difficult intubation. Drug Des Devel Ther. 2014;8: 909–12.
37. Bergese SD, Patrick bender S, Mcsweeney TD, Fernandez S, Dzwonczyk R, Sage K. A comparative study of dexmedetomidine with midazolam and midazolam alone for sedation during elective awake fiberoptic intubation. J Clin Anesth. 2010;22(1):35–40.
38. Amin HM, Sopchak AM, Esposito BF, et al. Naloxone-induced and spontaneous reversal of depressed ventilatory responses to hypoxia during and after continuous infusion of remifentanil or alfentanil. J Pharmacol Exp Ther. 1995;274(1):34–9.
39. Machata AM, Gonano C, Holzer A, et al. Awake nasotracheal fiberoptic intubation: patient comfort, intubating conditions, and hemodynamic stability during conscious sedation with remifentanil. Anesth Analg. 2003;97(3):904–8.
40. Ryu JH, Lee SW, Lee JH, Lee EH, Do SH, Kim CS. Randomized double-blind study of remifentanil and dexmedetomidine for flexible bronchoscopy. Br J Anaesth. 2012;108(3):503–11.
41. Eipe N, Fossey S, Kingwell SP. Airway management in cervical spine ankylosing spondylitis: between a rock and a hard place. Indian J Anaesth. 2013;57(6):592–5.
42. Asai T, Shingu K. Difficulty in advancing a tracheal tube over a fibreoptic bronchoscope: incidence, causes and solutions. Br J Anaesth. 2004;92(6):870–81.

43. Park CD, Lee HK, Yim JY, Kang IH. Anesthetic management for a patient with severe mento-sternal contracture: difficult airway and scarce venous access: a case report. Korean J Anesthesiol. 2013;64(1):61–4.
44. Agarwal P. Safe method for release of severe post burn neck contracture under tumescent local anaesthesia and ketamine. Indian J Plast Surg. 2004; 37:51–4.
45. Sarkar M, Puri V, Rahul V, Chaudhari S. The use of ketamine for release of post-burn neck contracture. Bombay Hosp J. 2007;4902:306–9.
46. Sheridan RL, Ryan DP, Fuzaylov G, Nimkin K, Martyn JA, Case Records of the Massachusetts General Hospital Case 2-2008. Case 5-2008. An 18-month-old girl with an advanced neck contracture after a burn. N Engl J Med. 2008;358(7):729–35.

Breathing

4

Tina L. Palmieri

Introduction

Approximately 7–10 % of burn center admissions have concomitant inhalation injury [1]. Inhalation injury both increases the mortality associated with burn injury and is associated with burn size (i.e., the larger the burn, the more likely that inhalation injury will be present) [2, 3]. Timely diagnosis and treatment of inhalation injury is the key to improving survival. However, the diagnosis of inhalation injury is not always straightforward. The first question that arises is: "What is inhalation injury?" In practice, inhalation injury is used to define multiple different mechanisms of airway injury, each requiring unique diagnostic paradigms and treatment algorithms. There are three different types of airway injury that occur after exposure to fire and smoke: (1) effects of inhaled gases, (2) upper airway injury/edema (addressed in another chapter), and (3) lower airway injury [4]. Each of the different types of smoke inhalation injury has a different cause, pathophysiology, treatment, and prognosis. This chapter addresses factors that impact breathing: inhaled toxins and lower airway injury due to the effects of smoke and provides a roadmap to effectively navigate the diagnosis and treatment of inhaled toxins and smoke effects on lung parenchyma.

Effects of Inhaled Toxins

When fires burn they consume oxygen and generate toxic chemicals. As such, inhalation of toxic by-products of combustion accounts for 80 % of fire-related deaths [5]. Several changes in the composition of gases in the environment occur as the result of combustion of flammable objects, and the person exposed to these gases is subject to their effects. The changes induced by the fire environment include consumption of oxygen as well as generation of toxic gases such as carbon monoxide (CO), cyanide, and other systemic poisons.

Hypoxia

When flames engulf a room, they consume oxygen and decrease the fraction of inspired oxygen (FIO_2) in the room to <10 %, causing tissue hypoxia and asphyxia. Hence, one of the leading causes of death at the fire scene is hypoxia, not burns. Identification of patients at risk for hypoxia relies heavily on the history of the incident.

T.L. Palmieri, M.D., F.A.C.S., F.C.C.M. (✉)
Firefighters Burn Institute Burn Centre, University of California, Davis, Sacramento, CA, USA

Shriners Hospital for Children Northern California, 2425 Stockton Blvd, Suite 718, Sacramento, CA 95817, USA
e-mail: tlpalmieri@ucdavis.edu

D.G. Greenhalgh (ed.), *Burn Care for General Surgeons and General Practitioners*,
DOI 10.1007/978-3-319-29161-1_4

Clinicians should consider risk factors with respect to scene characteristics (house fire, multiple other deaths at the scene, loss of consciousness), patient exposure to smoke (prolonged period of time in flame-filled room, returning to a burning building), and injury characteristics (burns of the face and neck, large burns, confusion). Addressing hypoxia should be an essential component of any inhalation injury treatment strategy. As such, patients with suspected inhalation injury should receive initial administration of 100 % oxygen via face mask at the scene, during transport, and upon hospital arrival. Patients should be monitored for status changes, and oxygen should be continued until there is objective evidence (blood gas) that hypoxia and carbon monoxide poisoning do not exist.

Carbon Monoxide Poisoning

Carbon monoxide (CO) toxicity is a frequent cause of morbidity and mortality in patients who sustain inhalation injury. Each year CO causes an estimated 15,000 emergency room visits and 500 unintentional deaths [6]. CO decreases both the oxygen-carrying capacity and the delivery of oxygen to tissue because it has an affinity with hemoglobin 200–250 times that of oxygen [7]. The increased oxygen affinity shifts the oxyhemoglobin disassociation curve to the left, interfering with oxygen transport at the cellular level and impairing electron transport within the cells, resulting in tissue hypoxia [8]. CO also interferes with hepatic cytochromes, myoglobin binding, and peroxidation of cerebral lipids [7]. Finally, CO interacts with the hematologic system by altering leukocyte, platelet, and vascular endothelial function [9]. Injury severity is dependent on the duration of exposure, inhaled CO concentration, and patient baseline health status. The amount of CO needed to cause toxicity is small: exposure to a 0.1 % CO concentration can result in a carboxyhemoglobin (COHb) level of 50 % [4].

The risk factors for CO toxicity are similar to those for hypoxia. Confused or combative patients with a history of significant smoke exposure should initially be treated with oxygen.

Table 4.1 Symptoms associated with carbon monoxide exposure

Carboxyhemoglobin level (%)	Symptom
0–10	No significant physiologic changes
10–30	Throbbing, headache, blood vessel dilatation
30–40	Fatigue, nausea/emesis, disorientation, vision change
41–60	Combativeness, hallucinations, coma, shock
>60	Cardiorespiratory depression, seizure, mortality

Although initial symptoms of CO toxicity are primarily neurologic and correlate with COHb level [10] (Table 4.1), physical examination does not accurately predict the incidence of CO toxicity. The classically described rosy red cheeks and nose associated with CO toxicity are generally not present in inhalation injury due to hypoxia and soot. Hence, the use of skin color as a diagnostic modality for CO exposure is problematic. Standard oxygen monitoring tools are also unreliable: pulse oximetry does not accurately reflect systemic oxygenation in CO toxicity and should *not* be used in isolation to assess oxygenation after burn/smoke exposure. Cooximetry, which delineates the impact of COHb, in association with an arterial blood gas, should be used.

Suspected CO toxicity is confirmed by measuring plasma COHb levels. If inhalation injury is suspected, supplemental oxygen should be administered. Oxygen displaces CO from the hemoglobin molecule and can facilitate the restoration of oxygen transport. Although the duration of the hypoxic state is a marker for CO injury severity, COHb levels do not correlate with the severity of poisoning, predict prognosis, or determine choice of a specific therapy [8].

Patients with a COHb >10 % should continue to receive supplemental oxygen, and COHb levels repeated every hour until <10 %. Patients who are awake and alert should receive 100 % FIO_2 via face mask. The use of 100 % oxygen for 6 h after COHb levels at <10 % may facilitate elimination of COHb from tissues. Intubation should be utilized for obtunded patients, patients who cannot protect their airway, patients with uncontrollable agitation requiring significant sedation, and patients with severe face burns. After intubation, mechanical ventilation with 100 % inspired oxygen is optimal. The use of 100 % FIO_2 will decrease the half-life of COHb to 40–60 min [11]. Hyperbaric oxygen can be considered if the COHb level is >25 % despite aggressive oxygen therapy. Hyperbaric oxygen, however, is not a panacea; the half-life of COHb is only decreased to 30 min by hyperbaric oxygen [12]. Multiple studies have assessed the efficacy of hyperbaric oxygen to improve outcomes in CO poisoning. Unfortunately, four of six studies evaluating outcomes in 1335 patients randomized to either hyperbaric or normobaric oxygen demonstrated no improvement in neurologic sequelae with hyperbaric oxygen treatment [13–17]. Hyperbaric oxygen therapy has multiple potential complications, including tympanic membrane rupture, seizure, and lack of patient accessibility; hence, it should be reserved for patients with documented CO exposure (COHb>25 %) who fail to improve on normobaric oxygen therapy [4, 10].

Other Poisons

Hypoxia and CO poisoning are not the only concerns after prolonged exposure to smoke. Other substances, such as plastics, generate toxic combustibles. Table 4.2 contains a listing of toxic combustibles in smoke and their sources. As such, every person who sustains smoke inhalation injury will have a unique exposure to a variety of different toxins which cannot be identified or treated. Housing construction and room décor, which have changed over the years, have resulted in changes in the fire milieu [18].

Table 4.2 Toxic gases in house fire smoke

Gas	Source	Effect
Carbon monoxide	Organic matter	Tissue hypoxia
Hydrogen cyanide	Wool, silk, nylons	Headache, coma, respiratory failure
Aldehydes	Wood, cotton, paper	Severe mucosal, lung damage
Benzene	Petroleum plastics	Mucosal irritation, coma
Ammonia	Nylon	Mucosal irritation
Hydrogen chloride	Plastics	Severe mucosal irritation
Nitrogen dioxide	Wall paper, wood	Pulmonary edema, dizziness

One of the toxic agents in smoke that can be identified and treated is cyanide. Cyanide is generated by combustion of natural or synthetic household materials including synthetic polymers, polyacrylonitrile, paper, polyurethane, melamine, wool, and silk [19–24]. Cyanide has been detected both at the fire scene and in the blood of smokers and fire victims [19, 25–29]. Blood cyanide levels can range from 0.3 mg/L in nonsmokers to 0.5 mg/L in smokers. A blood cyanide level of 3 mg/L is generally defined as fatal, although both lower and higher levels have been cited [30–33]. Unfortunately, blood cyanide levels are not readily measured in hospitals and must be sent to specialized laboratories. As such, the test results generally are not available for 2–3 days post-injury, which makes them unhelpful in the acute treatment phase.

The first-line treatment for cyanide is appropriate resuscitation. Metabolic acidosis in a burn patient should initially be assumed to be due to under-resuscitation, carbon monoxide toxicity, missed associated traumatic injury, or a combination of these events. The use of antidotes for cyanide toxicity should be restricted to patients with a persistent metabolic acidosis after appropriate resuscitation is confirmed, carbon monoxide levels have normalized, and traumatic injury has been ruled out.

Recent literature suggests that early use of hydroxocobalamin therapy may be efficacious in cyanide poisoning. Hydroxocobalamin has been used to prevent cyanide toxicity associated with intravenous nitroprusside and to treat the toxic amblyopia and optic neuritis caused by tobacco smoke, which contains cyanide [34]. A cyanocobalamin dose of 100 mg/kg should be used in suspected cyanide toxicity. Although hydroxocobalamin therapy is generally well tolerated, side effects include headache, allergic reaction, skin and urine discoloration, hypertension, or reflex bradycardia [35, 36]. The urine color change (purple) can cause consternation among hospital providers, and hydroxocobalamin may interfere with the accuracy of cooximetry or autoanalyzer colorimetric blood assays (frequently used to assess liver enzymes, electrolytes, and minerals) for several days [35]. Anaphylactic reactions have also been documented [36]. Hence, treatment using hydroxocobalamin is not without risk. Patients with cyanide poisoning will gradually demonstrate an improvement in status with appropriate resuscitation and administration of hydroxocobalamin. Other antidotes, such as amyl nitrite, sodium nitrite, and sodium thiosulfate (formerly named the cyanide antidote kit), are being replaced by hydroxocobalamin, which has a better safety profile.

Effects of Smoke on Lung Function

Effects on Burn Prognosis

Inhalation injury with associated cutaneous burn injury results in increased mortality compared to burn injury alone [3, 37]. Survival after inhalation injury has increased from 56 % in 1986 to 27 % in 2010 and has been reported as low as 12 % [38, 39]. The improvement in survival can be attributed to a better understanding of the underlying pathophysiology of burns, changes in ventilation strategies, and newly developed ventilator technologies.

Pathophysiology and Diagnosis of Smoke Injury

Lower airway inhalation injury is due to the effects of the toxic products of combustion and the burn injury on lung parenchyma and blood flow. Casts and proteinaceous material accumulate in the airway, causing bronchoconstriction and airway hyperreactivity. Lower airway inhalation injury also results in increased capillary permeability, both in the lung and in the distal airway [40–42]. The inflammatory damage to the alveolar-capillary barrier seen in inhalation injury results in the release of proteinaceous fluid into the alveolar space, causing impaired gas exchange [43]. The bronchoconstriction that accompanies inhalation injury further impairs gas exchange. As such, inhalation injury may be viewed as a special form of acute lung injury (ALI), which may progress to the acute respiratory distress syndrome (ARDS).

The diagnosis of lower airway injury after smoke exposure is similar to that used for upper airway injury. History (with attention to high-risk scenarios) and physical examination (including inspection of the oropharynx for soot, edema, or ulceration) should be performed [44]. Further tests, including arterial blood gases, COHb levels, and a chest X-ray, should be obtained. Elevated levels of COHb are associated with an increased incidence of lower airway injury [19]. Although helpful to establish a baseline, normal arterial blood gases and chest X-ray do not exclude lower airway injury. Laryngoscopy may be helpful to diagnose upper airway edema; however, the provider should be prepared to intubate at the time of laryngoscopy, as it can precipitate airway obstruction. Bronchoscopy should be used to visualize the extent of lower airway injury as it provides valuable information with respect to airway anatomy and obstruction. Multiple grading systems have been proposed to diagnose inhalation injury, but none have been universally adopted [45, 46]. Current multicenter trials are evaluating the utility of computed tomography scanning and inflammatory markers in the diagnosis and grading of inhalation injury.

Treatment of Inhalation Injury

Treatment of Uncomplicated Inhalation Injury

Not all patients with inhalation injury require mechanical ventilation. Patients with a patent upper airway (absence of stridor), burn size <40 % TBSA, intact mental status, the ability to clear secretions, and adequate oxygenation and ventilation ($PO2>60$ mmHg, $PCO2<55$ mmHg in the absence of chronic obstructive pulmonary disease) may often be safely managed without mechanical ventilation. These patients should be placed on humidified oxygen therapy and be admitted to an intensive care unit for close monitoring. Treatment should focus on clearance of secretions; hence, early mobility, incentive spirometry, intrapulmonary percussive ventilation (IPV), and encouragement are keys to successful management. If COHb toxicity is present, an arterial line will facilitate testing and may be helpful. Arterial line insertion should be reserved for patients who have demonstrated hypoxia or hypercarbia. Intravenous steroids are not indicated in inhalation injury [1]. There is no evidence that steroids improve outcomes. Likewise, prophylactic antibiotics are not indicated, as they may predispose patients to more virulent infections.

Treatment of Inhalation Injury Requiring Intubation

Patients with severe face burns, significant hypoxia or hypercarbia (PO2 < 60 mmHg or PCO2 > 55 mmHg), altered mental status, inability to protect the airway, or massive burns (>40 % TBSA) should be intubated and placed on mechanical ventilation. The most experienced practitioner should intubate the patient with suspected inhalation injury, as anatomy is often distorted and edema may severely limit visualization of vital structures. In severe inhalation injury associated with ulceration or airway sloughing, bronchoscopy may be necessary to remove debris and facilitate oxygenation for days after injury. Securing the airway can pose a challenge in face burns, as tape will not adhere to a blistered face. The use of a tracheostomy tie in both the horizontal and vertical planes may be helpful. The ties should be checked regularly for evidence of erosion into soft tissue structures. The ventilator circuit should be humidified to prevent drying of secretions. Inhaled albuterol may be beneficial in patients with bronchospasm [47]. *N*-acetyl cysteine has also been used in conjunction with albuterol to facilitate secretion removal. Nebulized heparin, when used with either FFP or antithrombin III, may also be used to decrease the formation of airway casts [48].

One of the emerging challenges in inhalation injury is the patient who sustains face burns while smoking on home oxygen. These patients present with burns of the nose tip and nares. The burn is generally limited to the nose and/or midface, and the patient rarely sustains any significant inhalation injury. Unfortunately, people on home oxygen have a preexisting hypoxic and/or hypercarbic state (otherwise they would not be on home oxygen); hence, the decision on whether or not to intubate is not always straightforward. In general, intubation in home oxygen burns should be avoided unless there is evidence that the respiratory status has changed from baseline (i.e., development of stridor, respiratory acidosis, hypoxia compared to baseline) [49]. Intubation prolongs hospital stay and may increase mortality. Initial treatment with oxygen and saline nasal spray usually suffices.

Basic Ventilator Strategies

Treatment of patients with lower airway inhalation injury requiring mechanical ventilation is largely supportive. Lung epithelium and airway casts may slough in the first 3–7 days post-injury. Meticulous pulmonary hygiene, including frequent suctioning, is vital to maintain airway patency and to prevent pneumonia. Humidified oxygen should be utilized to keep secretions moist and prevent endotracheal tube obstruction from dry and hard secretions. In the early phases of injury, when a patient is markedly edematous, an obstructed endotracheal tube can be a deadly problem. Sedation should be limited to enable the patient to assist in secretion removal via coughing and position changes.

There is no consensus on the best form of mechanical ventilation for lower airway inhalation injury. However, several basic principles apply. Maintaining a "perfect" blood gas (pH of 7.40, PCO2 of 40 mmHg, PO2 of 100 mmHg) is not appropriate. The objective is to support lung function while minimizing the complications of mechanical ventilation. Hence, the goal is to maintain adequate oxygenation and ventilation while minimizing barotrauma and volutrauma. In patients intubated with minor inhalation injury or purely for edema, pressure support with positive end expiratory pressure of 5 mmHg may be sufficient. For patients with severe hypoxia, however, using protocols designed for ARDS may be helpful. A seminal randomized prospective trial in ARDS reported a 22 % decrease in mortality, utilizing a pressure- and volume-limited approach (tidal volume 6 ml/kg and pressure <30 mmHg) compared to a higher tidal volume (12 ml/kg) [50]. This philosophy has been applied to severe inhalation injury (patients with ventilation/perfusion ratios of <200) and has likely contributed to the decrease in mortality. Likewise, the use of permissive hypercapnia (not treating pCO2 until pH is <7.2) also limits ventilator pressures and decreases lung injury.

A multitude of different traditional ventilator modes have been used in inhalation injury, including pressure control, volume control, airway pressure release ventilation (APRV), high-frequency ventilation, and liquid ventilation. However, none of these has clearly demonstrated outcome superiority in inhalation injury [51]. One form of ventilation, volumetric diffusive ventilation, may improve outcomes. The volumetric diffusive respirator, a time-cycled pressure limited ventilator, has been shown to decrease the incidence of pneumonia and improve mortality after inhalation injury [52]. However, this mode of ventilation has not been tested against a low-tidal-volume ventilation strategy or some of the newer forms of mechanical ventilation such as airway pressure release ventilation or oscillatory ventilation. The type of ventilation used is less important than the philosophy of airway management.

One final adjunct for the management of severe burn with ARDS is tracheostomy. Tracheostomy can improve laminar air flow, prevent pressure ulcers from endotracheal tube tying, decrease ventilator pressures, facilitate weaning, and allow for easier pulmonary toilet [53]. Tracheostomy is indicated if the patient has been intubated for 2 weeks and is not improving. In addition, tracheostomy may be beneficial in the early phase of burn injury in patients with extensive face burns, massive burn injury (>50 % TBSA), patients who cannot be electively intubated, and patients with severe lung injury.

Complications of Smoke Injury

Smoke inhalation injury not only markedly complicates medical management of the burn patient, but also increases mortality. Pulmonary complications contribute to 77 % of burn-related deaths [54]. Two particular complications of smoke inhalation injury are frequently encountered: pneumonia and the acute respiratory distress syndrome.

Pneumonia

Pneumonia is a common complication of inhalation injury. Pneumonia occurs twice as often in burn with inhalation injury compared to burn injury alone and increases mortality 40–60 % [55]. The incidence of pneumonia in the burn inhalation patient has been reported as high as 46 % and accounted for 75 % of cases of pneumonia in 1 unit [56]. The high rate of pneumonia is multifactorial: (1) The airway casts and debris from the initial injury can cause airway obstruction. (2) The mucociliary apparatus is impaired from the initial insult, making secretion removal problematic. (3) Patients have concomitant wound colonization, which can infect airways. (4) Burn patients are hypermetabolic, which increases the work of breathing and subsequent pulmonary failure. (5) Burns >20 % have decreased cell-mediated, natural killer cell, and macrophage responses.

Diagnosis of pneumonia requires a high index of suspicion. In patients with a fever, leukocytosis, and purulent secretions bronchoscopy with washing or protected brush sampling may provide the most accurate diagnosis. Patients should be aggressively treated with intravenous antibiotics and pulmonary hygiene measures. In recurrent cases, inhaled antibiotics may be required.

Acute Respiratory Distress Syndrome

Smoke inhalation injury is caused by breathing toxic smoke from the products of combustion. Severe cases of smoke inhalation can result in either acute lung injury (ALI) or acute respiratory distress syndrome (ARDS) The traditional definition of ALI includes an alveolar-arteriolar gradient of <300; for ARDS the alveolar-arteriolar gradient is <200. The Berlin definition of ARDS has modified those criteria to include (1) timing (must occur within 1 week of a known clinical insult), (2) chest imaging (bilateral opacities not explained by other causes), (3) origin of edema (not explained by cardiac failure or fluid overload), and (4) oxygenation (defined as mild, moderate, or severe based on alveolar oxygen gradient and PEEP) [57]. Regardless of the definition, ARDS is characterized by increased permeability of pulmonary capillary endothelial cells and alveolar epithelial cells, leading to hypoxemia that is refractory to oxygen therapy.

Patients with smoke inhalation injury can develop ARDS in different phases of illness. During the acute phase (first days after injury), patients can develop severe hypoxemia and impaired pulmonary function from the smoke toxins. This represents a direct parenchymal injury. A second cause of ARDS in the early phase of burn injury is the burn wound itself. The burn injury induces the development of a systemic inflammatory response syndrome and subsequent ARDS. After the first several days of injury, the development of ARDS is multifactorial and similar to other ICU populations. Both direct injury (pneumonia, aspiration) and indirect (sepsis, blood transfusion) mechanisms can cause ARDS in the weeks after a burn injury. Analysis of outcomes in patients with combined burn/inhalation injury is consistent with this bimodal pattern [3].

The treatment of ARDS is generally supportive, as described above. However, for ARDS occurring in the early phase (first 1–2 days post-injury), early excision of the burn wound, which is associated with decreased mortality, may be helpful [58]. The burn wound itself can be the source of a severe inflammatory response; removing the wound removes the source and may decrease the associated capillary leak and alveolar arterial gradient.

Smoke inhalation injury with ARDS is associated with increased mortality. A recent military experience demonstrated a fourfold increase in mortality with moderate ARDS and a ninefold increase in mortality with severe ARDS [59]. Appropriate early resuscitation, meticulous pulmonary hygiene, early excision, and aggressive treatment of infection may help decrease the incidence of ARDS after smoke inhalation injury.

Conclusion

Smoke inhalation injury significantly contributes to burn morbidity and mortality due to the direct toxicity from products of combustion as well as the subsequent inflammatory response. Identification and early aggressive treatment are keys to minimizing the morbidity associated with inhalation injury.

References

1. American Burn Association National Burn Repository 2012 Report. American Burn Association NBR Advisory Committee. Chicago, IL.
2. Chen MC, Chen MH, Wen BS, et al. The impact of inhalation injury in patients with small and moderate burns. Burns. 2014;40(8):1481–6. doi:10.1016/j.burns.2014.06.016.
3. Taylor SL, Sen S, Greenhalgh DG, et al. A competing risk analysis for hospital length of stay in patients with burns. JAMA Surg. 2015;150(5):450–6.
4. Traber DL, Herndon DN, Soejima K. The pathophysiology of inhalation injury. In: Total burn care. 2nd ed. London: W.B. Saunders; 2002. p. 221–231.
5. Birke MM, Clarke FB. Inhalation of toxic products from fires. Bull NY Acad Med. 1981;57:997–1013.
6. Centers for Disease Control and Prevention. Carbon monoxide-related deaths-United States, 1999–2004. 2007;56:1309–10.
7. Weaver LK. Carbon monoxide poisoning. Crit Care Clin. 1999;15:297–317.
8. Hardy KR, Thom SR. Pathophysiology and treatment of carbon monoxide poisoning. J Clin Tox. 1994;32(6):613–29.
9. Jasper BW, Hopkins RO, Duker HV, Weaver LK. Affective outcome following carbon monoxide poisoning: prospective longitudinal study. Cogn Behav Neur. 2005;18(2):127–34.

10. Demling RH. Burn care in the immediate resuscitation period. In: New York: Scientific American Surgery; 1995. p. 1–16.
11. Crapo RO. Smoke inhalation injuries. JAMA. 1981;246(18):1694–6.
12. Hart GB, Strauss MB, Lennon PA, Whitcraft III D. Treatment of smoke inhalation by hyperbaric oxygen. J Emerg Med. 1985;3:211–5.
13. Mathieu D, Wattel F, Mathieu-Nolf M, Durak C, et al. Randomized prospective study comparing the effect of HBO vs. 12 hours NBO in non-comatose CO-poisoned patients: results of the preliminary analysis. Undersea Hyperbar Med. 1996;23(Suppl):7. abstract.
14. Raphael JC, Elkharrat D, Jars-Guincestre M-C, Chastang C, et al. Trial of normobaric and hyperbaric oxygen for acute carbon monoxide intoxication. Lancet. 1989;2:414–9.
15. Raphael JC, Chevret S, Driheme A, Annane D. Managing carbon monoxide poisoning with hyperbaric oxygen (abstract). J Toxicol-Clin Tox. 2004;42:455–6.
16. Scheinkestel CD, Bailey M, Myles PS, Jones K, et al. Hyperbaric or normobaric oxygen for acute carbon monoxide poisoning: a randomized controlled clinical trial. Med J Austral. 1999;170:203–10.
17. Thom SR, Taber RL, Mendiguren II, Clark JM, et al. Delayed neurologic sequelae after carbon monoxide poisoning: prevention by treatment with hyperbaric oxygen. Ann Emer Med. 1995;25:474–80.
18. Bwalya A, Lougheed G, Kashef A, Saber H. Survey results of combustible contents and floor areas in Canadian multi-family dwellings. Fire Technol. 2011;47:1121–40.
19. Clark CJ, Campbell D, Reid WH. Blood carboxyhaemoglobin and cyanide levels in fire survivors. Lancet. 1981;1:1332–5.
20. Woolley WD. Nitrogen containing products from the thermal decomposition of flexible polyurethane foams. Br Polymer J. 1972;4:27–43.
21. Bell RH, Stemmer KL, Barkley W, Hollingsworth LD. Cyanide toxicity from the thermal degradation of rigid polyurethane foam. Am Ind Hyg Assoc J. 1979;40:757–62.
22. Terrill JB, Montgomery RR, Reinhardt CF. Toxic gases from fires. Science. 1978;200:1343–7.
23. Cahalane M, Demling RH. Early respiratory abnormalities from smoke inhalation. JAMA. 1984;251: 771–3.
24. Fein A, Leff A, Hopewell PC. Pathophysiology and management of the complications resulting from fire and the inhaled products of combustion: review of the literature. Crit Care Med. 1980;8:94–8.
25. Burgess WA, Treitman RD, Gold A. Air contaminants in structural firefighting. Springfield, VA: National Technical Information Service Publication PB 299017, US Dept of Commerce, 1979.
26. Silverman SH, Purdue GF, Hunt JL, Bost RO. Cyanide toxicity in burned patients. J Trauma. 1988;28: 171–6.
27. Wetherell HR. The occurrence of cyanide in the blood of fire victims. J Forensic Sci. 1966;11:167–73.
28. Barillo DJ, Goode R, Rush BF, Lin RL, Freda A, Anderson EJ. Lack of correlation between carboxyhemoglobin and cyanide in smoke inhalation injury. Curr Surg. 1986;43:421–3.
29. Barillo DJ, Rush BF, Goode R, Lin RL, Freda A, Anderson EJ. Is ethanol the unknown toxin in smoke inhalation injury? Am Surg. 1986;52:641.
30. Gettler AO, Baine JO. The toxicology of cyanide. Am J Med Sci. 1938;195:182–98.
31. Graham DL, Laman D, Theodore J, Robin ED. Acute cyanide poisoning complicated by lactic acidosis and pulmonary edema. Arch Intern Med. 1977;137: 1051–5.
32. Jones J, McMullen MJ, Dougherty J. Toxic smoke inhalation: cyanide poisoning in fire victims. Am J Emerg Med. 1987;5:317–21.
33. Hartzell GE. Combustion products and their effects on life safety. In: Cote AE, Linville JL, editors. Fire protection handbook. 17th ed. Quincy, MA: National Fire Protection Association; 1991.
34. Cottrell JE, Casthely P, Brodie JD, Patel K, Klein A, Turndorf H. Prevention of nitroprusside-induced cyanide toxicity with hydroxocobalamin. N Engl J Med. 1978;298:809–11.
35. Hall AH, Dart R, Bogdan G. Sodium thiosulfate or hydroxocobalamin for the empiric treatment of cyanide poisoning? Ann Emerg Med. 2007;49:806–13.
36. DesLauriers CA, Burda AM, Whal M. Hydroxocobalamin as a cyanide antidote. Am J Therapuetics. 2006;13:161–5.
37. Smith DL, Cairns BA, Ramadan F, et al. Effect of inhalation injury, burn size, and age on mortality: a study of 1447 consecutive burn patients. J Trauma. 1994;37:655–9.
38. Edelman DA, White MT, Tyburski JG, Wilson RF. Factors affecting prognosis of inhalation injury. J Burn Care Res. 2006;27:848–53.
39. Colohan SM. Predicting prognosis in thermal burns with associated inhalational injury: a systematic review of prognostic factors in adult burn victims. J Burn Care Res. 2010;31:529–39.
40. Carvajal HF, Linares HA, Brouhard BH. Relationship of burn size to vascular permeability changes in rates. Surg Gynecol Obstet. 1979;149:193–202.
41. Harms BA, Bodai BI, Kramer GC, Demling RH. Microvascular fluid and protein flux in pulmonary and systemic circulations after thermal injury. Microvasc Res. 1982;23:77–86.
42. Ward PA, Till GO. Pathophysiologic events related to thermal injury of skin. J Trauma. 1990;30:S75–9.
43. Wyncoll DL, Evans TW. Acute respiratory distress syndrome. Lancet. 1999;354:497–501.
44. American Burn Association. Airway management and smoke inhalation injury. In: Advanced burn life support manual. Chicago: American Burn Association; 2004. p. 16–20.
45. Mosier MJ, Pham TN, Park DR, Simmons J, et al. Predictive value of bronchoscopy in assessing the

severity of inhalation injury. J Burn Care Res. 2012;33(1):65–73.
46. Oh JS, Chung KK, Allen A, Batchinsky AI, et al. Admission chest CT complements fiberoptic bronchoscopy in prediction of adverse outcomes in thermally injured patients. J Burn Care Res. 2012;33:532–8.
47. Palmieri TL. Use of beta-agonists in inhalation injury. J Burn Care Res. 2009;30(1):156–9.
48. Miller AC, Elamin EM, Suffredini AF. Inhaled anticoagulation regimens for the treatment of smoke inhalation-associated acute lung injury: a systematic review. Crit Care Med. 2014;42:413–9.
49. Murabit A, Tredget EE. Review of burn injuries secondary to home oxygen. J Burn Care Res. 2012; 33(2):212–7.
50. The Acute Respiratory Distress Syndrome Network. Ventilation with lower tidal volumes as compared with traditional tidal volumes for acute lung injury and the acute respiratory distress syndrome. N Engl J Med. 2000;342:1301–8.
51. Dries DJ. Key questions in ventilator management of the burn-injured patient. J Burn Care Res. 2009;30:211–20.
52. Carman B, Cahill T, Warden G, et al. A prospective, randomized comparison of the volume diffusive respirator vs conventional ventilation for ventilation of burned children. J Burn Care Rehabil. 2001;13:444–8.
53. Palmieri TL, Jackson W, Greenhalgh DG. Benefits of early tracheostomy in severely burned children. Crit Care Med. 2002;30(4):922–4.
54. Darling GE, Keresteci MA, Ibanez D, Pugash RA, Peters WJ, Neligan PC. Pulmonary complications in inhalation injuries with associated cutaneous burn. J Trauma. 1996;40:83–9.
55. La Cal MA, Cerda E, Garcia-Hierro P, et al. Pneumonia in patients with severe burns: a classification according to the concept of the carrier state. Chest. 2001;119:1160–5.
56. Still J, Newton T, Friedman B, Furhman S, Law E, Dawson J. Experience with pneumonia in acutely burned patients requiring ventilator support. Am Surg. 2000;66:206–9.
57. The ARDS Definition Task Force. Acute respiratory distress syndrome: the Berlin definition. JAMA. 2012;307:2526–33.
58. Ong YS, Samuel M, Song C. Meta-analysis of early excision of burns. Burns. 2006;32(2):145–50.
59. Belenkiy SM, Buel AR, Cannon JW, Sine CR, et al. Acute respiratory distress syndrome in wartime military burns: application of the Berlin criteria. J Trauma Acute Care Surg. 2014;76:821–7.

Circulation: Burn Shock Resuscitation

5

Soman Sen

Introduction

Burn shock is a consequence of massive inflammation from the depth and extent of burn injury and evaporative loss from the destruction of the cutaneous barrier (skin). This leads to progress intravascular volume depletion leading to reduced organ perfusion and ultimately organ failure. Left unabated, burn shock will ultimately lead to death. The primary goal of burn shock resuscitation is to restore and maintain adequate intravascular volume to provide adequate organ perfusion. Although formulas and algorithms have been developed over past few decades for resuscitation of the severely burn-injured patient, management of the resuscitation of burn shock is a complex process that requires not only constant monitoring but also evaluation of alternative and adjunctive therapies. Burn shock resuscitation is a key component of the initial management of a severely burned patient; however several patient and injury-related factors have to be considered during resuscitation. In this chapter, we will introduce burn shock management algorithms, calculation of fluid requirements, monitoring of resuscitation, special considerations that may alter fluid resuscitation, and adjunctive resuscitative therapies.

S. Sen, M.D., F.A.C.S. (✉)
Division of Burn Surgery, Department of Surgery, University of California, Davis, 2425 Stockton Blvd., Suite 718, Sacramento, CA 95817, USA
e-mail: somsen@ucdavis.edu

Pathophysiology of Burn Shock

Severe burn injury results in an extensive amount of tissue damage producing a massive systemic inflammation. At the tissue level, necrotic and damaged cells trigger an inflammatory response with release of cytokines and other pro-inflammatory agents (histamine, bradykinins, prostaglandins, thromboxanes) [1–3]. The release of these pro-inflammatory agents causes the activation and mobilization of leukocytes (neutrophils, dendritic cells, and macrophages). In addition, the pro-inflammatory agents also cause vasodilation and widening of capillary gap junctions to allow for egress of leukocytes into the interstitial space [4]. The activated leukocytes then cause production of oxygen free radicals through the release of hydrogen peroxide from activated neutrophils and consumption of adenosine triphosphate (ATP). ATP is consumed by the leukocytes and is not replenished adequately due to the relative hypoxia of the damaged tissue and results in increased levels of adenosine monophosphate (AMP). The increased tissue AMP is then catabolized to hypoxanthine, which is then converted to xanthine, which is further metabolized into uric acid and hydrogen peroxide and superoxide. The increased tissue

D.G. Greenhalgh (ed.), *Burn Care for General Surgeons and General Practitioners*,
DOI 10.1007/978-3-319-29161-1_5

hydrogen peroxide and superoxide cause lipid peroxidation generating oxygen free radicals. These free radicals cause cellular damage through direct DNA damage, which causes more inflammatory stimulation resulting in more leukocyte migration and increased plasma depletion from the systemic circulation. In addition, oxygen free radicals alter myocardial cell wall membranes resulting in deceased cardiac contractility [1, 5].

The extensive damage to the skin following severe burn injury also results in significant evaporative losses. The evaporative water loss from a burn injury can range from 146 to 176 ml/m^2/h [6, 7]. For example, a patient with a surface area of 2 m^2 who has suffered a 50 % total body surface area partial- and full-thickness burn injury would expect to lose approximately 150 ml of water per hour through evaporation. Thus, in a matter of a few hours, a significant portion of the patients circulating plasma volume will be depleted. Combined, the intravascular-volume depletion from both the systemic inflammation and evaporative water loss significantly compromises a burn patient's hemodynamic status.

The ongoing volume loss from the intravascular space through evaporation and inflammation ultimately results in reduced venous return to the heart. If not restored, the reduced intravascular volume causes a reduced end systolic volume ultimately leading to a lower cardiac output. With the increasing oxygen demands from leukocytes in the damaged tissues and low intravascular volume, tachycardia ensues to maintain or increase cardiac output. However, with falling intravascular volume, tachycardia is not sufficient to meet the cardiac output demands and tissue perfusion is compromised. Ultimately, reduced tissue perfusion results in cellular hypoxia and cell death with the end result of organ failure. Thus, the hallmark of burn shock resuscitation is restoration of adequate intravascular volume to prevent organ failure [8].

Venous Access

During the initial assessment of a severely burned patient, venous access sites should be evaluated and prompt establishment of venous access should ensue. Because of the potential emergent need for venous access for stabilization of the airway or breathing, peripheral venous access is appropriate for the initial management. Optimally, the largest bore peripheral catheter should be placed in the most accessible vein. This includes areas where burned skin overlies the vein. This will ensure a large enough venous access for both medication administration and initial fluid resuscitation.

In some cases, peripheral venous access cannot be established quickly and alternative strategies for venous access should be initiated. If the patient's airway and breathing are stable, it may be safe to proceed with placement of a central venous catheter. However, if there is any concern about airway or breathing stability or hemodynamic status, then an intraosseous catheter should be placed. Intraosseous catheters can be placed in both adults and children with burn injuries and can be place quickly in both populations. Unlike the peripheral vascular space, the intraosseous space is a noncollapsible space and provides immediate access to the systemic circulation. Interosseous catheters are often placed in the anterior surface of the tibia, distal femur, humerus, sternum, calcaneus, and distal radius and provide circulatory access for medications, resuscitative fluids, and diagnostic laboratory measurements. However, intraosseous lines are contraindicated in sites that are fractured [9]. Although, resuscitative fluid can be given through an intraosseous catheter safely, care must be taken as to the volume of fluid administered per hour. For large burn injuries, intraosseous lines should only be used for initial vascular access until a central venous catheter can be placed.

Central venous catheters are necessary for most severely burned patients in order to establish safe and secure vascular access. While large amount of resuscitative fluid can be administered through large-bore peripheral intravenous (IV) catheters, these catheters do not provide a secure vascular access point for many burn patients. Dislodgement of peripheral IV catheters can leave a severely burned patient without vascular access at a critical point in resuscitation for burn shock.

Central venous catheters can be placed in any central vein (jugular, subclavian, and femoral) to provide adequate vascular access. In choosing the appropriate site for central venous access, several considerations need to be made. First, choose a site that is not burned. Burned skin is already compromised to the environment and is at high risk for bacterial infections, and placing a catheter through burned skin may increase the risk of a catheter infection. Additionally, securing a central venous catheter to burned skin is problematic. Because of the injury to the dermis in severely burned skin, the tensile strength of the underlying tissue is much less than noninjured skin. This creates an increased risk of catheter dislodgement. Second, the subclavian and jugular veins are safe locations with respect to infections. Femoral venous catheters have the highest risk of infection; however if the skin is intact overall the femoral vein and is burned over the subclavian and jugular vein, then the femoral site is probably a more ideal site [10]. Third, the risk of thrombosis is likely higher in adult patients with femoral central venous catheters [11]. For pediatric burn patients, however, the risk of complications from a femoral CVC is not higher than either a subclavian or jugular CVC [12]. Finally, while placing a CVC in an ideal location is the optimal treatment, establishing a secure CVC in the most efficient and expedited manner prevents any delays in starting resuscitative fluids for burn shock.

Formulas for Initiation of Fluid Resuscitation

In the 1960s and 1970s, Dr. Charles Baxter developed a resuscitation formula for severe burn injury at Parkland Hospital in Dallas, Texas. Over the next few decades, Dr. Baxter's formula of fluid resuscitation (known commonly as the Parkland formula) has become a standard in the resuscitation of severely burned patients [13]. In the original Parkland formula, 4 ml per kilogram (kg) of weight per % TBSA (total body surface area of burned skin) of intravenous fluid is administered over the first 24 h following injury. Half of this volume is administered in the first 8 h and the other half in the ensuing 16 h. Following this, in the next 24-h period, dextrose- and potassium-containing fluid is administered to maintain vascular volume (standard maintenance fluid plus evaporative loss), and colloid-containing fluid is administered at 20–60 % of calculated plasma volume [14].

In practice, however, the Parkland formula is used as a starting point for resuscitation. Guidelines for the management of fluid titration have been developed to reduce the rate of fluid administration hourly based on urine output [15]. For adults this means that fluid rate is reduced about 10–20 % per hour if the urine output target is above 0.5 ml/kg (ideal body weight)/h, and in children (under 30 kg of weight), fluid rate is decreased if the urine output target is above 1 ml/kg/h [16]. The fluid titration should continue until the infusion rate reaches the rate for maintenance fluid plus evaporative losses [17]. For children under 30 kg, adjustments should be made to increase the volume of fluid administered due to the high body surface area to weight ratio and immature kidneys that are not as efficient at absorbing water [18]. Similar to resuscitation of an adult burn patient, a similar strategy should be employed for fluid titration; however during resuscitation, weight-based maintenance fluid should be added to the resuscitative fluid rate to account for the increased fluid needs in children.

Over the past few years, several studies have noted that many burn patients are receiving more fluid in the first 24 h than was calculated using the Parkland formula [19]. The reasons for this have not been fully solved; however some evidence suggests that the excessive fluid administration (fluid creep) is due to increased opioid and sedative administration [20]. Additionally, other factors such as excessive fluid administration in pre-burn center hospitals and delays in fluid titration have probably contributed to the above predicted fluid administration [21]. As a result of this observation, and a concern about over-resuscitation, many other burn resuscitation formulas have been developed. The most commonly used one in practice, other than the Parkland formula, is the modified Brooke formula. In the formula, originally developed by Dr. Artz at the Army Burn Center, fluid resuscitation is initiated at 2 ml per kg per % TBSA for adults and 3–4 ml

Table 5.1 Commonly used burn resuscitation formulas

Adult burn injury resuscitation formulas	*24 h fluid calculation formula*
Parkland	4 ml per kg per TBSA%
Modified Brooke	2 ml per kg per TBSA%
Pediatric burn injury resuscitation formulas	*24 h fluid calculation formula*
Galveston	5000 ml/m^2 burn + 2000 ml/m^2 (BSA)
Shriner's	4 ml per kg per %TBSA + 1500 ml/m^2 (BSA)

TBSA% percentage of total body surface area burned, *BSA* body surface area

per kg per % TBSA for children in the first 24 h. In the second 24 h, colloid is administered at 0.3–0.5-ml/kg/% TBSA in addition to maintenance fluid [22]. In comparison to the Parkland formula, the Brooke formula may lead to less fluid administration and fewer complications of over-resuscitation [23]. Regardless of the choice of formula to follow, the key tenant of burn shock resuscitation is to provide adequate fluid administration to maintain organ perfusion while avoiding both the consequences of under- and over-resuscitation. This involves not just the initial administration of fluid but also constant (hourly) adjustments of fluid rate based on urine output goals (Table 5.1).

Choice of Fluid for Resuscitation

As mentioned in a previous section, a severe burn injury produces a constant loss of fluid from the intravascular space through a massive inflammation and on-going evaporative losses. Because of this, the recommended and most common choice of fluid for burn shock resuscitation is an isotonic fluid that can restore plasma volume. Lactated Ringer's is the common fluid used in the initial resuscitation of burn injury [24]. Unlike normal saline, lactated Ringer's is an isotonic solution that is not administered as large as sodium and chloride load. For resuscitation purposes, administration of lactated Ringer's as compared to normal saline maintains a higher plasma pH and less pulmonary edema [25]. For pediatric patients under 10 kg, dextrose is often added to lactated Ringer's solution during burn shock resuscitation due to the decreased glycogen storage in small children [26]. If feedings are initiated early, then adding dextrose is not necessary.

While the use of isotonic crystalloid during burn resuscitation is standard therapy for burn shock, many burn centers administer colloid fluids in the form of albumin. Overall, albumin administration for hypovolemia has not shown any survival benefit compared to crystalloid administration [27]. However, albumin administration during burn shock may reduce fluid requirements in burn patients who are receiving a higher than expected rate of fluid infusion. In both pediatric and adult burn patients, administration of 5 % albumin along with lactated Ringer's was initiated in patients whose fluid rate was adjusted to a level higher than originally calculated using the Parkland formula. The input and output ratios were measured for these patients and were compared to patients who received only crystalloid fluids. Patients who received albumin predictably had a higher input/output ratio in the first 14 h following the initiation of resuscitation fluids; however by the fourteenth hour, the input/output ratios returned to baseline and were not different than the crystalloid patients [28, 29]. Other colloids such as fresh frozen plasma (FFP) have historically been a part of burn shock resuscitation formulas (i.e., Brooke, Parkland). However, due to the higher costs and risks of infection and anaphylaxis, most burn centers do not use FFP for burn resuscitation [30].

Concerns about excessive resuscitation have led to the exploration into the use of hypertonic crystalloid solutions for burn shock. A prospective randomized trial of pediatric and adult burn patients was recently undertaken to compare hypertonic saline (HS) to lactated Ringer's (LR) solutions for burn shock. In this study the overall mortality was 9 % for both groups. The HS group had a higher fluid and sodium load in the first hour of resuscitation. However, in the subsequent 23 h, the HS group had a slightly lower, but not significant, fluid administration rate than thc LR group. Overall, there was not a difference in the amount of fluid administered between both groups; however net fluid retention was significantly less in the HS group [31]. In another retrospective study of resuscitation of burn shock using hypertonic lactated saline (HLS), overall fluid administration was significantly less. Additionally, the HLS group had significantly fewer cases of abdominal compartment syndrome compared to the LR group [32]. Currently, due to the lack of further prospective studies, hypertonic crystalloid solutions for burn shock resuscitation are not recommended [17].

Guidelines for Adjusting Fluids

Despite the significant fluid shifts from the intravascular space, most hemodynamic parameters do not change significantly during resuscitation. Parameters such as mean arterial pressure and heart rate either do not change or are unreliable measures for guiding burn shock resuscitation [33]. Additionally, preload measurements such as central venous pressure also do not exhibit any significant changes in the first few hours of burn shock resuscitation and are a poor guide to adjust fluids [34]. More invasive hemodynamic monitoring may give more information about a patient's cardiac function, but most studies have not shown that invasive hemodynamic monitoring to maximize cardiac function and intravascular volume is an effective guide for burn shock resuscitation. A prospective study of 50 burn patients compared invasive thermodilution (TDD) monitoring in goal-directed fluid resuscitation to resuscitation using the Baxter (Parkland) formula. Patients who were resuscitated using the TDD goal-directed method received significantly more fluid than the patients who were resuscitated with the Baxter formula. However, patients on the goal-directed resuscitation did not have improved intravascular volume or cardiac function [35].

Acid-base balance has also been touted as a potential guide for burn shock resuscitation. Elevated serum lactate has been associated as a potential marker for mortality following burn shock. Early measurements of serum lactate were found to be associated with increased risk of dying, and it was thought that titration of resuscitation to normalize lactate levels may be beneficial [36, 37]. Base deficit was also thought to be a potential maker of resuscitation. Elevated base deficits in burn patients are associated with increased risk of dying and may be related to poor organ perfusion [38]. Despite the evidence for acid-base disorders indicating poor resuscitation, goal-directed therapy for burn shock to resolve acidosis and lactate levels has shown mixed results. In one study, burn shock resuscitation guided by TDD monitoring and lactate failed to show any overall benefit. Additionally, the patients whose resuscitation was guided by TDD monitoring and lactate received a higher volume of fluid than patients whose resuscitation was guided by the Parkland formula [39]. Another study in which burn resuscitation was also guided by TDD monitoring and lactate showed that with less restrictive hemodynamic goals, this method is effective to normalize lactate and maintain organ perfusion without administering excessive fluid [40].

Despite the ongoing controversy about the guidelines of burn resuscitation, maintaining an adequate hourly urine output is the current standard guideline for burn shock resuscitation [41, 42]. Maintaining a urine output of either 30–50 ml/h or 0.5 ml/kg/h for adult patients has been established as the standard goal of effective burn shock resuscitation [43]. For pediatric patients under 30 kg, urine output of 1 ml/kg/h is the standard goal [44]. Titration of resuscitative fluids should start early and fluids should be adjusted to meet adequate urine output [15]. A recommended strategy for the titration of fluids is to increase or decrease fluids by 10 or 20 %, respectively, if urine output is below or above the target goal [16].

Maintenance Fluids

After the first 24 h of resuscitation, the patient should be transitioned to maintenance fluid. During the resuscitative phase (first 24 h), fluid

Table 5.2 Maintenance fluid formulas for 24-h fluid requirements are calculated by adding daily basal fluid requirements and evaporative fluid losses

Weight	Hourly formula (ml)
<20 kg	(2000 × BSA)/24 h +([35 + %TBSA] × BSA)
>20 kg	(1500 × BSA)/24 h +([25 + %TBSA] × BSA)

%TBSA percentage of total body surface area burned, *BSA* body surface area

Table 5.3 Example of resuscitation and maintenance fluid requirements for an adult

Example: 20-year-old male who suffered a 50 % TBSA burn injury
Weight: 80 kg
Height: 183 cm
BSA = 2 m^2
Parkland formula resuscitation = 4 × 80 × 50 = 16,000 ml/h
Hourly maintenance fluid = (1500 × 2)/24 + ([25+50] × 2) = 275 ml/h

should be titrated to a maintenance goal rate. The goal rate should include both the patient's weight-based daily fluid and salt requirements and additional fluid to account for the ongoing environmental fluid loss from the areas of burned skin (evaporative loss) [45]. Evaporative water loss from burned skin can be calculated for the following equations: for patients that weigh less than 20 kg, hourly evaporative loss = (35 + %TBSA) × BSA (m^2), and for patients that weigh greater than 20 kg, hourly evaporative loss = (25 + % TBSA) × BSA (m^2) [6, 7, 46, 47]. Patients should be maintained at this fluid rate (basal fluid plus evaporative fluid loss) until the burn skin has healed or skin grafts have fully engrafted (Tables 5.2 and 5.3).

Management of the Complications of Resuscitation

Due to the massive fluid shifts following a severe burn injury, complications can occur during resuscitation that can lead to life-threatening consequences. Prompt recognition and treatment of these complications can reverse or mitigate organ ischemia and prevent death. The majority of complications due to burn shock resuscitation result from excessive (more than predicted) fluid administration [48].

A major life-threatening complication during burn shock resuscitation is abdominal compartment syndrome (ACS). The inciting cause is usually excessive fluid administration during burn shock resuscitation. Patients that receive greater than 250 ml/kg of fluid in the first 24 h after injury are at the highest risk of developing abdominal compartment syndrome [49]. ACS during burn resuscitation is considered secondary ACS. The diagnosis is made based on the following findings: sustained elevated intra-abdominal pressure (>20 mmHg) and organ dysfunction or failure (acute renal failure, progressive pulmonary failure, decreased cardiac output) [50]. A classic finding of ACS from burn shock is elevated intra-abdominal pressure, oliguria, and decreased tidal volumes. Intra-abdominal pressure can be measured via bladder pressures and repeated regularly if the concern for ACS is high [41]. Once the diagnosis is confirmed, a prompt decompressive laparotomy should be performed [51]. During the laparotomy, the bowels and intra-abdominal organs should be inspected for any injuries. The abdominal compartment should be left open and not closed. A temporary non-adhesive cover (silicone silastic sheet) should be sewn to the midline fascia or skin to protect the abdominal viscera. The patient typically improves urine output, ventilation, and hemodynamic stability within hours. We have found that the abdomen may often be closed within the next few days.

Excessive fluid administration can also lead to extremity compartment syndromes. The most at risk areas of the body are areas that have suffered from a circumferential full-thickness burn injury; however areas of near circumferential injuries are at risk as well. For the extremities, a prophylactic escharotomy can prevent compartment syndrome and limb-threatening ischemia from developing. Escharotomies of the extremities are performed with the patient's arms or legs in the anatomic position. Using cautery or a knife, an incision is made on the lateral and medial aspect of the extremity and carried down to the subcutaneous tissue level. The incision should run the entire length of the circumferential burn wound

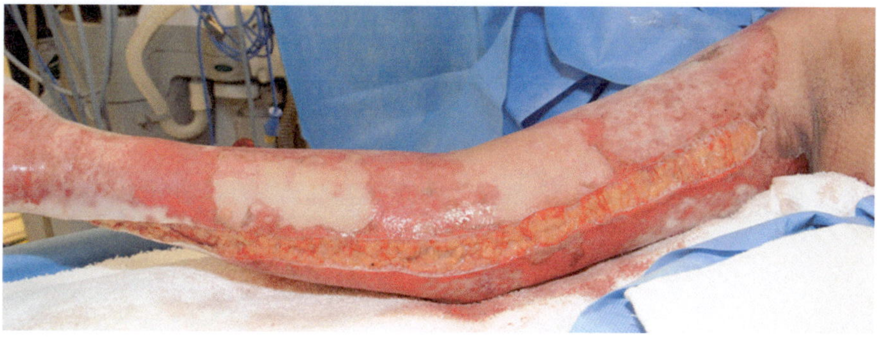

Fig. 5.1 Escharotomies of the upper extremity should be placed with hand supinated and along the lateral and medial aspect of the extremity

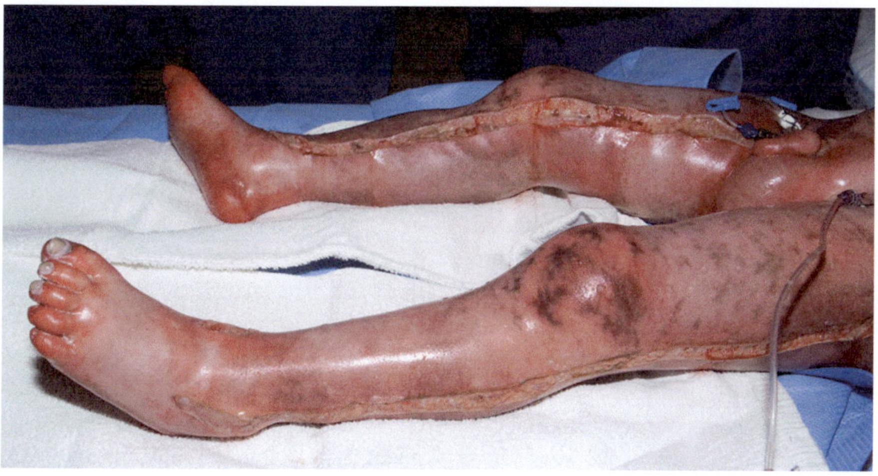

Fig. 5.2 Escharotomies of the lower extremity should be placed both laterally and medially

(Figs. 5.1 and 5.2). If a compartment syndrome persists, then the patients should undergo a fasciotomy of the relevant muscle compartment (Fig. 5.3). For the forearms this involves the volar muscle compartments and for legs this involves the four compartments of the calf. The anterior compartment is at greatest risk for compartment syndrome and is followed by the lateral compartment. For thermal burns, the posterior compartments are at less risk for problems. For concerns about circumferential burn wounds of the trunk, an escharotomy should be performed in a similar manner. The incisions should start on both sides of the trunk at the level of the anterior axillary lines [52].

For patients with severe burn injuries who are not mechanically ventilated, burn shock resuscitation can increase airway edema leading to acute respiratory failure. Patients who are spontaneously ventilating should be monitored closely for airway edema in the first 24 h after injury. Any signs of respiratory decline should prompt immediate airway evaluation. Tracheal intubation is easier before the airway edema increases and if there is any concern for acute respiratory failure, then the patient should be intubated [53].

Excessive fluid administration during burn resuscitation can also lead to many long-term complications such as pneumonia, organ failure,

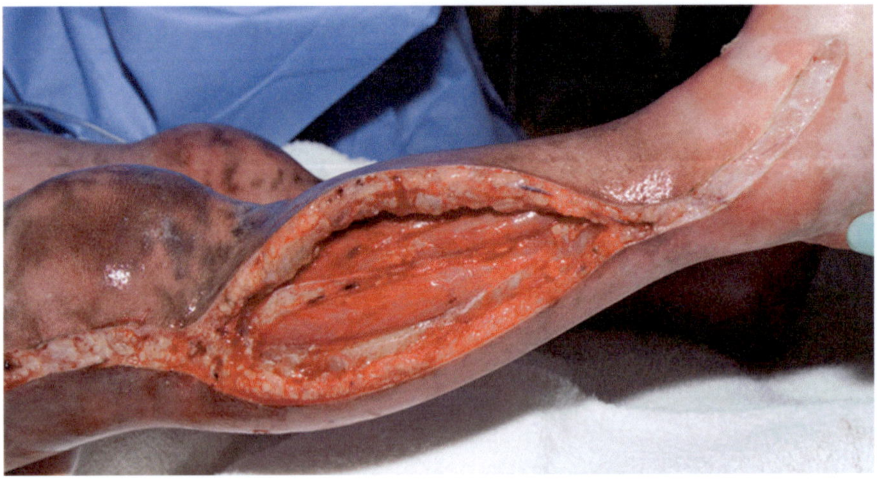

Fig. 5.3 The pressures in the anterior and lateral leg compartments were still high so fasciotomies were performed in both compartments

and infections [49]. To offset these occurrences, fluid management goals should include the addition of strategies to prevent excessive fluid administration. One major strategy is to avoid continuous infusion of opioids during burn shock resuscitation. "Fluid creep" is a phenomenon that has been increasingly prominent over the last decade. "Fluid creep" is the observation that both the volume of fluid administered for burn shock and the dosage of opioid administered during burn shock resuscitation have been going up over the last three decades [20, 21]. This association has caused many burn physicians to alter the initial opioid strategy. Hourly intermittent doses of opioid should be given if the patient appears to be in pain; however, continuous opioid infusion should be avoided in order to limit the dosage administered.

Another strategy to avoid excessive fluid administration is starting antioxidant therapy. A severe burn injury causes the release of peroxides that eventually lead to the peroxidation of lipids and the formation of free radicals. These lipid free radicals cause further cellular damage resulting in increased inflammation, vascular permeability, and eventually decreased intravascular volume [5]. In order to mitigate this process, high-dose antioxidant therapy is effective. In a randomized trial of high-dose ascorbic acid in during burn shock, patient who received high-dose ascorbic acid required significantly less fluid and had less tissue edema [54]. High-dose ascorbic acid infusion is started at 66 mg/kg/h. The solution is mixed into 1 l of lactated Ringer's and is infused for 24 h. Titration of fluids proceeds as per previously described. Care must be taken when interpreting glucose results from glucometers. Due to the redox reaction used by most glucometers to test glucose levels, glucose readings are falsely elevated during high-dose ascorbic acid infusion [55].

Summary

Prompt and accurate resuscitation of the burn patient is important to prevent complications of under- or over-resuscitation. Formulas should only be used to initiate resuscitation. All other adjustments in fluid should be based on the physiologic response of the patient—especially urine output. Other indicators of the adequacy of resuscitation are still lacking. On occasion, the burn surgeon must deal with the complications of resuscitation—compartment syndromes, renal failure, and acute respiratory distress syndrome.

References

1. Ahrns KS, Harkins DR. Initial resuscitation after burn injury: therapies, strategies, and controversies. AACN Clin Issues. 1999;10(1):46–60.
2. Carvajal HF, Brouhard BH, Linares HA. Effect of antihistamine-antiserotonin and ganglionic blocking agents upon increased capillary permeability following burn trauma. J Trauma. 1975;15(11):969–75.
3. Rantfors J, Cassuto J. Role of histamine receptors in the regulation of edema and circulation postburn. Burns. 2003;29(8):769–77.
4. Pitt RM, Parker JC, Jurkovich GJ, Taylor AE, Curreri PW. Analysis of altered capillary pressure and permeability after thermal injury. J Surg Res. 1987;42(6): 693–702.
5. Horton JW. Free radicals and lipid peroxidation mediated injury in burn trauma: the role of antioxidant therapy. Toxicology. 2003;189(1–2):75–88.
6. Lamke LO, Nilsson GE, Reithner HL. The evaporative water loss from burns and the water-vapour permeability of grafts and artificial membranes used in the treatment of burns. Burns. 1977;3:159–65.
7. Lamke LO, Liljedahl SO. Evaporative water loss from burns, grafts and donor sites. Scand J Plast Reconstr Surg. 1971;5(1):17–22.
8. Baxter CR, Shires T. Physiological response to crystalloid resuscitation of severe burns. Ann N Y Acad Sci. 1968;150(3):874–94.
9. Dev SP, Stefan RA, Saun T, Lee S. Videos in clinical medicine. Insertion of an intraosseous needle in adults. N Engl J Med. 2014;370(24):e35.
10. Ciofi Silva CL, Rossi LA, Canini SR, Goncalves N, Furuya RK. Site of catheter insertion in burn patients and infection: a systematic review. Burns. 2014;40(3):365–73.
11. Ge X, Cavallazzi R, Li C, Pan SM, Wang YW, Wang FL. Central venous access sites for the prevention of venous thrombosis, stenosis and infection. Cochrane Database Syst Rev. 2012;3:CD004084.
12. Goldstein AM, Weber JM, Sheridan RL. Femoral venous access is safe in burned children: an analysis of 224 catheters. J Pediatr. 1997;130(3):442–6.
13. Greenhalgh DG. Burn resuscitation: the results of the ISBI/ABA survey. Burns. 2010;36(2):176–82.
14. Baxter CR, Marvin JA, Curreri PW. Early management of thermal burns. Postgrad Med. 1974;55(1): 131–9.
15. Blumetti J, Hunt JL, Arnoldo BD, Parks JK, Purdue GF. The Parkland formula under fire: is the criticism justified? J Burn Care Res. 2008;29(1):180–6.
16. Faraklas I, Cochran A, Saffle J. Review of a fluid resuscitation protocol: "fluid creep" is not due to nursing error. J Burn Care Res. 2012;33(1):74–83.
17. Pham TN, Cancio LC, Gibran NS. American Burn Association practice guidelines burn shock resuscitation. J Burn Care Res. 2008;29(1):257–66.
18. Diver AJ. The evolution of burn fluid resuscitation. Int J Surg. 2008;6(4):345–50.
19. Cartotto RC, Innes M, Musgrave MA, Gomez M, Cooper AB. How well does the Parkland formula estimate actual fluid resuscitation volumes? J Burn Care Rehabil. 2002;23(4):258–65.
20. Saffle JI. The phenomenon of "fluid creep" in acute burn resuscitation. J Burn Care Res. 2007;28(3):382–95.
21. Cartotto R, Zhou A. Fluid creep: the pendulum hasn't swung back yet! J Burn Care Res. 2010;31(4):551–8.
22. Alvarado R, Chung KK, Cancio LC, Wolf SE. Burn resuscitation. Burns. 2009;35(1):4–14.
23. Pruitt Jr BA, Goodwin Jr CW. Current treatment of the extensively burned patient. Surg Annu. 1983;15: 331–64.
24. Shirani KZ, Vaughan GM, Mason Jr AD, Pruitt Jr BA. Update on current therapeutic approaches in burns. Shock. 1996;5(1):4–16.
25. Sakka SG. Resuscitation of hemorrhagic shock with normal saline versus lactated Ringer's: effects on oxygenation, extravascular lung water, and hemodynamics. Crit Care. 2009;13(2):128.
26. Schweer L. Pediatric trauma resuscitation: initial fluid management. J Infus Nurs. 2008;31(2):104–11.
27. Alderson P, Bunn F, Li Wan Po A, Li L, Blackhall K, Roberts I, Schierhout G. Human albumin solution for resuscitation and volume expansion in critically ill patients. Cochrane Database Syst Rev. 2011(10): CD001208.
28. Lawrence A, Faraklas I, Watkins H, et al. Colloid administration normalizes resuscitation ratio and ameliorates "fluid creep". J Burn Care Res. 2010;31(1):40–7.
29. Faraklas I, Lam U, Cochran A, Stoddard G, Saffle J. Colloid normalizes resuscitation ratio in pediatric burns. J Burn Care Res. 2011;32(1):91–7.
30. Fodor L, Fodor A, Ramon Y, Shoshani O, Rissin Y, Ullmann Y. Controversies in fluid resuscitation for burn management: literature review and our experience. Injury. 2006;37(5):374–9.
31. Belba MK, Petrela EY, Belba GP. Comparison of hypertonic vs isotonic fluids during resuscitation of severely burned patients. Am J Emerg Med. 2009;27(9):1091–6.
32. Oda J, Ueyama M, Yamashita K, et al. Hypertonic lactated saline resuscitation reduces the risk of abdominal compartment syndrome in severely burned patients. J Trauma. 2006;60(1):64–71.
33. Bak Z, Sjoberg F, Eriksson O, Steinvall I, Janerot-Sjoberg B. Cardiac dysfunction after burns. Burns. 2008;34(5):603–9.
34. Bak Z, Sjoberg F, Eriksson O, Steinvall I, Janerot-Sjoberg B. Hemodynamic changes during resuscitation after burns using the Parkland formula. J Trauma. 2009;66(2):329–36.
35. Holm C, Mayr M, Tegeler J, et al. A clinical randomized study on the effects of invasive monitoring on burn shock resuscitation. Burns. 2004;30(8):798–807.
36. Jeng JC, Jablonski K, Bridgeman A, Jordan MH. Serum lactate, not base deficit, rapidly predicts survival after major burns. Burns. 2002;28(2):161–6.

37. Kamolz LP, Andel H, Schramm W, Meissl G, Herndon DN, Frey M. Lactate: early predictor of morbidity and mortality in patients with severe burns. Burns. 2005; 31(8):986–90.
38. Andel D, Kamolz LP, Roka J, et al. Base deficit and lactate: early predictors of morbidity and mortality in patients with burns. Burns. 2007;33(8):973–8.
39. Berger MM, Que YA. A protocol guided by transpulmonary thermodilution and lactate levels for resuscitation of patients with severe burns. Crit Care. 2013;17(5):195.
40. Sanchez M, Garcia-de-Lorenzo A, Herrero E, et al. A protocol for resuscitation of severe burn patients guided by transpulmonary thermodilution and lactate levels: a 3-year prospective cohort study. Crit Care. 2013;17(4):R176.
41. Latenser BA. Critical care of the burn patient: the first 48 hours. Crit Care Med. 2009;37(10):2819–26.
42. Paratz JD, Stockton K, Paratz ED, et al. Burn resuscitation – hourly urine output versus alternative endpoints: a systematic review. Shock. 2014;42(4): 295–306.
43. Pruitt Jr BA. Advances in fluid therapy and the early care of the burn patient. World J Surg. 1978;2(2): 139–50.
44. Warden GD. Burn shock resuscitation. World J Surg. 1992;16(1):16–23.
45. Namdar T, Stollwerck PL, Stang FH, Siemers F, Mailander P, Lange T. Transdermal fluid loss in severely burned patients. Ger Med Sci. 2010;8:Doc28.
46. Lamke LO. Evaporative water loss from burns under different environmental conditions. Scand J Plast Reconstr Surg. 1971;5(2):77–81.
47. Gwosdow AR, Cunningham JJ, Lydon M, Rascati R, Berglund LG. Evaporative water losses through a temporary wound dressing under simulated wound conditions. J Burn Care Rehabil. 1993;14(4):450–4.
48. Dulhunty JM, Boots RJ, Rudd MJ, Muller MJ, Lipman J. Increased fluid resuscitation can lead to adverse outcomes in major-burn injured patients, but low mortality is achievable. Burns. 2008;34(8): 1090–7.
49. Klein MB, Hayden D, Elson C, et al. The association between fluid administration and outcome following major burn: a multicenter study. Ann Surg. 2007; 245(4):622–8.
50. De Laet IE, Ravyts M, Vidts W, Valk J, De Waele JJ, Malbrain ML. Current insights in intra-abdominal hypertension and abdominal compartment syndrome: open the abdomen and keep it open! Langenbecks Arch Surg. 2008;393(6):833–47.
51. Meldrum DR, Moore FA, Moore EE, Franciose RJ, Sauaia A, Burch JM. Prospective characterization and selective management of the abdominal compartment syndrome. Am J Surg. 1997;174(6):667–72. discussion 663–672.
52. Orgill DP, Piccolo N. Escharotomy and decompressive therapies in burns. J Burn Care Res. 2009;30(5): 759–68.
53. Baxter CR. Problems and complications of burn shock resuscitation. Surg Clin North Am. 1978;58(6): 1313–22.
54. Tanaka H, Matsuda T, Miyagantani Y, Yukioka T, Matsuda H, Shimazaki S. Reduction of resuscitation fluid volumes in severely burned patients using ascorbic acid administration: a randomized, prospective study. Arch Surg. 2000;135(3):326–31.
55. Kahn SA, Lentz CW. Fictitious hyperglycemia: point-of-care glucose measurement is inaccurate during high-dose vitamin C infusion for burn shock resuscitation. J Burn Care Res. 2015;36(2):e67–71.

Metabolic Response to Burn

6

Steven E. Wolf

Pathophysiology of Hypermetabolism and Catabolism

Severe burns significantly disrupt all normal metabolic processes, resulting in massive changes in systems generating and expending energy and those supporting critical bodily functions. Presumably these changes occur in an effort to respond favorably to the wounding process, which includes wound closure but also efforts to stave off microorganisms and protect from the external environment while the wound heals. A genomic storm ensues from the initial inflammatory response to wounding with significant changes in over 80 % of the genome in circulating cells [1]. The effects are massive changes in endocrine signaling and inflammatory mediator activity resulting in the condition referred to as "hypermetabolism." This is highlighted by the finding that all nutritional substrates are heavily utilized for energy production, both effective for reestablishing tissue integrity and ineffective through futile substrate cycling. Metabolically active tissues such as the muscle and liver are then compromised as these are used for substrate and as the engines of the metabolic response. Finally, the above events are compounded by the effects of treatment, which often include bedrest, and has its own effect to change metabolism and result in loss of muscle tissue and catabolism.

The condition of hypermetabolism persists until the wound is converted to scar, and even thereafter for up to 1 year until homeostasis is finally reached [2]. The challenge for the burn care provider then is to maximize and accelerate the beneficial effects of metabolism in the wound healing process while minimizing the long-term effects of catabolism. This is done through source control with rapid wound closure, nutritional management to provide substrate in excess of utilization, considerations for pharmacological manipulation of the hypermetabolic state to maximize benefit and attenuate risk, and generation of normal mobility to minimize the effects of bedrest and disuse. These efforts are often intense and prolonged.

Hormone Changes

One of the hallmarks of the response to injury is the dramatic changes that occur in hormone secretion and activity. Classically, this response was divided into "ebb" and "flow" phases in accordance with two distinct equilibria

S.E. Wolf, M.D. (✉)
Department of Surgery, University of Texas—Southwestern Medical Center, 5323 Harry Hines Blvd, Dallas, TX 75390-9158, USA
e-mail: steven.wolf@utsouthwestern.edu

D.G. Greenhalgh (ed.), *Burn Care for General Surgeons and General Practitioners*,
DOI 10.1007/978-3-319-29161-1_6

established at sequential time points [3]. Immediately after injury, the metabolic systems are relatively hypometabolic with diminished cardiac activity and absence of robust inflammation. After 3–5 days, increased secretion of catecholamines, cortisol, and glucagon/insulin and inflammatory genetic changes are associated with the hyperinflammatory condition referred to as hypermetabolism ("flow" state). Increased catecholamine activity appears to be central to this response [4] as does increased cortisol activity [5] (though this appears to be pale in comparison to the effects of hypercatecholaminemia).

Catecholamines act directly to induce increased hepatic gluconeogenesis and glycogenolysis and increased lipolysis which will be described in depth below. Activation of beta-adrenergic receptors favors the release and activity of glucagon in comparison to insulin due to concurrent alpha-adrenergic inhibition of insulin release, further augmenting the response. Glucocorticoid hormones also increase probably through central mechanisms related to pain and inflammation having similar actions to that of the catecholamines on substrate metabolism, thus augmenting the above responses.

Substrate Changes

Severe burns are characterized by hormone and inflammatory mediator activity to induce mobilization of available substrates for energy production. Excess carbohydrate in the form of hepatic glycogen is rapidly exhausted, and new glucose from dietary sources and conversion from other substrates are burned for energy production as well as futile cycling into lactate and back to glucose (Fig. 6.1). Increased lactate concentration is common following a severe burn which was thought to be due to some limitation in pyruvate dehydrogenase that limits entry of glucose metabolites into the Kreb's cycle; since pyruvate cannot be adequately metabolized, it is shunted to production of lactate. Further, inadequate microcirculation and oxygen abundance might be thought to cause shunting to lactate and anaerobic metabolism. However, studies have shown that pyruvate dehydrogenase activity is increased by up to 300 % after severe burn; thus the increase in lactate and subsequent futile cycling into and from glucose appears to be from massively increased glycolysis rather than some downstream limitation from oxygen availability [6]. Thus, increased lactate concentrations are not necessarily from an increase in anaerobic metabolism but could be

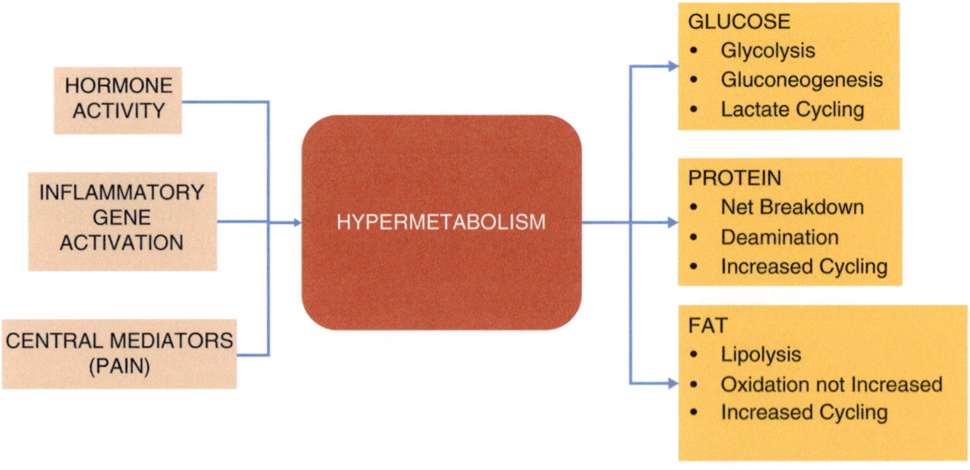

Fig. 6.1 Schematic of the causes of hypermetabolism and the effects on substrate metabolism. The burn wound induces hormone changes, inflammation, and central effects associated with pain to induce all the metabolic components of substrate hypermetabolism

seen simply as a result of the injury and the metabolic consequences. The cycling process uses energy generated from these metabolic processes in futile substrate processing and generates heat. This heat is clearly related to hyperpyrexia common in the severely burned.

As increased glucose cycling is established, muscle proteolysis also ensues from an increase in protein breakdown that is increased by up to 50 % in well-controlled studies [7]. Human studies in the severely burned corroborate these findings [8] which is paradoxically associated with an increase in protein synthesis. However, the increase in synthesis is insufficient to meet the increased protein breakdown, yielding a negative net balance of protein in the muscle. When this condition of negative net balance of protein in the muscle persists for weeks to months, muscle mass is lost with consequent decrease in strength and function [9].

The amino acids liberated from increased proteolysis reach the circulation and are deaminated for energy production as well as building blocks for other uses. Structural and constitutive proteins that were degraded to amino acids then enter into (1) the TCA cycle for energy production, (2) the liver to be used as substrate for gluconeogenesis, (3) the synthesis of new acute-phase proteins, or (4) cycling back to the same types of protein in protein synthesis. Most available body protein for this process is located in the musculature, thus depleting the muscle of its basic building blocks. Eighteen of the 20 amino acids are glucogenic and thus can be used for glucose synthesis. The processes surrounding these are not static, and continue in the background, with amino acids that are used for protein synthesis only to cycle back to protein breakdown; all of this requires energy and further results in production of heat. In particular, glutamine is mobilized from the muscle with decreases by more than 50 % in the tissue as well as plasma. One potential benefit for the glutamine mobilization may be as a nontoxic nitrogen donor as much of the glutamine appears to be used by inflammatory cells [10]. This provides a rationale for glutamine supplementation during recovery from injury; however, parenteral delivery of glutamine in critically ill surgical patients (not severe burns) was associated with no benefit [11]. Enteral sources appear to be more beneficial [12], particularly in burns, and a large multicenter trial has now commenced to determine potential improvements in outcomes.

Mobilization of fat is also a hallmark of the response to severe burn. Lipolysis is massively increased through augmented catecholamine signaling [6]. The free fatty acids that are generated are transported to the liver and muscle and re-esterified into triglyceride. In the case of the liver, these triglycerides are packaged into very low-density lipoprotein (VLDL) complexes and transported back to the periphery, again with cycling to and fro in an energy-requiring process. However, production of VLDL particles to transport fat out of the liver is insufficient to meet the increased delivery of free fatty acids, yielding fatty infiltration of the liver [13]; a similar process occurs in the muscle. To add further dysfunction, beta-oxidation rates of fat is also not appreciably increased after injury in response to the greater availability, yielding "ectopic" sites of fat in sites other than adipose tissue [14]. It has been proposed that the presence of this ectopic fat may be a key mediator in insulin resistance seen after severe burn and argues against the use of exogenous fat through the diet, since this source is inadequately utilized and only adds to the cycling problem.

Body Mass Changes

Severe burns have long been noted to have significant changes in body composition related to the substrate changes mentioned above. When the hypermetabolic state of futile substrate cycling and increased net proteolysis is prolonged, the result is loss of lean body mass which can be up to 40 % of the pre-injury condition and is commonly at least 10 % even in those with burns between 20 and 40 % total body surface area (TBSA) [15]. Studies using dual-image X-ray absorptiometry during acute hospitalization for severe burn confirm that muscle mass is lost both centrally and in the periphery, but curiously, fat mass is not particularly decreased [16]. Further, these changes are prolonged and in severely burned children do not go back to normal states of growth for at least 9 months after the initial injury [2]. Therefore, the effects of burn on metabolic states are dramatic with significant consequences.

Genetic Changes

The Glue Grant sponsored by the National Institute for General Medical Sciences led us to much greater understanding of the response to severe burn related to inflammation and associated changes in metabolism (www.gluegrant.org). These investigators found massive changes throughout the genome in the severely burned, with over 80 % of genes significantly up or downregulated in circulating cells [17]. Almost all genes associated with innate immunity were upregulated, while those associated with adaptive responses were downregulated. Further, the genetic responses seen were not related to the subsequent clinical outcomes when these were categorized. Finally, the genetic responses were 95 % congruent to those with other severe injuries, suggesting a common pathway of response [18]. Many years ago, Dr Basil Pruitt called severe burn the "universal trauma model" because of the similarity of responses to other severe injuries, and burns in particular are relatively easily quantitated by total body surface area burned, making study of this condition easier to categorize and compare [19]. This is particularly relevant in terms of metabolism and the expected responses.

The relation of the findings of the Glue Grant to metabolism is principally that responses to burn are similar to that of other injured patients with prolonged care. The massive genomic changes are indeed correlated with the significant changes in the metabolic systems that are also common between severe burns and those with other severe injuries. This is associated with massive changes throughout the genome with associated inflammation with correlated metabolic changes. It is likely that this inflammation induces, at least in part, the metabolic changes described above.

Changes Associated with Treatment

One of the factors that is not commonly considered in hypermetabolism and associated catabolism is the effect of treatment, namely, bedrest and disuse. Severely burned patients are often confined to bed due to pain from movement and to minimize shearing of grafts. This condition often lasts for days to weeks. It is well known that disuse of muscle leads to atrophy [20], exactly what is seen in the severely burned. We are only now beginning to appreciate the impact of disuse in the metabolic changes seen after burn. It is common for efforts to be made to increase mobility; however, these are difficult to control and more importantly difficult to measure. Recently, a rodent model was devised combining severe burn with disuse through a hind limb suspension model [21]. This model found that severe burn did induce muscle loss, but the effect was relatively short-lived and not congruent with the clinical condition. However, when disuse was added, catabolism was greater particularly over a prolonged period similar to what is seen in burned patients. These studies showed that the burn effect was more prominent in type I fast-twitch muscle, while the effects of disuse were higher in type II or slow-twitch fibers [22, 23]. This finding is plausible since type II muscle fatigues more slowly and might be more closely linked to routine mobility such as standing and walking. Further, these studies showed that the muscle mass losses were also associated with decreased muscle function [24], another finding common in the severely burned. It seems that we may have found a preclinical model that recapitulates the clinical condition more closely, and importantly this model includes injury as well as disuse. Further studies with this model could be used to define the effects of exercise in a measureable way as well as more closely mimic the effects of pharmacologic treatments.

Resolution

Common teaching suggests that once treatment for the wounds is complete, beginning the phase of convalescence, hypermetabolism resolves leading to a phase of anabolism. However, data suggest that this is not the case in severe burns, at least in the first year. Severely burned children were studied in a time course after injury for changes in metabolic markers [25] as well as muscle metabolism [2], and these investigators found that catabolism continued for up to 9 months from injury well after wound closure was secure and convalescence commenced. Only after a year from injury were these children found to be at a level to that of normal controls. Investigators found that some inflammatory mediators remained significantly elevated over this time period as well. Potential reasons for the prolonged period of catabolism may lay with the inflammation that persists due to immature scars, as the time periods coincide with scar maturation. Thus, significant whole-body inflammation persists even after wound closure continuing the metabolic changes described above. Further, mobility is impaired associated with scar formation and continued painful motion, oftentimes of the neuropathic type. This leads to lack of anabolic signals for muscle growth and thus the effect.

Interestingly, clinical observation found that at about the 9 month to 1-year point after injury, body mass begins to return to normal; however, this is commonly fat mass rather than lean mass. This idea has not been described in any detail; however, this might suggest that the return of fat metabolism to a more normal state is the precursor to generalized muscle anabolism under current regimens of recovery. This observation should clearly be investigated more fully.

Nutrition Support

A universal finding after severe burn is an increase in energy expenditure related to injury severity [8]. Both resting and total energy expenditure are increased which is associated with energy for wound healing as well as futile substrate cycling as described above. Regardless of the cause, increased energy expenditure should be met with an increase in energy provision through increasing the delivery of exogenous substrate from the diet. What is very clear is that failure to deliver adequate nutrition in the severely injured is associated with poorer outcomes, particularly in severe burns [26]. Thus, early feeding of the burned patient, generally through enteral means due to cost and safety, is the clear and established standard of care throughout the world. The question then is not whether to provide an adequate diet but instead "how much is enough" since dangers are also present with overfeeding [27]. Investigators found that the provision of calories above resting energy expenditure in the form of protein and carbohydrate did not in fact increase lean mass any further but only added to fat mass [16]. These findings highlight the general notion that nutrition should be given to the severely burned, but too much might not have further benefit. Therefore many approaches have been developed to provide some guidelines for nutritional provision.

Nutritional Recommendations

Nutrition has been recognized as an important treatment for the severely burned. Many formulae exist that provide guidelines for nutritional delivery in the severely burned (Table 6.1). One of the first of these was the Curreri formula which is expressed as 25 kcal/kg + 40 kcal/% TBSA burned and was derived from nine patients [28]. This formula has been found to generally overestimate caloric utilization when compared to indirect calorimetry measurements [29]. Another commonly used formula is a derivation of the Harris-Benedict equation, which was developed in the year 1919 using whole-body calorimetry in normal volunteers. For burns, a multiplicative modifier of 1.5 for burns 20–50 % TBSA and 2.1 for burns over 50 % TBSA. This formula also overpredicts utilization, leading some to recommend lower modifiers [30]. Other formulae were subsequently developed and include that from [31–35]. Of all of these, many investigators have found that no formula is particularly predictive of calorie production measured by energy expenditure because of variability within the population [36], but each provides a reasonable estimate that

Table 6.1 Nutritional formulae used in burns

Curreri	25 × wt (kg) + 40 × TBS burned
Harris-Benedict	Men: [66 + (13.7 × wt (kg)) + (5 × ht (cm)) – (6.8 × age (y))] × injury factor × activity factor
	Women: [655 + (9.6 × wt (kg)) + (1.8 × ht (cm)) – (4.7 × age (y))] × injury factor × activity factor
	Activity factor 1.5–2.1 for burn
Ireton-Jones	Mechanically ventilated: 1784 – 11[age (y)] + 5 [wt (kg)] + 244 (males) + 239 for injury + 804 for burn
	Not ventilated: 629 – 11[age (y)] + 25 [wt (kg)] – 609 (females)
Zawacki	1440 × TBSA burned (m^2)
Carlson	Basal metabolic rate (Harris-Benedict) × [0.89142 + (0.01335 × TBSA burned)] + [body surface area (m^2) × 24] × activity factor
Xie	[1000 × body surface area (m^2)] + (25 × TBSA burned)
Milner	Basal metabolic rate (Fleisch equation) × (0.274 + 0.0079 × TBSA burned – 0.004 × day after burn)

could be used clinically. I recommend that any might be used for initial estimates recognizing the variability that is found between patients. In addition, the bulk of this should be given enterally, as supplementing enteral feeding with parenteral has been tested and was not shown to be of benefit and was actually harmful [37].

Some have recommended that caloric delivery might be individualized based upon actual energy expenditure. In severe burns, total energy expenditure is estimated to be 1.2 times measured resting energy expenditure [38], and to account for vagaries and insure underfeeding does not occur, 1.4 times resting energy expenditure has been recommended [39]. This approach might be used when indirect calorimetry is used to monitor energy expenditure, but it comes with caveats. Increased feeding will itself increase energy expenditure associated with the energy utilized for digestion and handling substrate. Much of the futile substrate cycling mentioned above is probably associated with caloric delivery rather than solely related to the injury. This was shown in severely burned children who were not aggressively fed, and the results indicated that resting energy was actually much lower than predicted in the absence of feeding [40]. These findings then imply that we do have some control over resting energy expenditure, and feeding more calories will likely induce an increase in energy expenditure. Therefore the use of indirect calorimetry to measure resting energy expenditure as a target for caloric delivery must be seen in this light.

Another issue to consider is delivery of protein. Delivery of this substrate is clearly beneficial given the changes in utilization and the need for availability. Like that of caloric delivery, studies have shown that no particular amount is indicated once a threshold is reached. Most practitioners suggest that at least 1–2 g/kg is needed to support protein metabolism in the severely burned.

Substrate

Carl von Voit, a German chemist and physiologist in the late 1800s, explored the metabolic implications of protein, fat, and carbohydrate delivery. He observed that when dogs maintained on a protein diet alone were given fat, it only led to increased fat stores. Furthermore, he noted that carbohydrates were preferentially oxidized for energy regardless of volume administered [41]. This notion is congruent with the findings of metabolism after severe burn, in that beta-oxidation of fat is not increased after injury [6]; protein is not a desirable source of energy as amino acids might be better utilized for production of functional protein, leaving carbohydrate as the preferred fuel source. The association and significance of von Voit's work to the predominant notions of nutritional support and management of critically ill patients today cannot be overstated. I therefore recommend that caloric sources should be primarily carbohydrate for the severely burned to spare protein and fat, recognizing that some fat should be given to minimize essential fatty acid deficiency.

Handling Hypermetabolism

Addressing hypermetabolism after injury is a difficult problem with no clear solutions other than attempts at control of the source of hypermetabolism (the burn wound), dietary support, perhaps some pharmacologic manipulation of metabolism for benefit, and early mobilization and exercise. Control of the source of hypermetabolism is paramount, as sepsis that develops in the background of severe burn clearly increases energy expenditure and catabolism [8]. Early excision of the burn wound has been shown to decrease catabolism and is a practice that should be followed in addition to aggressive treatment of infection.

Pharmacologic Interventions

Upon examining the model of increased muscle proteolysis associated with injury (Fig. 6.2), the effects of hypermetabolism on the muscle might be limited mechanistically in a number of ways. The first is to increase amino acid availability in the cell through increased inward transport of amino acids by increasing the interstitial fluid concentration. This is partially the reason that dietary protein is given; however, this approach has been found to be ineffective in affecting net balance once a threshold is reached [16]. This threshold is likely reached through any of the available feeding formulae. A second strategy might be to stimulate protein synthesis, using the available intracellular amino acids from increased inward transport and those from increased protein breakdown. This could be considered increased protein synthetic efficiency since more amino acids within the cell go back into protein rather than leaving the cell. This response can be induced pharmacologically with a number of agents that I will describe below. A third strategy would be to inhibit protein breakdown within the cell through affecting the cellular protein breakdown machinery, such as inhibition of ubiquitin and other breakdown actors. However, this possibility remains speculative at this point, as none of the agents used to manipulate clinical metabolism have been shown to affect this pathway.

Stimulation of Anabolism

Pharmacologic adjuncts are often utilized to diminish catabolism to improve net protein synthesis. While they may reach this point on their own, these therapeutic interventions can shorten

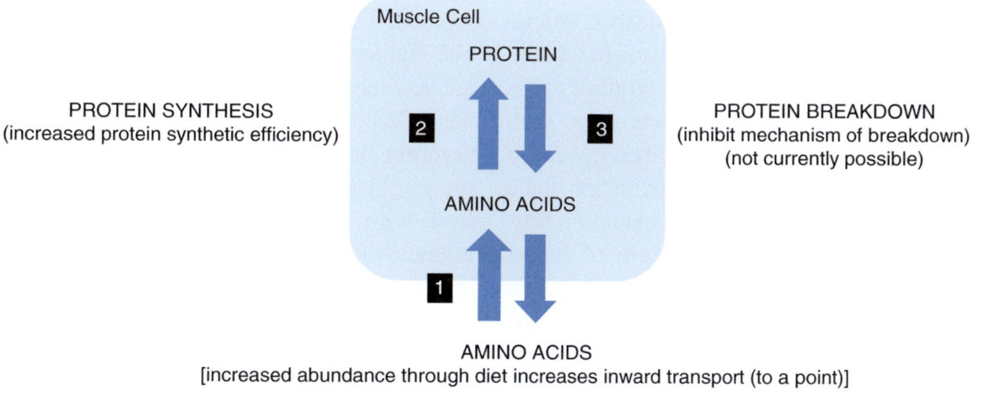

Fig. 6.2 Pictorial description of the flow of amino acids into and out of the cell and into and out of protein. Strategies to increase protein abundance would be to (1) increase intracellular concentration through dietary means, (2) increase the signals for protein synthesis which utilizes amino acids from both inward transport *and* from protein breakdown, (3) or inhibit protein breakdown. Efforts to increase inward transport through the diet are effective only to a point, and this point is commonly reached using the current diet formulas, and the anabolic agents regardless of class all work through the second strategy to increase protein synthetic efficiency of available amino acids. The final strategy has no known effective agents

the infirm period and improve recovery. The adjuncts can be broken into three major classes, soluble protein hormones, anabolic steroids, and beta-blockade.

Soluble Proteins

Many hormones are known to induce anabolic activity in cells, and most are related to growth factor activity through the phosphoinositol-3 related pathways. Growth hormone was the first agent used clinically to affect metabolism after injury. Sir David Cuthbertson used doses of growth hormone to improve protein balance in a leg fracture model [42], and investigators showed in 1991 using protein kinetics data measured in an isolated limb that burned adolescents given recombinant human growth hormone (rhGH) increased net protein synthesis in the muscle. This study also showed that insulin, by itself, had a similar effect [43]. However, enthusiasm for the use of growth hormone to treat hypermetabolism was severely diminished by the findings that the use of growth hormone in critically ill adults was associated with increased mortality [44]. This was not found to be the case in burns [45]; however, the emergence of other safer modalities has further dampened use.

Insulin-like growth factor-1 (IGF-1) is another agent that is in fact induced by growth hormone and is thought to be the principal actor in its anabolic effects. IGF-1 can be given to produce anabolism without some of the effects seen with growth hormone alone. IGF-1, when given to burned patients, decreased protein oxidation and a promoted glucose uptake while not changing resting energy expenditure [46]. The use of IGF-1 alone is plagued by induction of hypoglycemia through its effects on glucose transport into the cell. This effect can be diminished by giving IGF-1 with its principal binding protein insulin-like growth factor-1 binding protein-3 (IGFBP-3), which retained its anabolic effect on leg muscle, and was most profound in those who were the most catabolic [47]. A similar effect was seen in adults given IGF-1/IGFBP-3, but several of these subjects developed peripheral neuropathies, again quelling any enthusiasm for widespread use of this agent [48].

Insulin is in fact the most potent anabolic agent for muscle anabolism. When given in sustained doses even in those with insulin resistance, it induced improved protein net synthesis in the severely burned [49]. The first of these studies was done with high doses of insulin (>30 units/h) given for 3–5 days and demonstrated dramatic effects on protein synthesis, making even those patients who were at bedrest anabolic (net addition of muscle protein). This was associated with an increase in inward transport of amino acids as well as improved protein synthesis by more than 200 %. Other studies with lower doses were also effective in increasing net protein synthesis but had no effect on inward transport. When this dose of insulin was given for the entire hospital stay, it increased lean body mass and decreased length of hospital stay without increased caloric delivery. Interestingly, it also had dramatic effects on fat mass perhaps through inhibition of lipolysis [50].

Androgenic Steroids

Testosterone is the representative androgenic steroid normally produced in higher quantities in men, but a small amount is also produced in women. There are other derivatives of testosterone that have anabolic properties, but all of these are severely decreased after severe injury and illness. When testosterone itself was given to severely burned men to normalize these levels, protein synthetic efficiency improved over two-fold with a decrease in whole-body protein breakdown. The authors concluded that testosterone could be used to ameliorate muscle catabolism after injury; however, the androgenic properties such as potential for hirsutism must be considered [51].

Oxandrolone is an analogue of testosterone with only 1/6th of its androgenic potency, and this compound has been in common use to treat muscle wasting in severe burns. Many studies have been done to demonstrate the safety of oxandrolone, and its mechanism of action has been shown as an increase in protein synthesis using intracellular amino acids [52, 53]. It is effective in both children and adults [15]. When given over the entire hospitalization in a multicenter randomized clinical trial, it was shown to decrease length of hospital stay without significant side effects [54]. The investigators found some increase in hepatic transaminases; however, this was not associated with any clinical signs or symptoms. This was also associated with a decreased number of operations for wound closure. These findings have subsequently been corroborated in meta-analyses of extant data [55, 56].

Beta-Blockade

Several studies have been done in the severely burned to demonstrate the beneficial effects of propranolol on metabolism in the severely burned. Initial studies were done to decrease heart rate, showing benefit for overall cardiac work [57]. Further studies using a dose that decreased heart rate by 20 % in children demonstrated effects on fat metabolism to decrease lipolysis with beneficial effects on fat cycling and decreasing fatty infiltration of the liver [58]. In addition, beta-blockade is likely one of the few available means to decrease energy expenditure and thus could decrease minute ventilation in those with high ventilator pressures. Perhaps most intriguingly, propranolol effects on muscle were examined, and significant increases in net protein synthesis were demonstrated that resulted in improved lean body mass [59]. The effect was again through improved muscle protein synthetic efficiency and not through decreased protein breakdown as was expected. It is still confusing as to how a catecholamine inhibitor *increases* protein synthesis, implying that catecholamines have an action to decrease synthesis even when it is above normal levels. Further work will be done to investigate this finding. Large clinical trials are currently underway to further show effects of beta-blockade in adults, and we look forward to the results.

Anabolic Agents Summary

A summary of the information above suggests that the most effective and safe anabolic agents for use include insulin, oxandrolone, and propranolol. All of these are in common use in most burn centers.

Critical Care

A number of advances in critical care have occurred in the past several years, and the metabolic ramifications of these treatments have not been well studied. Among these are new ventilator techniques and the growing use of continuous renal replacement therapies. It has been known for some time that mechanical ventilation induces an increase in energy expenditure, but much of the work demonstrating this finding was done before the advent of low-pressure ventilation strategies and open-lung strategies common in burn centers [60]. It might be presumed that these newer methods that are more comfortable and less stressful to the patient might decrease energy utilization; however, we cannot know for sure. Whether recommendations for dietary provision should change is also not known.

Renal replacement therapies in the ICU are now a commonplace and for burns in particular have significantly improved outcomes [61, 62]. However, the effects on hypermetabolism after severe injury have not yet been described. The continuous filtration of the plasma is likely to have effects to decrease some of the inflammatory mediators that partly drive the hypermetabolic response as one example. Further, filtration of amino acids is also likely to occur, resulting in a loss of protein. Whether changes in dietary provision should be considered is not known.

Increased Activity

As stated previously, the effects of bedrest and disuse atrophy in burned patients have not been fully recognized until recently. The solution to this problem is to increase activity through mobilization and exercise. However, bedrest was never the desired condition for burn care providers, but resistance to aggressive physical activity was tempered by the negative consequences of graft loss due to shearing forces and the empiric belief that exercise is not possible during the critical illness phase of treatment or even during convalescence. Both of these concerns have now been drawn into question, as several have shown that graft loss does not appreciably increase with mobilization [63] and further that exercise is indeed possible during hospitalization and in convalescence, even in children [64, 65]. Recently, a trial was begun on the effects of a directed exercise program in burned patients while in the ICU as well as in convalescence, and the early results are showing benefit. We await the results of these trials and complete description of the effects.

Conclusion

Almost all burned patients develop the condition termed "hypermetabolism" for a variety of reasons which have been known for some time. The effect is profound and long-lasting and most visibly results in lean mass catabolism and wasting. Interventions to diminish the effects of this condition include attention to closing the wound and control of sepsis complications, provision of diet, and more recently considered increased activity.

References

1. Xiao Y, Hsiao TH, Suresh U, Chen HI, Wu X, Wolf SE, et al. A novel significance score for gene selection and ranking. Bioinformatics. 2014;30(6):801–7. PubMed Pubmed Central PMCID: 3957066.
2. Hart DW, Wolf SE, Mlcak R, Chinkes DL, Ramzy PI, Obeng MK, et al. Persistence of muscle catabolism after severe burn. Surgery. 2000;128(2):312–9. PubMed.
3. Moore FD. Bodily changes in surgical convalescence. I. The normal sequence observations and interpretations. Ann Surg. 1953;137(3):289–315. PubMed Pubmed Central PMCID: PMC1802509.
4. Wilmore DW, Long JM, Mason Jr AD, Skreen RW, Pruitt Jr BA. Catecholamines: mediator of the hypermetabolic response to thermal injury. Ann Surg. 1974;180(4):653–69. PubMed Pubmed Central PMCID: PMC1344163.
5. Vaughan GM, Becker RA, Allen JP, Goodwin Jr CW, Pruitt Jr BA, Mason Jr AD. Cortisol and corticotrophin in burned patients. J Trauma. 1982;22(4):263–73. PubMed.
6. Wolfe RR, Herndon DN, Jahoor F, Miyoshi H, Wolfe M. Effect of severe burn injury on substrate cycling by glucose and fatty acids. N Engl J Med. 1987;317(7):403–8. PubMed.
7. Clark AS, Kelly RA, Mitch WE. Systemic response to thermal injury in rats. Accelerated protein degradation and altered glucose utilization in muscle. J Clin Invest. 1984;74(3):888–97. PubMed Pubmed Central PMCID: PMC425244.
8. Hart DW, Wolf SE, Chinkes DL, Gore DC, Mlcak RP, Beauford RB, et al. Determinants of skeletal muscle catabolism after severe burn. Ann Surg. 2000;232(4):455–65. PubMed Pubmed Central PMCID: 1421178.
9. Grisbrook TL, Elliott CM, Edgar DW, Wallman KE, Wood FM, Reid SL. Burn-injured adults with long term functional impairments demonstrate the same response to resistance training as uninjured controls. Burns. 2013;39(4):680–6. PubMed.
10. Soeters PB, Grecu I. Have we enough glutamine and how does it work? A clinician's view. Ann Nutr Metab. 2012;60(1):17–26. PubMed.
11. Ziegler TR, May AK, Hebbar G, Easley KA, Griffith DP, Dave N, et al. Efficacy and safety of glutamine-supplemented parenteral nutrition in surgical ICU patients: an American multicenter randomized controlled trial. Ann Surg. 2015;22. PubMed.
12. van Zanten AR, Dhaliwal R, Garrel D, Heyland DK. Enteral glutamine supplementation in critically ill patients: a systematic review and meta-analysis. Crit Care. 2015;19:294. PubMed Pubmed Central PMCID: PMC4539709.
13. Aarsland A, Chinkes DL, Sakurai Y, Nguyen TT, Herndon DN, Wolfe RR. Insulin therapy in burn patients does not contribute to hepatic triglyceride production. J Clin Invest. 1998;101(10):2233–9. PubMed Pubmed Central PMCID: PMC508811.
14. Cree MG, Wolfe RR. Postburn trauma insulin resistance and fat metabolism. Am J Physiol Endocrinol Metab. 2008;294(1):E1–9. PubMed.
15. Demling RH, DeSanti L. The rate of restoration of body weight after burn injury, using the anabolic agent oxandrolone, is not age dependent. Burns. 2001;27(1):46–51. PubMed.
16. Hart DW, Wolf SE, Herndon DN, Chinkes DL, Lal SO, Obeng MK, et al. Energy expenditure and caloric balance after burn: increased feeding leads to fat rather than lean mass accretion. Ann Surg. 2002;235(1):152–61. PubMed Pubmed Central PMCID: 1422407.
17. Xiao W, Mindrinos MN, Seok J, Cuschieri J, Cuenca AG, Gao H, et al. A genomic storm in critically injured humans. J Exp Med. 2011;208(13):2581–90. PubMed Pubmed Central PMCID: PMC3244029.
18. Seok J, Warren HS, Cuenca AG, Mindrinos MN, Baker HV, Xu W, et al. Genomic responses in mouse

models poorly mimic human inflammatory diseases. Proc Natl Acad Sci U S A. 2013;110(9):3507–12. PubMed Pubmed Central PMCID: PMC3587220.
19. Pruitt Jr BA. The universal trauma model. Bull Am Coll Surg. 1985;70:2–13.
20. Cree MG, Paddon-Jones D, Newcomer BR, Ronsen O, Aarsland A, Wolfe RR, et al. Twenty-eight-day bed rest with hypercortisolemia induces peripheral insulin resistance and increases intramuscular triglycerides. Metabolism. 2010;59(5):703–10. PubMed Pubmed Central PMCID: PMC2856785.
21. Wade CE, Baer LA, Wu X, Silliman DT, Walters TJ, Wolf SE. Severe burn and disuse in the rat independently adversely impact body composition and adipokines. Crit Care. 2013;17(5):R225. PubMed Pubmed Central PMCID: 4057079.
22. Saeman MR, DeSpain K, Liu MM, Carlson BA, Song J, Baer LA, et al. Effects of exercise on soleus in severe burn and muscle disuse atrophy. J Surg Res. 2015;198(1):19–26. PubMed Pubmed Central PMCID: 4542145.
23. Wu X, Wolf SE, Walters TJ. Muscle contractile properties in severely burned rats. Burns. 2010;36(6):905–11. PubMed Pubmed Central PMCID: PMC2912951.
24. Wu X, Baer LA, Wolf SE, Wade CE, Walters TJ. The impact of muscle disuse on muscle atrophy in severely burned rats. J Surg Res. 2010;164(2):e243–51. PubMed Pubmed Central PMCID: PMC2991603.
25. Jeschke MG, Gauglitz GG, Kulp GA, Finnerty CC, Williams FN, Kraft R, et al. Long-term persistance of the pathophysiologic response to severe burn injury. PLoS One. 2011;6(7):e21245. PubMed Pubmed Central PMCID: PMC3138751.
26. Lyons M, Clemens LH. Energy deficits associated with nasogastric feeding in patients with burns. J Burn Care Rehabil. 2000;21(4):372–4. discussion 1. PubMed.
27. Wolf SE. Nutrition and metabolism in burns: state of the science, 2007. J Burn Care Res. 2007;28(4):572–6. PubMed.
28. Curreri PW, Richmond D, Marvin J, Baxter CR. Dietary requirements of patients with major burns. J Am Diet Assoc. 1974;65(4):415–7. PubMed.
29. Turner Jr WW, Ireton CS, Hunt JL, Baxter CR. Predicting energy expenditures in burned patients. J Trauma. 1985;25(1):11–6. PubMed.
30. Liusuwan RA, Palmieri TL, Kinoshita L, Greenhalgh DG. Comparison of measured resting energy expenditure versus predictive equations in pediatric burn patients. J Burn Care Rehabil. 2005;26(6):464–70. PubMed.
31. Zawacki BE, Spitzer KW, Mason AD Jr, Johns LA. Does increased evaporative water loss cause hypermetabolism in burned patients?. Ann Surg. 1970;171:236–40.
32. Carlson DE, Cioffi WG Jr, Mason AD Jr, McManus WF, Pruitt BA Jr. Resting energy expenditure in patients with thermal injuries. Surg Gynecol Obstet. 1992;174:270–6.
33. Ireton-Jones CS1, Turner WW Jr, Baxter CR. Nutritional considerations in recovered patients with burns. J Burn Care Rehabil. 1990;11(6):581–2.
34. Xie WG, Li A, Wang SL. Estimation of the calorie requirements of burned Chinese adults. Burns. 1993;19:146–9.
35. Milner EA, Cioffi WG, Mason AD, McManus WF, Pruitt BA Jr. A longitudinal study of resting energy expenditure in thermally injured patients. J Trauma. 1994;37:167–70.
36. Shields BA, Doty KA, Chung KK, Wade CE, Aden JK, Wolf SE. Determination of resting energy expenditure after severe burn. J Burn Care Res. 2013;34(1):e22–8. PubMed.
37. Herndon DN, Barrow RE, Stein M, Linares H, Rutan TC, Rutan R, et al. Increased mortality with intravenous supplemental feeding in severely burned patients. J Burn Care Rehabil. 1989;10(4):309–13. PubMed.
38. Goran MI, Peters EJ, Herndon DN, Wolfe RR. Total energy expenditure in burned children using the doubly labeled water technique. Am J Physiol. 1990;259(4 Pt 1):E576–85. PubMed.
39. Pereira C, Murphy K, Jeschke M, Herndon DN. Post burn muscle wasting and the effects of treatments. Int J Biochem Cell Biol. 2005;37(10):1948–61. PubMed.
40. Hart DW, Wolf SE, Chinkes DL, Beauford RB, Mlcak RP, Heggers JP, et al. Effects of early excision and aggressive enteral feeding on hypermetabolism, catabolism, and sepsis after severe burn. J Trauma. 2003;54(4):755–61. discussion 61–4. PubMed.
41. Sigerist HE. The history of dietetics. 1941. Gesnerus. 1989;46(Pt 3–4):249–56. PubMed.
42. Cuthbertson DP, Webster TA, Young FG. The anterior pituitary gland and protein metabolism. I. The nitrogen-retaining action of anterior lobe extracts. J Endocrinol. 1941;2:459–67.
43. Gore DC, Honeycutt D, Jahoor F, Wolfe RR, Herndon DN. Effect of exogenous growth hormone on whole-body and isolated-limb protein kinetics in burned patients. Arch Surg. 1991;126(1):38–43. PubMed.
44. Takala J, Ruokonen E, Webster NR, Nielsen MS, Zandstra DF, Vundelinckx G, et al. Increased mortality associated with growth hormone treatment in critically ill adults. N Engl J Med. 1999;341(11):785–92. PubMed.
45. Ramirez RJ, Wolf SE, Barrow RE, Herndon DN. Growth hormone treatment in pediatric burns: a safe therapeutic approach. Ann Surg. 1998;228(4): 439–48. PubMed Pubmed Central PMCID: 1191513.
46. Cioffi WG, Gore DC, Rue 3rd LW, Carrougher G, Guler HP, McManus WF, et al. Insulin-like growth factor-1 lowers protein oxidation in patients with thermal injury. Ann Surg. 1994;220(3):310–6. PubMed Pubmed Central PMCID: 1234384, discussion 6–9.
47. Herndon DN, Ramzy PI, DebRoy MA, Zheng M, Ferrando AA, Chinkes DL, et al. Muscle protein catabolism after severe burn: effects of IGF-1/

IGFBP-3 treatment. Ann Surg. 1999;229(5):713–20. PubMed Pubmed Central PMCID: 1420816, discussion 20–2.
48. Debroy MA, Wolf SE, Zhang XJ, Chinkes DL, Ferrando AA, Wolfe RR, et al. Anabolic effects of insulin-like growth factor in combination with insulin-like growth factor binding protein-3 in severely burned adults. J Trauma. 1999;47(5):904–10. discussion 10–1. PubMed.
49. Ferrando AA, Chinkes DL, Wolf SE, Matin S, Herndon DN, Wolfe RR. A submaximal dose of insulin promotes net skeletal muscle protein synthesis in patients with severe burns. Ann Surg. 1999;229(1):11–8. PubMed Pubmed Central PMCID: 1191603.
50. Sakurai Y, Aarsland A, Herndon DN, Chinkes DL, Pierre E, Nguyen TT, et al. Stimulation of muscle protein synthesis by long-term insulin infusion in severely burned patients. Ann Surg. 1995;222(3):283–94. PubMed Pubmed Central PMCID: 1234807, 94–7.
51. Ferrando AA, Sheffield-Moore M, Wolf SE, Herndon DN, Wolfe RR. Testosterone administration in severe burns ameliorates muscle catabolism. Crit Care Med. 2001;29(10):1936–42. PubMed.
52. Wolf SE, Thomas SJ, Dasu MR, Ferrando AA, Chinkes DL, Wolfe RR, et al. Improved net protein balance, lean mass, and gene expression changes with oxandrolone treatment in the severely burned. Ann Surg. 2003;237(6):801–10. PubMed Pubmed Central PMCID: 1514675, discussion 10–1.
53. Hart DW, Wolf SE, Ramzy PI, Chinkes DL, Beauford RB, Ferrando AA, et al. Anabolic effects of oxandrolone after severe burn. Ann Surg. 2001;233(4):556–64. PubMed Pubmed Central PMCID: 1421286.
54. Wolf SE, Edelman LS, Kemalyan N, Donison L, Cross J, Underwood M, et al. Effects of oxandrolone on outcome measures in the severely burned: a multicenter prospective randomized double-blind trial. J Burn Care Res. 2006;27(2):131–9. discussion 40–1. PubMed.
55. Cochran A, Thuet W, Holt B, Faraklas I, Smout RJ, Horn SD. The impact of oxandrolone on length of stay following major burn injury: a clinical practice evaluation. Burns. 2013;39(7):1374–9. PubMed.
56. Li H, Guo Y, Yang Z, Roy M, Guo Q. The efficacy and safety of oxandrolone treatment for patients with severe burns: a systematic review and meta-analysis. Burns. 2015;7. PubMed.
57. Herndon DN, Barrow RE, Rutan TC, Minifee P, Jahoor F, Wolfe RR. Effect of propranolol administration on hemodynamic and metabolic responses of burned pediatric patients. Ann Surg. 1988;208(4):484–92. PubMed Pubmed Central PMCID: 1493755.
58. Morio B, Irtun O, Herndon DN, Wolfe RR. Propranolol decreases splanchnic triacylglycerol storage in burn patients receiving a high-carbohydrate diet. Ann Surg. 2002;236(2):218–25. PubMed Pubmed Central PMCID: 1422568.
59. Herndon DN, Hart DW, Wolf SE, Chinkes DL, Wolfe RR. Reversal of catabolism by beta-blockade after severe burns. N Engl J Med. 2001;345(17):1223–9. PubMed.
60. Chung KK, Rhie RY, Lundy JB, Cartotto R, Henderson E, Pressman MA, et al. A survey of mechanical ventilator practices across burn centers in North America. J Burn Care Res. 2015;26. PubMed.
61. Chung KK, Juncos LA, Wolf SE, Mann EE, Renz EM, White CE, et al. Continuous renal replacement therapy improves survival in severely burned military casualties with acute kidney injury. J Trauma. 2008;64 Suppl 2:S179–85. discussion S85–7. PubMed.
62. Chung KK, Lundy JB, Matson JR, Renz EM, White CE, King BT, et al. Continuous venovenous hemofiltration in severely burned patients with acute kidney injury: a cohort study. Crit Care. 2009;13(3):R62. PubMed Pubmed Central PMCID: 2717417.
63. Lorello DJ, Peck M, Albrecht M, Richey KJ, Pressman MA. Results of a prospective randomized controlled trial of early ambulation for patients with lower extremity autografts. J Burn Care Res. 2014;35(5):431–6. PubMed.
64. Al-Mousawi AM, Williams FN, Mlcak RP, Jeschke MG, Herndon DN, Suman OE. Effects of exercise training on resting energy expenditure and lean mass during pediatric burn rehabilitation. J Burn Care Res. 2010;31(3):400–8. PubMed Pubmed Central PMCID: 3856323.
65. Suman OE, Spies RJ, Celis MM, Mlcak RP, Herndon DN. Effects of a 12-wk resistance exercise program on skeletal muscle strength in children with burn injuries. J Appl Physiol. 2001;91(3):1168–75. PubMed.

Infection and Sepsis

7

Sharmila Dissanaike, Samantha A. Moore, and Derek Yang

Introduction

Infection is a common complication of major burns, with over 24,000 reported cases of infections associated with burns in the USA over a 10-year period, as reported by the American Burn Association (ABA) 2015 National Burn Repository. They contributed towards the 6500+ burn patient deaths over the past 10 years [1], with leading cause of death after 24 h in severely burned patients being multiple organ dysfunction syndrome (MODS) secondary to sepsis [2].

The damage of our primary defense mechanism, skin, and our secondary defenses, cellular and humoral immunity, places burn patients at high risk for infection. A key treatment recommendation for sepsis is antimicrobial therapy, along with a focused, goal-directed approach to sepsis. Adherence to best practices in sepsis treatment may be a reason for the nationwide decline in mortality associated with sepsis from 1999 to 2008 [3]. Although antimicrobials have helped decrease mortality overall, extensive use has resulted in an increased incidence of multidrug-resistant (MDR) organisms and associated morbidity and mortality.

Many criteria and scoring systems have been developed to help identify infections and their extent of damage; however, burn patients are typically excluded during their development, rendering such systems less applicable to this population [2]. Since the systemic inflammatory response to burn is very similar to that seen in sepsis, distinguishing between these two entities is complex, and requires different definitions from those used in other populations. Reporting and following burn wound infection is difficult without standardized definitions of burn infection and sepsis. Thus, in 2007, the ABA held a consensus conference that set out to standardize definitions of infection in burns [2].

Here we discuss definitions and treatment options for common infectious complications seen in burn patients, including wound infection, ventilator-associated pneumonia (VAP), central line-associated bloodstream infection (CLABSI), urinary catheter-related infection (UTI), sepsis and septic shock.

Definitions

Burn Wound Infection

The progression of burn wound infection can be defined in three steps. The first is **wound colonization**, where there are bacteria present at

S. Dissanaike, M.D., F.A.C.S. (✉)
S.A. Moore, M.D., Ph.D. • D. Yang, B.S.
Department of Surgery, Texas Tech University Health Sciences Center, 3601 4th Street STOP 8312, Lubbock, TX 79430-8312, USA
e-mail: sharmila.dissanaike@ttuhsc.edu

D.G. Greenhalgh (ed.), *Burn Care for General Surgeons and General Practitioners*,
DOI 10.1007/978-3-319-29161-1_7

concentrations $<10^5$ bacteria/g tissue. The second step is **wound infection**, where the bacteria are present at concentrations $>10^5$ bacteria/g tissue. Finally, **invasive infection** is the diagnosis of a wound infection plus invasion or destruction of unburned areas (with or without sepsis as defined in "Sepsis").

There are both subjective and quantitative findings which may suggest the diagnosis of burn wound infection. Subjective findings include the symptoms of pain and the signs of erythema, color changes, change in wound appearance or depth, systemic changes, and early burn eschar separation. Early burn eschar separation signifies an invasive infection as the pathophysiology of the separation is due to bacterial digestion of underlying tissue. However, one obvious confounding factor is the need to distinguish changes secondary to infection from visible changes and symptoms resulting from the burn itself. Given the high overlap between subjective findings—symptoms and signs—from the burn itself and potential infection, there is a significant risk of false positive diagnoses; therefore, objective, quantitative confirmation of infection is very important in order to prevent overtreatment with antibiotics in cases where they may not be necessary. Quantitative studies may include quantitative cultures of tissue biopsy or tissue histology. Tissue diagnoses are more accurate when larger samples are obtained, with at least 1 cm^3 of tissue being ideal; however, a compromise must often be made between increased yield and the cosmetic deformity occasioned by the biopsy itself, which may vary depending on the anatomic location of the burn.

There are some characteristic clinical findings in burn wound infections which may guide our index of suspicion towards a particular pathogen. For example, a yellow/green exudate does not necessarily signify an invasive infection, but may represent a *Pseudomonas aeruginosa* infection. Were an infection invasive, it would present with black to purple, punched out areas and require immediate surgery. Also, yeast and molds may cause infection. If small, purulent papules are present, *Candida* spp. may be suggested. If gray-brown fungating masses are present, *Aspergillus* spp. may be suspected [2].

Ventilator-Associated Pneumonia (VAP)

Many patients suffering burns to the upper or lower airway—chemical or thermal inhalation injury—require intubation and mechanical ventilation to prevent airway compromise and/or respiratory failure. A significant proportion of patients with burns greater than 30 % TBSA also require prolonged intubation and mechanical ventilation due to high metabolic demand and need for repeated operations. Unfortunately, this life-saving therapy carries with it the risk of VAP, the incidence of which is currently estimated at 2–16 infections per 1000 ventilator days in all hospitalized patients [4, 5]. Although VAP in most critically ill populations is considered a nosocomial infection, there is some evidence that in patients with smoke inhalation the pathogenic organisms may be detected in endotracheal secretions on admission [6]; the damage to the bronchi and alveolar tissue from smoke inhalation likely accelerates the pathogenesis of VAP in these patients. Therefore, it may be advisable periodically to perform surveillance cultures of endotracheal aspirates [7] in patients presenting with signs of inhalation injury; the process of bronchoalveolar lavage (BAL) in these cases may also prove therapeutic to the burn patient suffering compromise of tracheal mucosal clearance. It is, of course, essential for all health care personnel to practice superior hand disinfection and equipment sterilization techniques and to keep all ancillary materials (ventilator hardware, tape, etc.) separate for each patient.

It is essential not to succumb to temptation prophylactically to dose each ventilated burn patient with antibiotics preemptively. In order that MDR organisms not be promoted through the extermination of beneficial, native flora, antimicrobials ought to be held as the patient is watched for clinical signs of infection and such therapy should be used only in response to positive microbiology results. In confirmed cases of VAP, as soon as samples have been obtained for culture, broad-spectrum empiric therapy should be initiated in accordance with local patterns of pathogenic prevalence and then the spectrum narrowed as culture results return [5, 8–10].

Diagnosis of pneumonia in burn patients should be based on clinical suspicion and then confirmed by microbiology. The clinical diagnosis of pneumonia requires two of the following: (1) Chest X-ray (CXR) with a new infiltrate, consolidation or cavitation, (2) sepsis (per definition later in this chapter), or (3) change in sputum or purulence [2]. Following clinical diagnosis, subsequent treatment should be guided by the results of microbiologic analysis, and pneumonia can be considered in three categories. (1) **Confirmed**: clinical diagnosis and positive microbiology, (2) **Probable**: clinical diagnosis with a negative microbiology, (3) **Possible**: mild clinical suspicion with abnormal CXR and positive microbiology. Positive microbiology is defined in one of three ways: (1) tracheal aspirate with $\geq 10^5$ total organisms, (2) bronchoalveolar lavage with $\geq 10^4$ total organisms, (3) protected bronchial brush with $\geq 10^3$ total organisms (Table 7.1).

Central Line Associated Blood Stream Infection (CLABSI)

The placement of central venous catheters often cannot be avoided in the burn critical care environment for necessary fluid resuscitation and intravenous drug delivery. However, each day of catheterization brings an increased risk of the patient's sustaining a CLABSI, with the highest rates of infection specifically associated with non-tunneled and pulmonary arterial catheters, and those placed at femoral sites [11]. Prevention of CLABSI begins with sufficient disinfection of the access site and introduction of the catheter under sterile conditions; surveillance and early recognition of cutaneous signs of inflammation may result in replacement of the catheter (preferably at a different site) before significant bacteremia or sepsis may develop. Tools such as checklists and implementation bundles when inserting lines, as well as strict use of aseptic technique, are helpful in avoiding these infections. Catheters with impregnated materials such as silver or antibiotic agents have been shown to reduce the incidence of CLABSI and are increasingly being used [12–14].

Blood stream infections (BSIs) are defined in one of three ways: (1) two or more blood cultures of a microorganism which is not usually a skin contaminant, (2) one blood culture with sepsis, or (3) sepsis with two or more blood cultures of a common skin contaminant with at least one culture from a venipuncture. Examples of skin contaminants are *Bacillus* spp., *Propionibacterium* spp., coagulase negative *Staphylococci*, and diphtheroids. BSIs are called primary if the microorganism has not caused an infection at another site, or secondary if it has already caused an infection at another site. Note that culture results are dependent both on techniques and on current use of antimicrobial agents.

Catheter-related infections are diagnosed when there was a central venous catheter in the patient 48 h before an infection, regardless of whether the catheter was removed before symptoms arose. If symptoms resolve within 24 hours after catheter removal, a central venous catheter infection should be considered as having been the source. Catheter infections can be localized, cause inflammation, or cause infection. **Localized catheter colonization** is diagnosed when there are >15 colony-forming units (CFU) at the catheter tip, subcutaneous segment of the catheter, or from the catheter hub. **Exit site inflammation** is diagnosed when there is any erythema or induration within 2 cm of the catheter exit site but the criteria for infection are not met. There cannot be signs of localized purulence. **Exit site infection** is diagnosed when there is tenderness, erythema, or induration >2 cm from the catheter exit site, and is also diagnosed if there is purulence or necrosis at the exit site. There cannot be a concurrent BSI or sepsis in order for exit site inflammation or infection to be diagnosed.

Central venous catheter infection (CVCI) is defined one of four ways: (1) any bacteremia or fungemia in a patient with a catheter that has at least one positive blood culture at a distant site from the catheter, clinical signs of infection, and no other source of infection, (2) bacteremia or fungemia with >15 CFU on semiquantitative culture analysis or $>10^3$ CFU on quantitative culture analysis, (3) simultaneous quantitative blood cultures from the catheter site and a distant site with

Table 7.1 Diagnosis of burn infections [2]

Burn wound infection	Pneumonia/VAP	CLABSI	UTI (1)	UTI (2)
		Any of the following where catheter has been in place for >2 days:	Any of the following where catheter has been in place for >2 days:	Any TWO of the following where catheter has been in place for >2 days:
Colonization: <10^5 organisms/g tissue	*Possible:* mild clinical suspicion, abnormal CXR, positive microbiology	Bacteremia/fungemia plus one positive blood culture at distant site, with no other source	Fever >39 °C with no other source of fever, Urinary urgency, frequency, dysuria, suprapubic tenderness	Fever >39 °C with no other source of fever; urinary urgency, frequency; dysuria, suprapubic tenderness
Infection: >10^5 organisms/g tissue	*Probable:* clinical diagnosis, negative microbiology	Bacteremia/fungemia with >15 CFU on semiquantitative or >10^3 CFU on quantitative culture analysis	PLUS urine cultures >10^5 CFU/ml	Positive dipstick for leukocyte esterase and/or nitrite
Invasive infection: infection plus destruction of unburned areas	*Confirmed:* clinical diagnosis, positive microbiology	5:1 Ratio of semiquantitative results from catheter–distant site cultures	–	≥10 WBC/μl or ≥3 WBC/hpf of unspun urine
–	–	Catheter culture grows organisms more than 2 h before culture from distant site	–	Two urine cultures with repeated isolation of ≥10^2 CFU/ml in a nonvoided specimen
–	–	–	–	Two urine cultures with ≥10^5 CFU/ml of a single uropathogen in patient being treated with appropriate antimicrobials

VAP: ventilator-associated pneumonia, *CLABSI:* central line-associated bloodstream infection, *UTI*: urinary tract infection, *CXR:* chest X-ray, *CFU:* colony forming units, *hpf:* high-power field, *WBC:* white blood cells

>5:1 ratio of organism counts at catheter–distant site, (4) if catheter blood grows pathogenic organisms more than 2 h before a separate site grows that organism. It has been shown that the high rate of skin colonization in burn patients may lead to a falsely elevated documentation of CLABSI, especially where automated electronic surveillance is used. Since this is an outcome tracked by the Centers for Medicare & Medicaid Services (CMS) and other agencies which maintain publicly reportable databases, it is essential that this diagnosis along with other nosocomial infections be carefully evaluated in the burn patient and confirmed based on clinical findings prior to documentation [15].

Due to the high risk of CLABSI in burn patients, a policy of routine line changes every 3 days is utilized in some burn centers. Recent evidence suggests no additional benefit from more frequent line changes of every 48 hours [16, 17].

Urinary Tract Infection (UTI)

Since urine output is the standard used to guide initial resuscitation in burn patients, most patients with major burns will receive urinary catheters upon admission if not sooner. However, the longer a catheter resides indwelling, the greater the risk for urinary tract infection to arise. Therefore, the goal should always be to remove urinary catheters as soon as possible; however, this may not be practical for weeks in a patient with major burns. Therefore, precautions ought to be taken when catheter lines are manipulated during dressing changes along with adherence to standard urinary catheter maintenance with daily chlorhexidine sterilization.

Although it is not usually a major cause of sepsis in burn patients, UTI can still cause sepsis. UTI diagnosis should be based on modified CDC criteria. A patient with any of the following is said to have a UTI: fever (>39 °C and no other source of fever), urgency, frequency, dysuria, suprapubic tenderness in addition to urine culture $\geq 10^5$ CFU/ml with ≤ 2 species of organisms. Note that burn patients may not exhibit these clinical symptoms as one might expect in an outpatient setting. Also, the diagnosis of UTI should be made if the patient has two of the following: fever (>39 °C and no other source of fever), urgency, frequency, dysuria, suprapubic tenderness in addition to one of the following: (1) positive dipstick for leukocyte esterase and/or nitrate, (2) ≥10 WBC/μl or ≥3 WBC/high-power field of unspun urine, (3) organisms seen on Gram's stain of unspun urine, (4) two urine cultures with repeated isolation of the same uropathogen with $\geq 10^2$ CFU/ml in a nonvoided specimen, (5) two urine cultures with $\geq 10^5$ CFU/ml of single uropathogens in a patient being treated with appropriate antimicrobial therapy (Table 7.1).

Treatment

All infections in burn patients should be assumed to be due to nosocomial pathogens unless proven otherwise (which simplifies the initial approach to treatment) with slight variations for type and site of infection which are considered individually here. Local antibiograms should be used in developing protocols for empiric antimicrobial coverage in the inpatient setting; however, consideration should be given to covering MDR organisms until results of cultures are available. In treating infections, it is important to also ensure proper nutrition, hydration, and oxygenation of the host, without which other therapies have a lesser chance of success.

In addition to strict adherence to universal precautions at dressing changes, all dressing materials such as gauze, bandages, and tape, as well as any creams and ointments, should be strictly isolated from one patient to the next so as to avoid the transfer of microorganisms. Topical ointments such as **silver sulfadiazine 1 %** (Sulfadene) and **mafenide acetate 11 %** (Sulfamylon) provide broad-spectrum coverage and are often used on burn wounds, as well as formulations of **mupirocin 2 %** (Bactroban) and **bacitracin/neomycin/polymyxin B** (Neosporin). Silver sulfadiazine, though broad-spectrum against gram-positive, gram-negative, and fungal species, can cause neutropenia and thrombocytopenia and patients should be monitored for these potential consequences; it also results in pseudoeschar formation, which may complicate wound care. Mafenide acetate, though providing good coverage for *Pseudomonas* and *Enterococcus*, can cause electrolyte imbalances and is less effective against fungal infection. It should not be used to cover more than 20 % TBSA due to risk of systemic metabolic acidosis. The biggest drawback to its use is that it causes significant pain on application on partial thickness burns. Topical mupirocin is suitable for *S. aureus* and *S. pyogenes* infections when these pathogens are known or specifically suspected to be causal, and the Neosporin formulation, while effective against a broad spectrum of organisms, may result in irritation or contact dermatitis in susceptible patients, especially with prolonged usage.

Topical soaks, such as **0.025 % sodium hypochlorite (Dakin's solution), 0.5 % silver nitrate, or 0/25 % acetic acid solutions** may also be applied. Each of these is highly effective against a broad range of pathogens, but sodium hypochlorite has cytotoxic effects and dressings must be changed frequently as the compound is inactivated by contact with proteins, either cellular or pathogenic. Silver nitrate is highly effective and is painless upon application, but has the disadvantage of turning wound surfaces gray to black, which can interfere with visual inspection and assessment of wound healing.

Although many of these agents are widely used as first-line wound care in uninfected burns in addition to their role in the treatment of established colonization or infection, evidence supporting the use of prophylactic topical antibiotics is limited. Although silver sulfadiazine may be considered the drug of choice for prophylaxis [18], Storm-Versloot *et al.* and Barajas-Nava *et al.* suggest that there is insufficient evidence for using silver-containing agents in preventing infection [19, 20]. The potential to increase multidrug-resistant organisms by liberal use of antimicrobial ointments in non-infected patients is a concern, and an area that deserves further study.

VAP, as soon as suspected with high certainty, will require empiric systemic antimicrobial therapy and immediate acquisition of cultures of involved organisms via bronchial lavage. Empiric therapy is directed primarily toward gram-negative organisms such as *Acinetobacter* and *Pseudomonas* spp. as well as methicillin-resistant staphylococcal organisms. Single-agent coverage is considered adequate first-line therapy for each organism, as multiple agent coverage has not been shown to be more effective and is only more likely to compound medication side effects [21]. Vancomycin and linezolid are each an appropriate choice for resistant *Staphylococcus* coverage, bearing in mind that daptomycin, another agent used for MRSA in the ICU setting, does not have lung penetration. Tigecycline will provide broad spectrum coverage including MRSA but has no pseudomonal coverage. A beta lactam-beta lactamase inhibitor combination will cover most gram negative organisms as well as gram positives; piperacillin-tazobactam is commonly used and has retained efficacy without significant resistance in most organisms despite many years of use. Aminoglycosides can also be used in combination with stronger gram positive agents. Carbapenems are considered first-line agents for *Acinetobacter* infections and also provide good broad-spectrum coverage; however, resistant *Acinetobacter* strains may be more susceptible to aminoglycosides or polymyxins. While there are many options as demonstrated above, we would like to reiterate that there is no substitute for carefully chosen empiric coverage based on the most prevalent organisms in a particular burn unit, and based on susceptibilities from the local antibiogram. Many units use antibiotics on a rotational schedule, whereby single-antimicrobial coverage is maintained while periodically varying the drug of choice. This has been shown to slow the evolution of drug-resistant mutations in microbial species while avoiding toxicities associated with prolonged use of a single agent [22].

In cases of CLABSI, the first step in treatment is to remove the catheter, reevaluate its necessity, and choose a new site if it is deemed essential. Cultures are to be drawn thrice from blood and also from the tip of the removed catheter device, and empiric therapy then initiated while awaiting sensitivity results. Since the primary organisms causal of CLABSI are expected to be gram positive cocci, MRSA, and *enterococci*, initial antimicrobial therapies are directed toward these organisms. Either vancomycin or daptomycin are appropriate single-agent bactericidal therapies for the most likely species. Linezolid has the benefit of an oral formulation; however, it is bacteriostatic rather than bactericidal. Patients who have been in the burn unit for an extended period or have other primary foci of infection are also at risk for gram negative bacteremia, which is associated with a higher mortality [3]. In these cases, empiric coverage should include gram negative agents as discussed in the section on VAP above. The most probable pathogens involved in nosocomial UTI are the same as those for the other nosocomial infections described above, with a higher incidence of gram negative organisms; steps to coverage should proceed in similar fashion.

In any of the types of infections described above, after the return of culture and sensitivity results, initial antimicrobial therapy should be either continued, escalated (with expanded coverage), or narrowed (with more specific coverage) accordingly. In choice of antimicrobial agents, the most specific coverage should always be used, with additional consideration for side effect profiles in the patient at hand, in order to minimize the development of resistant strains. If a patient with VAP proves to be a non-responder to drug therapy, one must begin to suspect empyema, intrapulmonary abscess, or other persistent collection of organisms. If other signs of resistance are encountered, repeat cultures may be in order as well as a diligent search for an additional site of infection.

Sepsis

Definitions of Sepsis and Septic Shock

Sepsis and septic shock are discussed here; the terms "SIRS" and "severe sepsis" are no longer used to describe burn patients for reasons specified by the ABA Consensus [2].

Sepsis is defined broadly as any "change in the burn patient that triggers concern for infection" [2]. Clinically, a septic patient may be recognized by symptoms such as hyperthermia, altered mental status, tachypnea, hyperglycemia, thrombocytopenia [23], and intolerance of enteral feeds [24]. The criteria for sepsis, in both burn and non-burn patients, are outlined in Table 7.2. Note that in the case of burns, it is imperative that an infection be present, since similar symptoms may be seen in virtually all severe burn patients and therefore must be attributable to an infection before sepsis may be diagnosed. As burn patients become hypermetabolic, their set points for respiration, heart rate, and temperature all become elevated, which is accounted for by the increased cutoffs for diagnosis. Sepsis mortality has been declining in the USA for all organisms [2]; however, sepsis and multiple organ dysfunction syndrome (MODS), which results therefrom, are still the two leading causes of morbidity and mortality in burn patients [25].

Table 7.2 Diagnosis of burn sepsis [2]

	Standard sepsis	Burn sepsis (adult)
Definition	*Two* of the following plus infection:	*Three* of the following plus documented infection:
Temperature	<36 °C >38.3 °C	<36.5 °C >39 °C
Heart rate	>90 BPM	>110 BPM
Respiratory rate	>20 BrPM	>25 BrPM (non-ventilated)
Blood cell counts	WBC <4 k/μl WBC >12 k/μl	Platelets <100 k/μl
Other criteria:	–	Hyperglycemia (absent DM): GLC >200 mg/dl
–	–	Insulin resistance: >7 units/h or >25 % increase in insulin requirements
–	–	Enteral feeding intolerance: residual equal to two times feeding rate
–	–	Uncontrolled diarrhea: >2500 ml/day

BPM: beats per minute, *BrPM:* breaths per minute, *WBC:* white blood cells, *DM:* diabetes mellitus, *GLC:* glucose

Sepsis can progress to septic shock, defined as sepsis in the presence of shock-like hemodynamic parameters. Clinically, it is defined as refractory hypotension despite volume resuscitation of 30 ml/kg of crystalloid [26]. Because septic shock has such a poor prognosis overall and is associated with a high mortality, early diagnosis is imperative [27]. Once diagnosed, source control, resuscitation, and appropriate antibiotic treatment are necessary, as improper or delayed treatment of septic shock has been consistently shown to result in poor outcomes [28].

Pathophysiology of Sepsis

The pathophysiology of sepsis in burn patients is important to understand in order to comprehend and treat sepsis and septic shock properly. This chapter, however, does not attempt to cover the entirety of a vast and ever-expanding body of knowledge on this topic, but rather only touches on concepts sufficient for our purpose here.

The first step in the pathophysiology begins with an inciting event. Here specifically the inciting even is a superimposed infection on a thermal, electrical, or chemical burn, which causes an acute release of pro-inflammatory cytokines, most notably interleukin-1 (IL-1), interleukin-6 (IL-6), and tumor necrosis factor-α (TNF-α). The release of TNF-α is predominantly mediated by transcription factor nuclear factor kappa-light-chain-enhancer of activated B cells (NF-κB), which also mediates the transcription of many other cytokines [29]. TNF-α may act locally and cause inflammation and tissue damage as well as systemically causing fever, vasodilation, further release of cytokines, and mounting of the acute phase response. IL-6 is the most notable mediator of the acute phase response, leading to amplification of inflammation as well as activation of the coagulation cascade, which may lead in turn to hypovolemia and interstitial edema. All of this can result in hypoxic organ damage, which is why adequate fluid resuscitation is imperative in treating septic patients. To counter, the host also mounts an anti-inflammatory response to suppress the pro-inflammatory mediators caused by infection and burn damage. Theoretically, promoting anti-inflammatory effects should suppress the progressively devastating effects of sepsis; however, exogenous modulation of these pathways has yet to be proven beneficial [29].

Measures of cytokine expression, however, have not been shown effective predictors of outcome. The two most commonly used predictors of sepsis outcome are procalcitonin (PCT) and C-reactive protein (CRP). Although some studies have shown the utility of procalcitonin [30–32], other studies have shown the opposite [33, 34]. Lavrentieva *et al.* show that daily consecutive measurements of PCT can be more valuable than those of CRP in following antibiotic effectiveness [32], but Jeschke *et al.* suggest that CRP may not be a predictor of sepsis [35]. Paratz *et al.* suggest a new marker, N-terminal pro-B-type natriuretic peptide (NT-proBNP), which may be superior to PCT in early detection of sepsis [33]. This novel marker may be important for scenarios in which early diagnosis is imperative (liver failure, transplant, and chronic renal replacement therapy patients), but is to be used with caution until further research validates this approach [36, 37].

Treatment

Broad-spectrum antimicrobial therapy should be initiated until blood culture and sensitivity results specify in which direction to narrow the scope of therapy. Physical exam findings such as hemodynamic parameters, cardiopulmonary exam, capillary refill time and responsiveness to passive leg raise can be augmented with quantitative measures such as central venous pressure (CVP), central venous oxygen saturation ($ScvO_2$) and bedside cardiovascular ultrasound. The patient should be assessed for the need for resuscitation as well. Assessment of fluid responsiveness can be performed with a 500 ml fluid bolus challenge. If fluid responsiveness is poor, or if there are signs of persistent hypotension or MAP <65 mmHg, pressors such as norepinephrine should be administered. Serum lactate and base deficit are commonly used parameters to monitor the success of resuscitative measures.

Intravenous empiric antimicrobial therapy should be given within the first hour of sepsis diagnosis, ensuring the coverage of all susceptible organisms. In addition to the empiric coverage of gram-positive and -negative organisms discussed in the previous section, empiric coverage against fungal infection may also be considered. Fluconazole may be used at a higher dose as a first-line agent; if there is a significant prevalence of non-albicans *Candida* species then an agent with extended coverage such as micafungin, caspofungin, or voriconazole may be used. Voriconazole is also first line therapy for aspergillosis; however, this is an uncommon infection and would not routinely be included in initiating empiric coverage. Patients with sepsis caused by *P. aeruginosa* should be given an extended-spectrum beta-lactam and either an aminoglycoside or a fluoroquinolone. Monotherapy with an aminoglycoside for *P. aeruginosa* sepsis should be avoided. Patients with *S. pneumoniae* infection should be given a beta-lactam and macrolide, and therapy should last 7–10 days for most patients. If the patient has neutropenia, immunologic deficiencies, or is slow to respond to therapy, a longer course of treatment may be necessary. Finally, source control is imperative for the treatment of sepsis and septic shock. If an intravascular device is the suspected as the source of infection, it should be removed. If the burn wound itself is the source, then this should be debrided to healthy tissue. On occasion, patients with major burns (especially with electrical injury) will develop intra-abdominal complications such intestinal perforation, which can manifest as occult sources of sepsis.

Conclusion

Infection remains a significant clinical problem in burn patients, representing an opportunity for health care professionals to improve outcomes and reduce mortality with timely and appropriate treatment. Recognizing the unique definition and presentation of infection in burn patients compared to all other populations ensures appropriate treatment while minimizing the drawbacks of overtreatment. The prevalence of MDR organisms present one of the most challenging aspects of work in this field, which will continue to evolve over ensuing decades.

Common Multidrug-Resistant Organisms in Burn Infections

Acinetobacter baumanii
Pseudomonas aeruginosa
Klebsiella pneumoniae
Methicillin-resistant *Staphylococcus aureus* (MRSA)

References

1. Bessey PQ, Phillips BD, Lentz CW, Edelman LS, Faraklas I, Finocchiaro MA, et al. Synopsis of the 2013 annual report of the national burn repository. J Burn Care Res. 2014;35 Suppl 2:S218–34.
2. Greenhalgh DG, Saffle JR, Holmes 4th JH, Gamelli RL, Palmieri TL, Horton JW, et al. American Burn Association consensus conference to define sepsis and infection in burns. J Burn Care Res. 2007;28(6):776–90.
3. Ani C, Farshidpanah S, Bellinghausen Stewart A, Nguyen HB. Variations in organism-specific severe sepsis mortality in the United States: 1999-2008. Crit Care Med. 2015;43(1):65–77.
4. Weber DJ, van Duin D, DiBiase LM, Hultman CS, Jones SW, Lachiewicz AM, et al. Healthcare-associated infections among patients in a large burn intensive care unit: incidence and pathogens, 2008-2012. Infect Control Hosp Epidemiol. 2014;35(10):1304–6.
5. Barbier F, Andremont A, Wolff M, Bouadma L. Hospital-acquired pneumonia and ventilator-associated pneumonia: recent advances in epidemiology and management. Curr Opin Pulm Med. 2013; 19(3):216–28.
6. Mosier MJ, Gamelli RL, Halerz MM, Silver G. Microbial contamination in burn patients undergoing urgent intubation as part of their early airway management. J Burn Care Res. 2008;29(2):304–10.
7. Luna CM, Bledel I, Raimondi A. The role of surveillance cultures in guiding ventilator-associated pneumonia therapy. Curr Opin Infect Dis. 2014;27(2): 184–93.
8. Diaz E, Munoz E, Agbaht K, Rello J. Management of ventilator-associated pneumonia caused by multiresistant bacteria. Curr Opin Crit Care. 2007;13(1): 45–50.
9. Karaiskos I, Giamarellou H. Multidrug-resistant and extensively drug-resistant Gram-negative pathogens: current and emerging therapeutic approaches. Expert Opin Pharmacother. 2014;15(10):1351–70.
10. Goutier JM, Holzmueller CG, Edwards KC, Klompas M, Speck K, Berenholtz SM. Strategies to enhance adoption of ventilator-associated pneumonia prevention interventions: a systematic literature review. Infect Control Hosp Epidemiol. 2014;35(8):998–1005.
11. Townsend CM, Beauchamp RD, Evers BM, Mattox KL, editors. Sabiston textbook of surgery: the biological basis of modern surgical practice. 19th ed. Philadelphia, PA: Elsevier Saunders; 2012.
12. O'Grady NP, Alexander M, Burns LA, Dellinger EP, Garland J, Heard SO, et al. Guidelines for the prevention of intravascular catheter-related infections. Clin Infect Dis. 2011;52(9):e162–93.
13. Pronovost P. Interventions to decrease catheter-related bloodstream infections in the ICU: the Keystone

Intensive Care Unit Project. Am J Infect Control. 2008;36(10):S171.e1–5.
14. Miller RS, Norris PR, Jenkins JM, Talbot 3rd TR, Starmer JM, Hutchison SA, et al. Systems initiatives reduce healthcare-associated infections: a study of 22,928 device days in a single trauma unit. J Trauma. 2010;68(1):23–31.
15. Venable A, Dissanaike S. Is automated electronic surveillance for healthcare-associated infections accurate in the burn unit? J Burn Care Res. 2013;34(6):591–7.
16. Kagan RJ, Neely AN, Rieman MT, Hardy A, Warner P, Bailey JK, et al. A performance improvement initiative to determine the impact of increasing the time interval between changing centrally placed intravascular catheters. J Burn Care Res. 2014;35(2):143–7.
17. Sacks GD, Diggs BS, Hadjizacharia P, Green D, Salim A, Malinoski DJ. Reducing the rate of catheter-associated bloodstream infections in a surgical intensive care unit using the Institute for Healthcare Improvement Central Line Bundle. Am J Surg. 2014;207(6):817–23.
18. Ungureanu M. Concepts in local treatment of extensive paediatric burns. J Med Life. 2014;7(2):183–91.
19. Storm-Versloot MN, Vos CG, Ubbink DT, Vermeulen H. Topical silver for preventing wound infection. Cochrane Database Syst Rev. 2010;3:CD006478.
20. Barajas-Nava LA, Lopez-Alcalde J, Roque i Figuls M, Sola I, Bonfill Cosp X. Antibiotic prophylaxis for preventing burn wound infection. Cochrane Database Syst Rev. 2013;6:CD008738.
21. Paul M, Benuri-Silbiger I, Soares-Weiser K, Leibovici L. Beta lactam monotherapy versus beta lactam-aminoglycoside combination therapy for sepsis in immunocompetent patients: systematic review and meta-analysis of randomised trials. BMJ. 2004;328(7441):668.
22. Kim S, Lieberman TD, Kishony R. Alternating antibiotic treatments constrain evolutionary paths to multidrug resistance. Proc Natl Acad Sci U S A. 2014;111(40):14494–9.
23. Housinger TA, Brinkerhoff C, Warden GD. The relationship between platelet count, sepsis, and survival in pediatric burn patients. Arch Surg. 1993;128(1):65–6. discussion 66–7.
24. Wolf SE, Jeschke MG, Rose JK, Desai MH, Herndon DN. Enteral feeding intolerance: an indicator of sepsis-associated mortality in burned children. Arch Surg. 1997;132(12):1310–3. discussion 1313–4.
25. Dellinger RP, Carlet JM, Masur H, Gerlach H, Calandra T, Cohen J, et al. Surviving Sepsis Campaign guidelines for management of severe sepsis and septic shock. Crit Care Med. 2004;32(3):858–73.
26. Dellinger RP, Levy MM, Rhodes A, Annane D, Gerlach H, Opal SM, et al. Surviving Sepsis Campaign: international guidelines for management of severe sepsis and septic shock, 2012. Intensive Care Med. 2013;39(2):165–228.
27. Harrison DA, Welch CA, Eddleston JM. The epidemiology of severe sepsis in England, Wales and Northern Ireland, 1996 to 2004: secondary analysis of a high quality clinical database, the ICNARC Case Mix Programme Database. Crit Care. 2006;10(2):R42.
28. Vazquez-Guillamet C, Scolari M, Zilberberg MD, Shorr AF, Micek ST, Kollef M. Using the number needed to treat to assess appropriate antimicrobial therapy as a determinant of outcome in severe sepsis and septic shock. Crit Care Med. 2014;42(11):2342–9.
29. Herndon DN. Total burn care. 4th ed. Philadelphia, PA: Elsevier Saunders; 2012.
30. Mann EA, Wood GL, Wade CE. Use of procalcitonin for the detection of sepsis in the critically ill burn patient: a systematic review of the literature. Burns. 2011;37(4):549–58.
31. Barati M, Alinejad F, Bahar MA, Tabrisi MS, Shamshiri AR, Bodouhi NO, et al. Comparison of WBC, ESR, CRP and PCT serum levels in septic and non-septic burn cases. Burns. 2008;34(6):770–4.
32. Lavrentieva A, Papadopoulou S, Kioumis J, Kaimakamis E, Bitzani M. PCT as a diagnostic and prognostic tool in burn patients. Whether time course has a role in monitoring sepsis treatment. Burns. 2012;38(3):356–63.
33. Paratz JD, Lipman J, Boots RJ, Muller MJ, Paterson DL. A new marker of sepsis post burn injury?*. Crit Care Med. 2014;42(9):2029–36.
34. Bargues L, Chancerelle Y, Catineau J, Jault P, Carsin H. Evaluation of serum procalcitonin concentration in the ICU following severe burn. Burns. 2007;33(7):860–4.
35. Jeschke MG, Finnerty CC, Kulp GA, Kraft R, Herndon DN. Can we use C-reactive protein levels to predict severe infection or sepsis in severely burned patients? Int J Burns Trauma. 2013;3(3):137–43.
36. Rousseau AF, Layios N. Serum markers of sepsis in burn patients: it takes more to convince! Crit Care Med. 2015;43(3):e100–1.
37. Honore PM, Jacobs R, De Waele E, Spapen HD. Biomarkers to detect sepsis: a "burning" issue but still a long way to go*. Crit Care Med. 2014;42(9):2137–8.

Wound Healing

8

David G. Greenhalgh

Introduction

Burns are the most extensive wounds that anyone will face. Whether the burn is massive or small, simple principles of wound healing apply to close the wound. The goal of any caregiver is to heal any wound as rapidly as possible while minimizing the extent of scar formation. There are several basic principles to optimize healing. The first principle is that optimizing the healing process the "first time" leads to a better outcome. If one believes that delaying the healing process and then hoping for some form of reconstructive surgery will optimize the ultimate outcome, then he/she will be greatly disappointed. A second principle is that if a wound heals within 2–3 weeks, then scarring is minimized. As described in the 1970s [1], the likelihood of developing hypertrophic scarring is greatly increased if it remains open for 2–3 weeks. As an example, this child suffered a typical scald burn to the chest (Fig. 8.1). All areas healed within 2 weeks except for the site on the upper chest where healing occurred in 3 weeks. All of the areas that healed before 2 weeks are perfectly flat, but the area of delayed closure developed significant hypertrophic scarring. Even more discouraging is the fact that after excising and closing the scar, it recurred. Some unknown "signal" in the wound at 2–3 weeks directs the cells to produce an excessive amount of scar. The "signal" that dictates this delayed and excessive scar formation is not known, but it is clear that the goal of treating a wound is to have it re-epithelialize within that 2–3 weeks period. If it will not re-epithelialize in 2 weeks, then consideration for grafting (which will be covered in the next chapter) is indicated. The goal of this chapter is to provide the basic principles of wound healing to allow the caregiver to develop a strategy for more rapid wound closure that will lead to a better chance for minimizing scar formation.

Severity of Burn Injury

How well a burn heals depends on the severity of injury. Clearly, superficial and small wounds do well no matter what we do to them. Very deep burns are much more difficult to manage and lead to more scarring. Severity is not only dependent upon depth, but also on the size of the burn injury. Clearly, a patient with 90 % total body surface area (TBSA) full-thickness burns is going to have a greater challenge to heal his/her wounds. As a wound becomes massive, the "burden" of the injury tends to slow the healing process as the

D.G. Greenhalgh, M.D. (✉)
Shriners Hospitals for Children Northern California
University of California, Davis Medical Center,
2425 Stockton Boulevard, Sacramento, CA 95817, USA
e-mail: dggreenhalgh@ucdavis.edu

D.G. Greenhalgh (ed.), *Burn Care for General Surgeons and General Practitioners*,
DOI 10.1007/978-3-319-29161-1_8

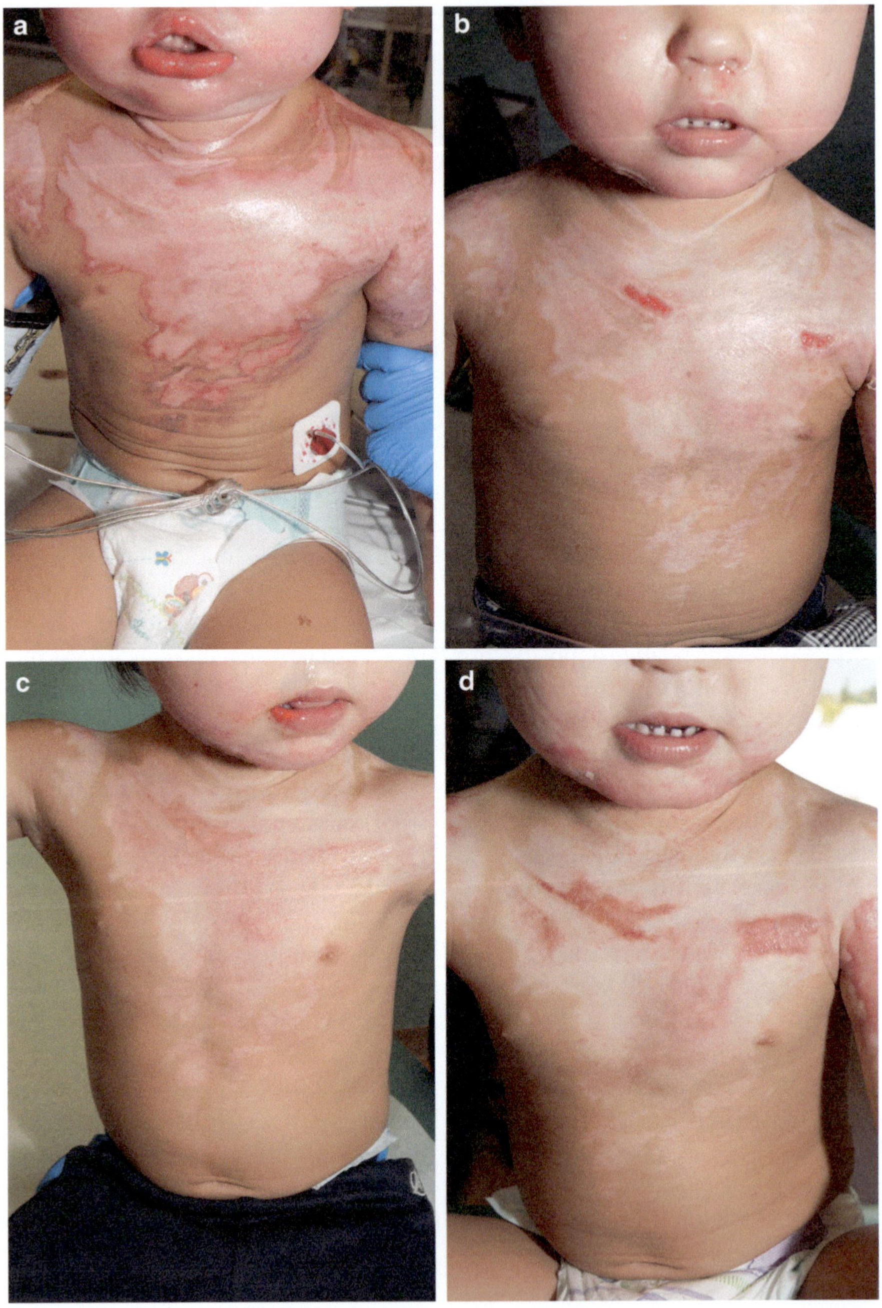

Fig. 8.1 This is a typical accidental scald burn for this child (**a**). The lower areas healed in less than 2 weeks, but there remained a couple of open areas that were open at 18 days (**b**). At 6 weeks, there are signs of hypertrophic scarring (**c**) that eventually became hypertrophic (**d**). The "signal" tying delayed epithelialization and hypertrophic scarring is unknown

"supplies" needed for repair become more limited. The stress of the massive injury and the need to develop a "defense" against the invading organisms also make healing more challenging.

Burn depth has traditionally been divided into first-, second-, third-, and fourth-degree injuries. These categories are based on how deeply the injury penetrates the skin and subcutaneous tissue. In simple terms, skin is divided into the outer "epidermis," which acts as a barrier, and the "dermis," which provides the strength of skin (Fig. 8.2). The skin covers the subcutaneous adipose tissue and the fat overlies the fascia, muscle, tendons, and bone. Depending on the depth of the burn, different strategies exist to close that injury with the least possible scarring.

The epidermis has several layers of cells (Fig. 8.3). The bottom layer of epithelial cells (called keratinocytes) is the "basal cell layer." These basal cells are the only keratinocytes with the potential for growth and migration. They are the cells that re-epithelialize any wound in the skin. During their lifespan, the basal cells eventually differentiate and migrate towards the surface to form the stratum spinosa and eventually produce keratin. The migration starts with undifferentiated basal cells at the basement membrane to fully differentiated keratin-containing mature cells toward the surface. They eventually undergo apoptosis (programmed cell death) to form the

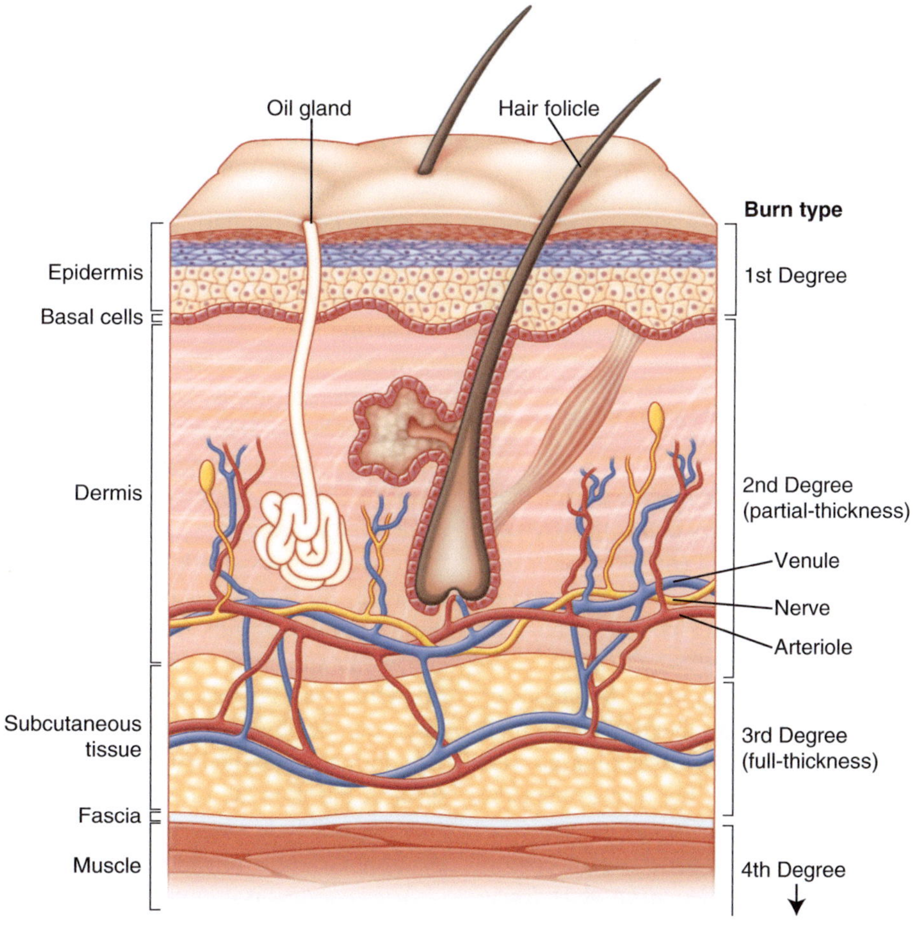

Fig. 8.2 In normal skin, the epidermis makes up the most superficial layer. It keeps fluid from escaping and prevents bacterial invasion. Any burn that does not penetrate the epithelium is called a *first-degree burn*. First-degree burns are dry since the epithelium maintains its barrier function. Any burn that penetrates into but not through the dermis is called a *second-degree or partial-thickness burn*. Since the barrier function of the epithelium is lost, it weeps fluid. Since the dermis has a plexus of nerves and blood vessels, it is painful and blanches with pressure. If the burn progresses through the dermis and into the subcutaneous fat, it is called a *third-degree or full-thickness burn*. Since the dermal plexus of blood vessels and nerves are destroyed, the burn does not blanch and there is less pain than for a second-degree burn. If a burn penetrates to the muscle, bone, or tendon, it is called a *fourth-degree burn*

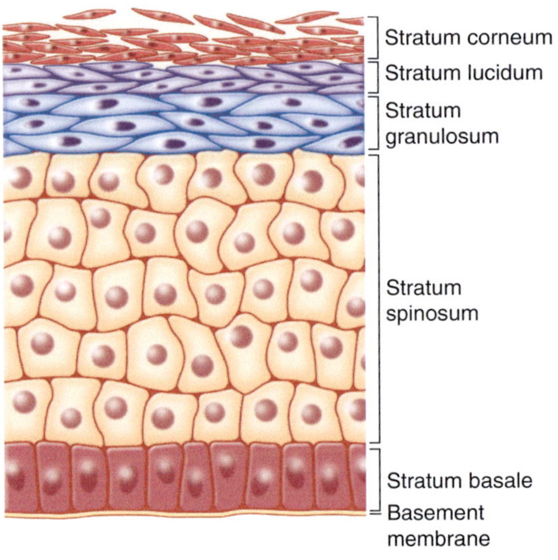

Fig. 8.3 *Epithelium anatomy*. The epithelium is classically divided into five layers. The bottom layer is the *stratum basale* or basal cell layer. This layer attaches to the basement membrane and is the least differentiated layer of the epidermis. This layer has the potential for migration and proliferation. The second layer is called the *stratum spinosum* where the cells start to differentiate but are still viable. The third layer is the *stratum granulosum* and the fourth layer is the *stratum lucidum*. The most superficial layer, called the *stratum corneum,* consists of several layers of dying and dead flattened cells that eventually flake off

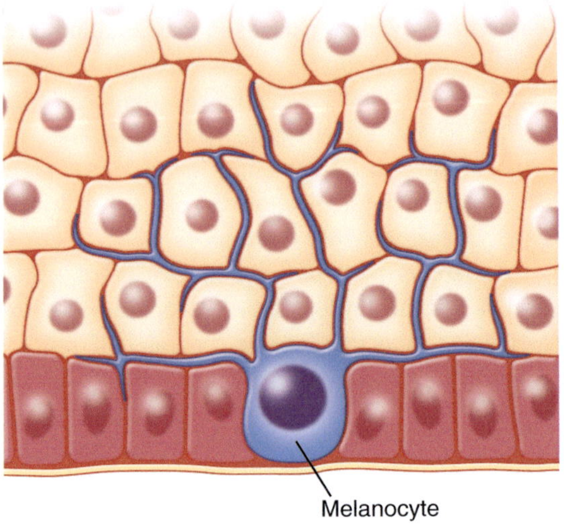

Fig. 8.4 Melanocytes live in the basal layer of the epidermis and spread dendrites to dozens of keratinocytes. These dendrites deliver melanosomes containing melanin to the keratinocytes to create the pigmentation of skin

top layer where the keratinocytes dry up and flake off. These dead keratinocytes create the dry skin that is common to dandruff and other skin diseases. Much of the dust in houses is the result of these same dried cells. Interspersed among the basal cells are "melanocytes" which create melanin—the main pigment of skin. Melanocytes have multiple dendritic arms that deliver the melanin pigment to the lower layers of keratinocytes to not only create pigment, but also protect the nuclei of the lower levels of keratinocytes (Fig. 8.4). Any burn that does not penetrate the epidermis is considered "first degree" (Fig. 8.5). Since the epidermis acts as a barrier to keep the moisture in and keep the bacteria out, all first-degree burns are dry, red, and painful. The pigment is maintained since the melanocytes are not destroyed. The epidermis contains other immune cells such as Langerhans cells and dendritic cells.

The epidermis is attached to the dermis through a basement membrane that is made of type IV collagen and laminin. There are also "anchoring fibers" that are made of type VII collagen which increase the strength of the attachment of the epidermis. Damage or loss to any of these proteins tends to weaken the epithelial layer bond and leads to blistering diseases. For instance, Stevens-Johnson syndrome or toxic epidermal necrolysis syndrome (TENS) result from lymphocytes attacking the basement membrane [2, 3]. *Staphylococcus* scalded skin syndrome involves results from a toxin that attacks at a higher site in the basement membrane [4, 5]. Epidermolysis bullosa results from defects in anchoring fibrils including type VII collagen [6]. The dermal–epidermal junction is not a smooth surface, but is made of hills and valleys called "rete pegs." Rete pegs reduce the chances for shearing the epidermis in normal skin.

The "dermis" is dominated by type I collagen and produces the real "strength" of skin. Several other forms of extracellular matrix proteins also exist in the dermis. The dermis has a lower population of cells than the epidermis, but it is dominated by fibroblasts and immune cells. Recent studies suggest that fibroblasts of the deeper dermis are different from those of the more superficial fibroblasts [7, 8]. The hypothesis is

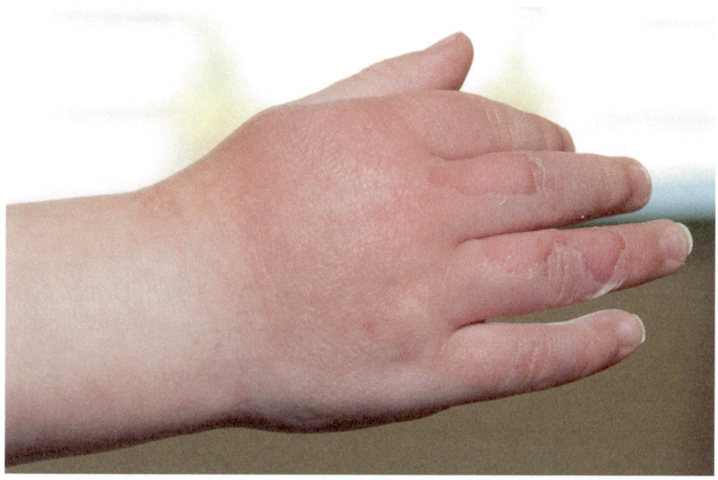

Fig. 8.5 A first-degree burn is observed on the hand that is red but dry since the epithelium remains viable. There is a small area of second-degree burn that is moist and red

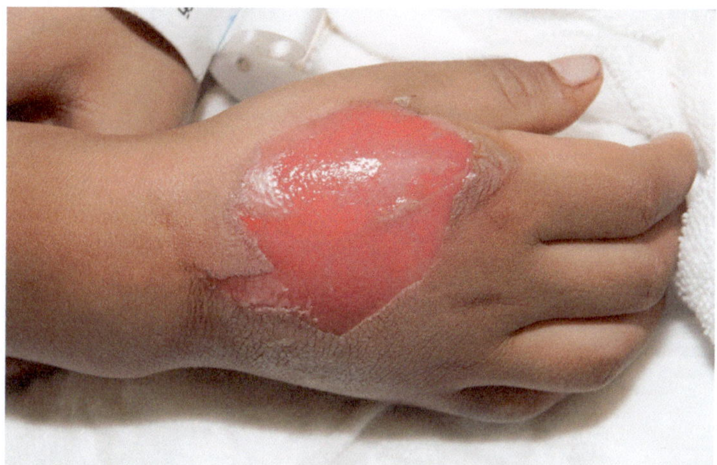

Fig. 8.6 A second-degree or partial-thickness burn is *red*, weeping and blanches with pressure

that the deeper cells contribute more to the formation of excessive scar formation than the more superficial ones. The dermis contains a plexus of capillaries and nerves that provide sensation (pain with exposure) and redness that blanches with pressure. Any second-degree burn or any injury that destroys the protective epidermal barrier leads to a weeping wound (Fig. 8.6). The fluid that leaks is essentially extracellular fluid and leaking serum. If the wound is exposed to air, the fluid dries to form a "scab" that consists of fibrin and other debris. Exposure of the plexus of nerves leads to severe "burning" pain, and since the vascular supply is intact, the wounds blanch with pressure. Blisters are also typical of these "partial-thickness" burns. Some people divide "partial-thickness" burns into "superficial" and "deep" burns. The superficial burns are those that heal within 2–3 weeks and the deep partial-thickness burns are those that heal over a longer period and thus are at risk for hypertrophic scarring. The dermis also contains numerous skin "adnexa" such as hair follicles, oil glands, sebaceous glands, and sweat glands. As will be discussed later, these skin adnexa are essential for re-epithelializing the wound.

A "third-degree" or "full-thickness" burn extends all the way through both the epidermis and dermis. These burns tend to be dry since they form an "eschar" that consists of coagulated

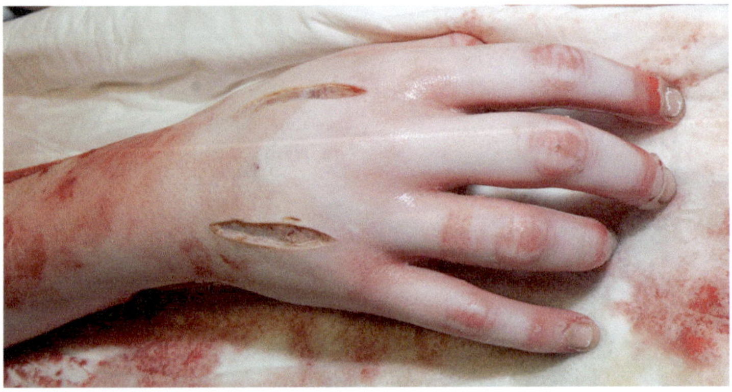

Fig. 8.7 Third-degree or full-thickness burns can be of multiple colors, but they do not blanch since the dermal plexus of blood vessels in the dermis are destroyed. This burn is white and does not blanch

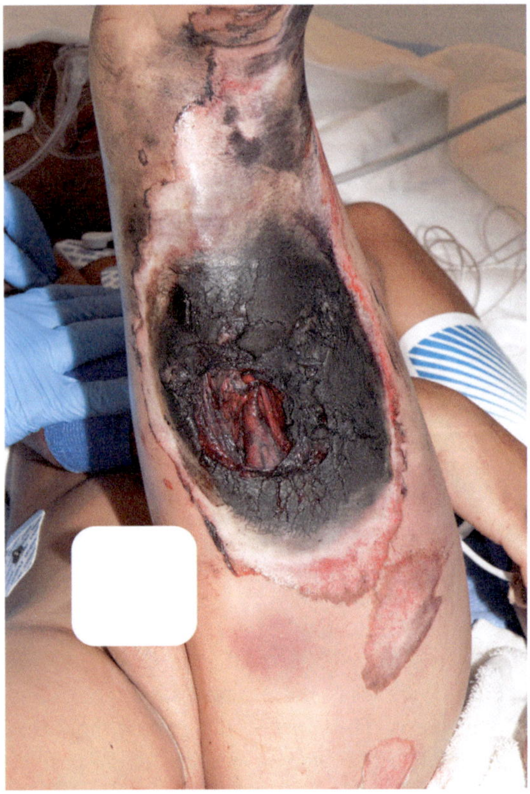

Fig. 8.8 Fourth-degree burns penetrate down to muscle. This deep contact burn was the result of prolonged contact with a hot item. The exposed muscle is easy to observe

proteins from the destroyed tissue. Since the dermal plexus of nerves and vessels are destroyed, the wound no longer blanches and has less pain, especially to exposure or touch. Full-thickness burns can be white, red, yellow, or black (Fig. 8.7). Third-degree burns also tend to be inelastic and thus will not stretch when the underlying tissues continue to swell. Therefore, circumferential, full-thickness burns often need to be released through escharotomies ("cuts through the eschar"). These wounds are usually treated with skin grafts.

A "fourth-degree" burn is one that involves any structure deeper than the subcutaneous fat. These burns involve fascia, muscle, bone, tendons, or deeper (Fig. 8.8). These wounds will not "take" a skin graft and thus need to be covered with different techniques such as flaps.

Basics of Wound Healing

Wound healing can be divided into three main forms—scar formation (recreation of the dermis), re-epithelialization (recreation of the barrier), and contraction (shrinking the wound). While the chapter is focused on healing in the skin, these same principles apply to healing of any tissue in the body. Understanding the principles of healing will allow any surgeon to optimize tissue repair to not only close the wound expeditiously, but also to minimize wounds that fail to heal or those that produce excessive scar.

Scar Formation

Traditionally, scar formation is divided into three phases—inflammatory (lag) phase, proliferative (collagen) phase, and maturation phase. These

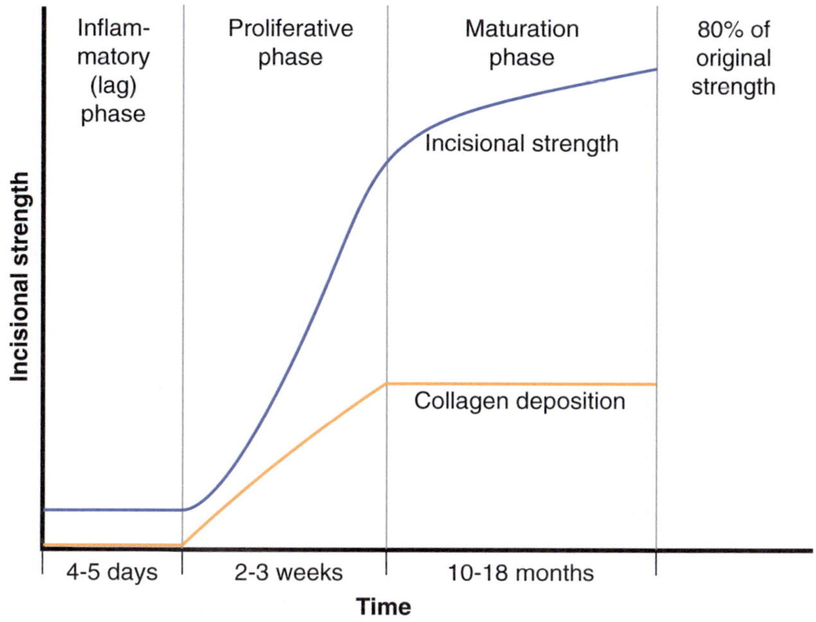

Fig. 8.9 For an incision, incisional strength can be plotted over time. The graph can be broken into three phases—the *inflammatory (or lag) phase* where there is little increase in wound strength, the *proliferative (or collagen) phase* where there is a rapid increase in incisional strength that correlates with an increase in collagen in the wound, and the *maturation phase* where the increase in strength continues without any change in the amount of collagen in the wound. In an incision, the inflammatory phase lasts 4–5 days, the proliferative phase lasts 2–3 weeks, and the maturation phase lasts 1–2 years

phases were originally described in studies that examined the breaking strength of an incision over time (Fig. 8.9). For the first 4–5 days, during the *inflammatory phase*, there is little increase in incisional strength (thus the alternative name - "lag" phase), which is why stitches are used for immediate closure. Fibrin may provide some adhesion but it is very ineffective. During this time, an inflammatory response is initiated, but there is no increase in extracellular matrix proteins. At around 5 days, the *proliferative phase* starts. During this phase, there is a rapid increase in strength as collagen and other extracellular proteins are deposited in increased concentrations. For an incision that is closed primarily, this proliferative phase lasts for 3–4 weeks. After that time, there is a prolonged *maturation phase* where there is no increase in collagen formation, but the breaking strength still continues to increase so that the incision has regained approximately 80 % of the original strength of skin. The maturation phase lasts for 12–18 months. Over the last several decades, a great deal has been learned about cellular processes and signaling that are involved in each one of these phases.

The *inflammatory phase* involves the signals that start the normal inflammatory response of an injury. Injury is detected by many cellular signals. Local nerves that initiate pain detect injury. All tissues have "sentinel" macrophages whose role is to detect any perturbations in the environment and respond to regain homeostasis [9]. They detect signals from pathogens or tissue damage through receptors called "pattern recognition receptors" (PRRs). For pathogens, they detect "pathogen-associated molecular patterns" (PAMPs), which are bacterial and viral products through these receptors. When cells are damaged, they release "damage-associated molecular patterns" (DAMPs). If there are just a few bacteria, the sentinel macrophages phagocytize them and the process stops. As there is more damage or pathogen invasion, the activation of the PAMPs leads to complex signaling to produce mediators that assist with the inflammatory response. The classic example is from lipopolysaccharide (LPS) of gram negative bacteria that binds to Toll-like Receptor-4 (TLR-4), which then initiates a complex signaling pathway through "nuclear factor-κB" (NF-κB) which then leads to production of many "cytokines" such as tumor necrosis factor-α (TNF-α), interleukin-1 (IL-1), and interleukin-6 (IL-6). For viral infections, foreign DNA or RNA is detected by other cytoplasmic PRRs. For cellular damage, the classic DAMP is the expelled mitochondria since these organelles originally evolved from bacteria.

These cytokines (there are hundreds) released by the sentinel macrophages diffuse into the local blood supply and are detected by the endothelial cells of the nearby vessels to induce activation of "adhesion" molecules that make the capillaries "sticky" for inflammatory cells. Inflammatory cells and other cells migrate towards the inflammatory signals (by *chemotaxis*) and are activated to produce adhesion molecules to adhere to the capillaries and venules near the site of injury and then enter (by *diapedesis*) into the site of injury. The inflammatory cells then assist with the destruction of pathogens in preparation for healing. To assist with this process, local cells release histamine and serotonin (plus other proteins—leukotrienes, cyclooxygenases) to cause vasodilation and increased permeability, which we know as the "edema" of injury.

Another initiator of these inflammatory signals occurs when cells in one compartment invade a "foreign" compartment. The classic example occurs when cells within blood vessels suddenly leak out and contact the proteins outside the vessel. Platelets inside the blood vessel are "content" until they are exposed to the damaged surroundings such as type I collagen. When contacting "foreign" proteins, they adhere and release their alpha granules, which contain many signals, especially "growth factors" that initiate the healing process. Growth factors are proteins released from one cell that stimulate migration and growth of other cells. The alpha granules contain, among many others, two important growth factors involved in tissue repair—platelet-derived growth factor (PDGF) and transforming growth factor-β (TGF-β). These growth factors attract both inflammatory cells and fibroblasts into the wound. Products of clotting, such as thrombin and fibrin, also act to attract cells required for healing. Finally, the compliment components C3a and C5a initiate the inflammatory response. These local processes are the major initial activity of the inflammatory phase. As is covered in Chap. 7, the same process when driven to excess leads to sepsis and if uncontrolled—"multiple organ dysfunction syndrome," which often ends in the patient's death.

Many studies from the past determined that many inflammatory cells have little role in the actual healing process. Neutrophils are essential for fighting infection, but healing proceeds normally in their absence [10]. Subsequent studies clearly demonstrated that macrophages are the main orchestrators of the healing process [11]. It is not clear whether the resident "sentinel" macrophages or migrating monocytes play this regulatory role, but is likely that both populations of macrophages are involved. The inflammatory response continues in any open wound until it has closed, but the arrival of the fibroblast starts the next phase of scar formation.

The next phase, the *proliferative phase,* involves two activities, the deposition of an extracellular matrix between wound edges and the development of a new blood supply to the wound (angiogenesis and vasculogenesis). Several growth factors, including PDGF and TGF-β, attract fibroblasts into the wound. Once they are present, fibroblasts produce collagen and other extracellular matrix proteins. The main strength of the wound is derived from collagen, which has a very complex biochemical pathway. All collagens consist of repeats of the amino acid triplets glycine, X and Y, where "X" is frequently proline and "Y" is either a proline or lysine that are hydroxylated to add a hydroxyl (–OH) group. The enzyme that hydroxylates proline or lysine is called "prolyl hydroxylase" or "lysyl hydroxylase." This step, which requires vitamin C, is required to produce the triple helix that produces the chains procollagen. If this step fails, such as in the vitamin C deficiency disease *scurvy,* collagen fails to form. Another essential step involves an enzyme called "lysyl oxidase," which creates intermolecular cross-links between collagen molecules. Failure to complete this step leads to impaired healing diseases such as "lathyrism." The rapid increase in collagen continues for 2–3 weeks in an incision and then there becomes a balance between collagen synthesis and breakdown that is the start of the maturation phase of healing.

The second component of the proliferative phase is the creation of a new blood supply. In essence, without nutrients, fibroblasts are unable to complete their job. The main form of blood vessel repair outside the embryo is called *angiogenesis* (Fig. 8.10). The signals that regulate angiogenesis are well-known [12, 13]. Resident macrophages can tolerate a relatively hypoxic environment. When oxygen is deficient, hypoxia-inducible factor-1 and -2 (HIF-1, HIF-2) is produced by the macrophages [14, 15]. These proteins stimulate the production of specific growth factors that stimulate angiogenesis. The two key growth factors that directly stimulate angiogenesis are fibroblast growth factor-2 (FGF-2, also known as basic fibroblast growth factor [bFGF]) and vascular endothelial growth factor (VEGF). Endothelial cells of post-capillary venules detect these angiogenic factors and release collagenases that digest the endothelial cell basement membrane. The endothelial cells

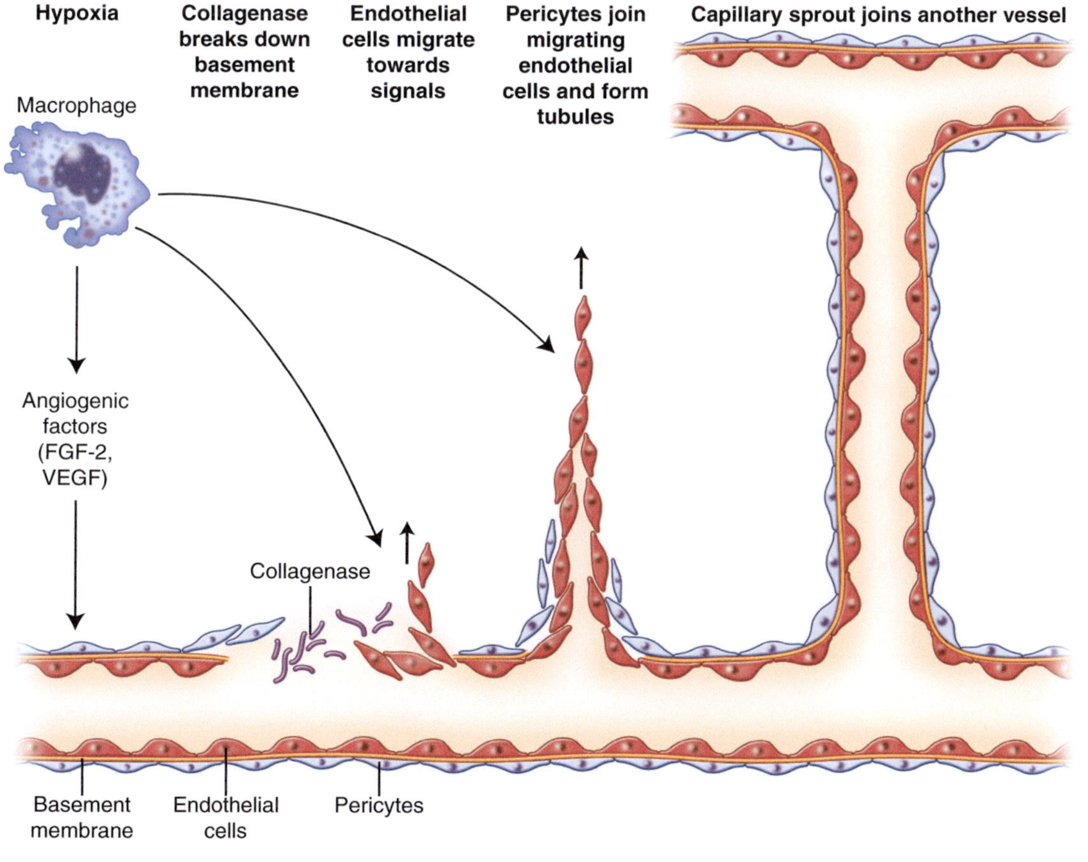

Fig. 8.10 *Angiogenesis*. A hypoxic environment stimulates macrophages to produce angiogenic factors such as fibroblast growth factor-2 (FGF-2) and vascular endothelial growth factor (VEGF). When the endothelial cells detect the angiogenic factors, they release collagenases to digest away the venule basement membrane and they migrate towards the angiogenic stimuli. The migrating cells eventually form tubules and local pericytes cover the new capillary. Eventually, they "hook" into other vessels to create a new blood supply

then migrate towards the angiogenic signal, form tubules, and join other vessels in the hypoxic environment. Other growth factors stimulate the pericytes that surround vessels to accompany the endothelial cells during their migration. The other method of blood vessel growth is called *vasculogenesis* where bone marrow-derived stem cells migrate to the wound to create new blood vessels. Vasculogenesis is very important during embryogenesis, but its role in wound healing is less clear.

The final phase of healing is called the *maturation phase*. During this phase, which can last up to 2 years, there is no increase in the amount of collagen in the wound, although wound strength continues to increase. In addition, there is a gradual resolution of inflammation and angiogenesis that results in a relatively avascular scar. The reason why there is no change in collagen content is that collagenases are induced to breakdown collagen at the same rate as collagen is synthesized. The wound continues to increase in strength because collagen is broken down in planes that do not require strength, while it is increased along lines of stress. At the same time, intercollagenous bonds are formed with the enzyme "lysyl oxidase" to further increase the strength of the incision. In normal healing, this balance leads to a wound that is 80 % as strong as the original tissue. Unfortunately, collagen synthesis and degradation may become unbalanced leading to pathologic healing. If there is decreased collagen synthesis relative to breakdown, such as with scurvy, lathyrism, or impaired blood supply, then chronic, nonhealing wounds result. If, on the other hand, the balance is shifted to produce too much collagen relative to collagen breakdown, hypertrophic scarring and fibrosis result. Once the balance between collagen synthesis and breakdown is altered, regaining the proper balance becomes very difficult. The treatment of excessive scar formation will be examined in greater detail in Chap. 20.

The previous description of scar formation really applies to the simple closure of an incision. Dealing with a larger wound, such as a burn, is significantly more complex. As long as the wound is exposed, all of the phases, including the inflammatory phase, persist (Fig. 8.11). There tends to be a blending of the phases so that on the exposed surface there is persistent inflammation. Beneath the exposed area, fibroblasts lay down collagen in an attempt to "wall off' the exposed

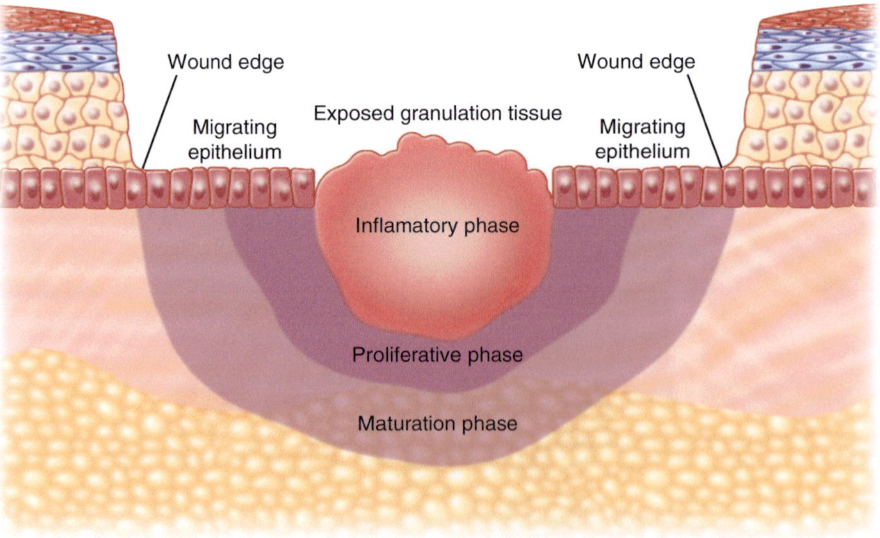

Fig. 8.11 In a wound that remains chronically open, all of the three phases of scar formation exist at the same time. The exposed tissue forms granulation tissue, which has some barrier function but not as much as a new epithelium

wound. At the edges, where the epithelium starts to migrate across the wound, there are signs of maturation. The red, moist tissue consisting of collagen, blood vessels, and inflammatory cells is known as "granulation tissue." Granulation tissue has some barrier function, but it is not as effective as a re-epithelialized wound.

A major role of the maturation phase is to "turn off" the processes of tissue repair. Several processes stop healing. First of all, eliminating exposure to the environment is required to stop the ongoing inflammatory stimuli. Therefore, eliminating exposure to the signals of pathogens (PAMPs) and damaged tissues (DAMPs) is required. The primary way to stop these inflammatory signals is to develop a new epithelium. It turns out that the epithelium releases signals that induce apoptosis (programmed cell death) in both inflammatory cells and fibroblasts [16, 17]. In addition, covering an open wound with a skin graft or flap induces apoptosis in the cells of tissue repair [18, 19]. Another factor that decreases the healing process is to eliminate tension in the wound. Tension is detected by fibroblasts and other cells, which in turn signal through the Rho pathway to produce more TGF-β1. TGF-β1 then stimulates more collagen production to "resist" the tension [20–22]. Releasing that tension, by simply performing a Z-plasty, will tend to slow down scar formation [23].

Re-epithelialization

The second form of healing involves recreating the *barrier* of skin—*re-epithelialization*. The bottom layer of the epithelium contains the "basal" cells that are the only keratinocytes that have the potential for epithelial growth. Normally, the basal cells are inhibited from proliferating by cell–cell contact inhibition. When juxtaposed, they differentiate and migrate to the surface to develop the multiple layers of the epithelium. Eventually, they undergo apoptosis (programmed cell death) to create the outer dead layer of skin. After wounding, there are at least three stimuli to initiate basal cell migration across the viable matrix of the wound (Fig. 8.12). First, loss of cell–cell contact inhibition stimulates migration. Second, several growth factors are released in the wound that stimulate epithelial proliferation and migration. The main growth factors that stimulate epithelial activity are epidermal growth factor (EGF), transforming growth factor-α (TGF-α), and keratinocyte growth factors 1 and 2 (KGF-1 and KGF-2). The final stimuli for cell migration are the actual proteins in the provisional matrix of the wound. Years ago, Woodley demonstrated that when keratinocytes are cultured on proteins found in the normal epithelial basement membrane, such as laminin or type IV collagen, they tend to be stationary. If they are cultured on proteins of the wound, such as type I collagen or fibronectin, they are stimulated to migrate [24–27].

The basal cells migrate across the wound surface as a continuous sheet with connection to the original epithelial edge. Basal cell proliferation takes place at the wound edge to replace cells that migrate across the wound bed. The migrating epithelium will only travel around 2 cm and then the rest of healing is from contraction in a full-thickness wound. For more superficial wounds (partial-thickness), there is a layer of dermis that remains. This dermis contains skin adnexa such as hair follicles, oil glands, sebaceous glands, and others. These adnexa are lined with keratinocytes, which migrate onto the wound surface and assist with re-epithelialization. Hair follicles have stem cells in the bulb and bulge, which are contributors to re-epithelialization. When there is a high density of hair follicles, re-epithelialization is very rapid. If one harvests scalp skin for a split-thickness skin graft, then the scalp will re-epithelialize within 4–5 days. In areas with fewer skin adnexa, such as on the lower leg, re-epithelialization is much slower—roughly 2–3 weeks. As people age, they tend to lose hair follicles. In the very elderly, hair follicles often disappear from areas such as the leg. When an older person suffers a very superficial scald, the loss of hair follicles prevents re-epithelialization so that they are often said to "convert" to a full-thickness wound. They really did not "convert" but, instead, without hair follicles, they did not have a chance to resurface the wound. Fortunately for the

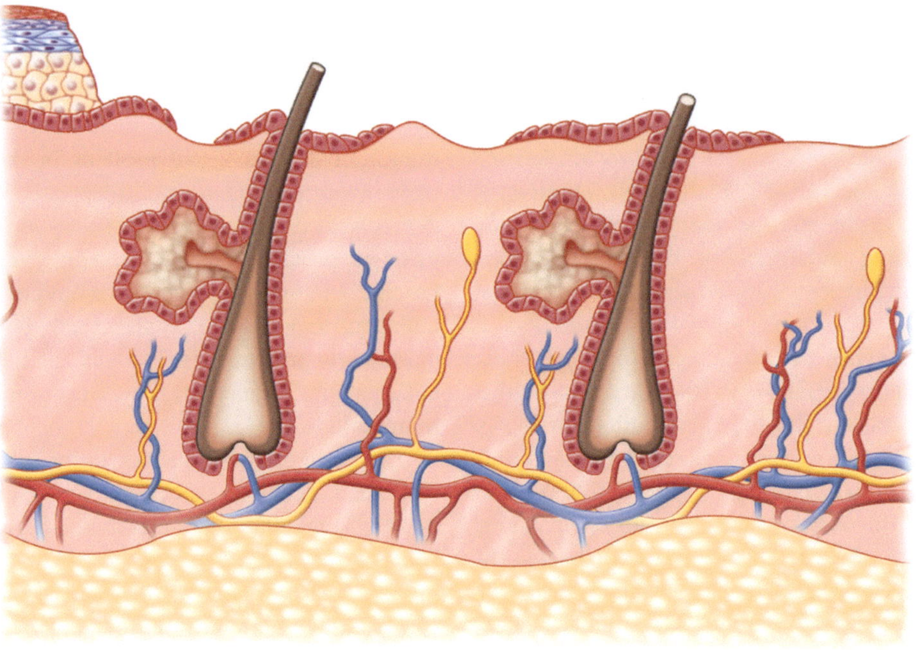

Fig. 8.12 At the edge of the wound, the basal cells are stimulated to migrate across the viable surface of the wound. The migrating cells are replaced by cellular proliferation at the base of the original wound. The migrating cells will only travel 1–2 cm, and if there are no skin adnexa, the rest of the closure depends on scar formation and wound contraction. If there are skin adnexa (hair follicles, oil glands, and other glands), the keratinocytes in those wounds migrate onto the wound surface to assist with closure. If the adnexa are close together, healing is faster

elderly, the laxity of skin may allow for contraction without contracture.

If the wound surface maintains a moist environment, the migrating keratinocytes receive little resistance with travel so that re-epithelialization proceeds rapidly. If, however, the wound is allowed to desiccate, the normal fluids that leak from the wound precipitate to form the "scab" we are familiar with. Scabs are made up of fibrin and other proteins that leak out of the wound. When the scab is covered with an ointment, it often appears as a white exudate. When the scab dries, it becomes darker and has a more leather-like appearance. Since migrating keratinocytes have to maintain contact with a viable wound surface, they have to "cut" through the scab by releasing proteases and fibrinolytic enzymes. Thus, they require more time to cover the wound. The keratinocytes eventually break out from beneath the scab to produce epithelial buds. Once these "epithelial buds" appear within the middle of the scab, the wound will likely heal within the next few days (Fig. 8.13). Allowing the wound to dry always slows the time to re-epithelialize compared to a wound that remains moist [28]. Clearly, if one tries to minimize scarring, then the wound must re-epithelialize within 2–3 weeks, so any wound that is allowed to desiccate retards closure and leads to a higher likelihood of forming a hypertrophic scar. There are techniques for treating a superficial wound that will maintain a moist environment. Simple application of an ointment will maintain a moist environment. Biologic dressings are designed to adhere to the wound and maintain the optimal moist surface. There are many choices of topical ointments or dressings that will allow more rapid re-epithelialization. These treatments will be covered later in the chapter.

Wound Contraction

The third type of tissue repair is *contraction*—where the wound edges are "pulled" together to close the wound. Wound contraction is an efficient compromise that rapidly closes the wound instead of replacing the original tissue. If one makes a large (1.5 × 1.5 cm) wound that covers around half of a mouse's back, that wound is "pulled" closed in around 10 days—leaving only a 1–2 mm central area that has formed a scar and has re-epithelialized. This efficient healing is essential for the survival of an animal that does not have the time that would be required to regenerate the lost skin. Contraction is the work of specialized fibroblasts, called "myofibroblasts," which lay down collagen, "grasp" that collagen, and then contract as though they were muscle cells (Fig. 8.14). Myofibroblasts contain α-actin and myosin, just like muscle cells, which create the force to shrink the edges of a wound. Since fibroblasts do not enter the wound for 4–5 days (during the "lag" period), there is little contraction until that period. Once myofibroblasts are present, however, contraction is relatively rapid. Also, in parallel with scar formation, there is a prolonged maturation phase where contraction persists for months.

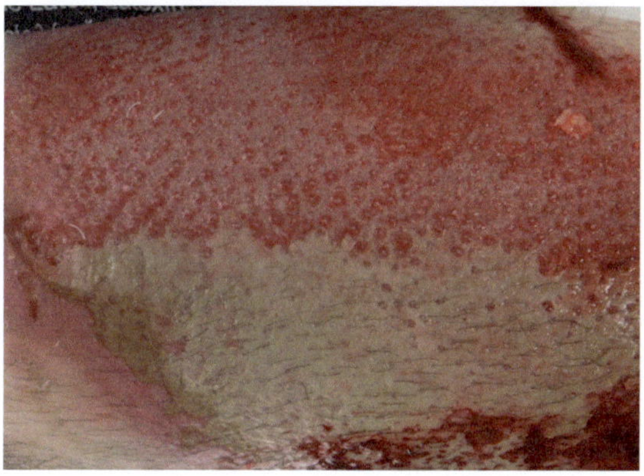

Fig. 8.13 Epithelial buds are visualized in this partial-thickness wound as pink islands that have digested away the "scab." Part of the "scab" remains in the lower part of the wound

Wound contraction is very helpful in many wounds. A gunshot wound to the buttocks will contract rapidly. The same process is helpful in

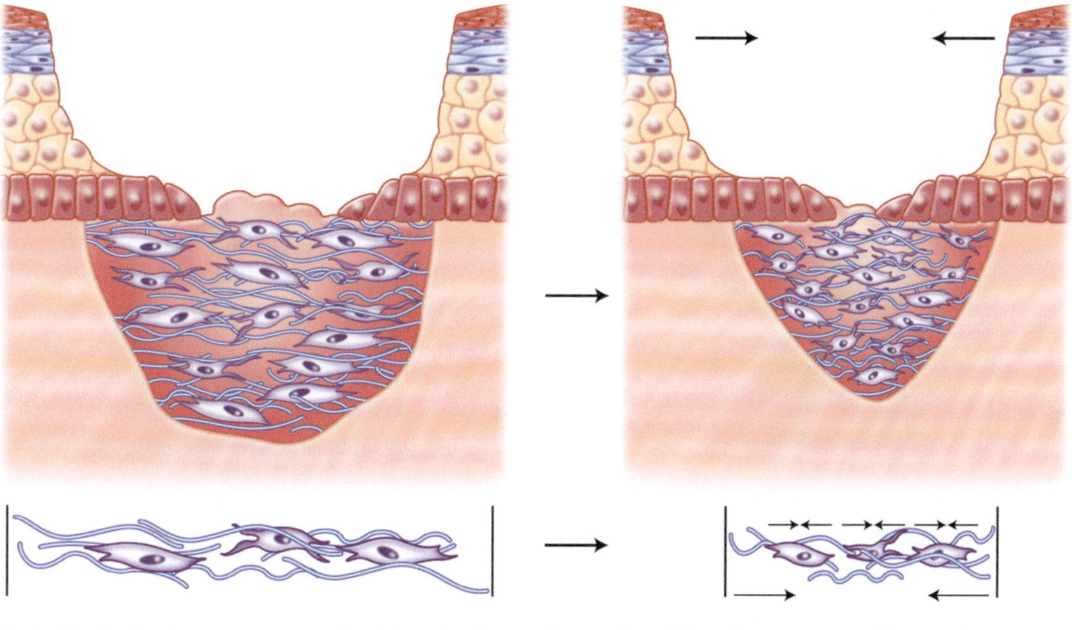

Fig. 8.14 Contraction occurs as myofibroblasts lay down collagen, "grab" it, and then contract like muscle cells

closing abdominal incisions left open to heal secondarily. Fingertip amputations will also contract nicely. It becomes clear that when the skin surrounding the wound is "loose," wound contraction is very effective. Unfortunately, contraction does not stop in instances where there is significant resistance to closure. While contraction is slower when resistance is higher, it does persist and the body will attempt to close any wound if given enough time. When contraction leads to functional or cosmetic deformity, it is called a *contracture*. An extreme example can be exemplified in a girl who sustained a full-thickness scald burn to her neck, chest, and abdomen. She was not treated for 16 months when she presented to us with her lip pulled onto her chest (Fig. 8.15). I have also seen toes pulled towards the ankle and fingers pulled into the palm. Clearly, over time the forces of wound contraction are incredibly strong.

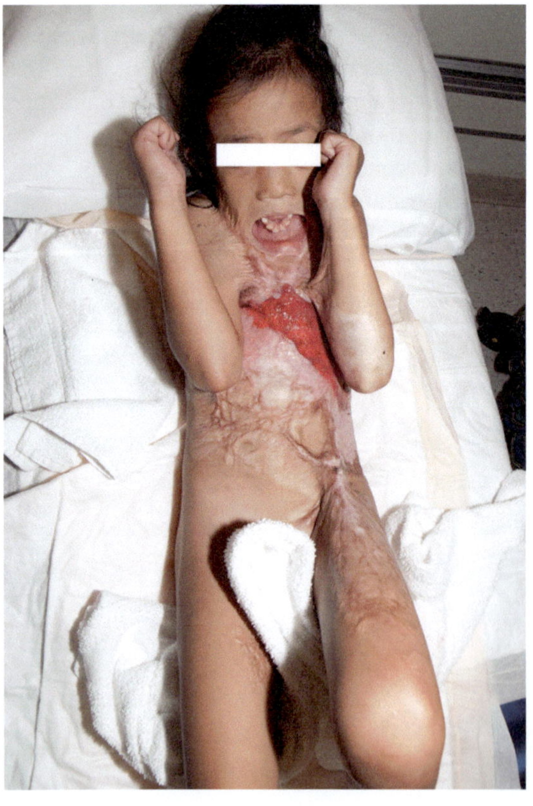

Fig. 8.15 This child had a scald burn to her neck, chest, and abdomen that was untreated for 16 months. The wound contracted to the point that her lip was on her chest. When the scar was removed the size of the original body was revealed. The area was resurfaced with a good result

The main role of occupational and physical therapists in the burn unit is to oppose these contractile forces. The contractile forces are persistent and frustrating. It is typical for a patient to make progress with stretching a fresh burn scar during the day and then after sleeping the contracture recurs. This is why splinting at night is very important. There is an ongoing "battle" between the shrinking scar and the stretching against the contractile forces. The process persists for months and gradually, after 4–6 months, the compliant patient will gain range of motion. If there is no resistance against the contracture, the new scar becomes less pliable and essentially becomes unresponsive to stretching. Thus, early therapy is essential. If the scar is allowed to mature, then reconstructive surgery may be required (see Chap. 11).

Pigmentation

Pigmentation changes after a burn injury are often not emphasized, but they can have profound effects on a burn survivor. Loss or gain of pigmentation in an otherwise perfectly healed area of skin is still very noticeable and may lead to social difficulties for that person. Any caregiver should always strive to allow a wound to regain as normal a pigment as possible. Unfortunately, very little is known about how to control pigmentation.

Skin pigmentation exists in the very superficial parts of the skin—the bottom of the epidermis [29]. The predominant physiologic role of pigment is to create a protective barrier to the harmful effects of the sun. The pigment blocks harmful ultraviolet rays from damaging the DNA of keratinocytes. It makes sense then that pigment is deposited above the nuclei in the bottom 2-3 cell layers of the epidermis. The superficial position of the pigmentation also means that even superficial second-degree burns lose pigment—leaving a pink wound base that initially lacks pigment with re-epithelialization. Re-pigmentation always lags behind re-epithelialization, but more superficial wounds tend to do better than deeper wounds.

The biology of pigmentation is somewhat complicated and has been recently reviewed in more detail [30]. The color of the skin is determined by four main pigments—*melanin* (brown/black), carotene (yellow), oxygenated hemoglobin (red), and reduced hemoglobin (blue). *Melanin* is the major pigment in skin and hair. Specialized cells called *melanocytes* produce melanin. They are derived from the neural crest during the second month of embryogenesis and migrate to the skin. These same neural crest cells are the source of neurons. Like neurons, melanocytes develop multiple dendrites that distribute melanin to around 40 keratinocytes in the bottom two to three layers of keratinocytes (Fig. 8.4). Melanin is stored in special organelles called *melanosomes* prior to transfer. The melanosomes are phagocytized by the keratinocytes and placed above the nucleus. In essence, they are strategically located as screens to protect the DNA from the harmful effects of ultraviolet light. There are specific receptors on the melanocyte, called melanocortin-1 receptors (MC1R), which stimulate pigment production. The pituitary gland produces a hormone precursor called proopiomelanocortin (POMC) that can divide into either α-melanocyte-stimulating hormone (α-MSH) or the hormone that stimulates cortisol production from the adrenal cortex—adrenocorticotropic hormone (ACTH). α-MSH is the main agonist for melanin synthesis by binding to MC1R. Melanin synthesis is also increased in response to ultraviolet light, which explains why pigmentation increases after sun exposure.

Any partial-thickness burn destroys the epithelium and therefore the pigment of the skin is lost. As stated above, skin initially re-epithelializes without pigment to produce a pink but unpigmented skin. Eventually, pigmentation appears at the same sites where skin adnexa had re-epithelialized the skin. The skin develops brown dots at hair follicles and other skin adnexa that eventually spread and coalesce into newly pigmented skin (Fig. 8.16). It is uncertain if the melanocytes migrate onto the skin surface after the keratinocytes or if they migrate with the

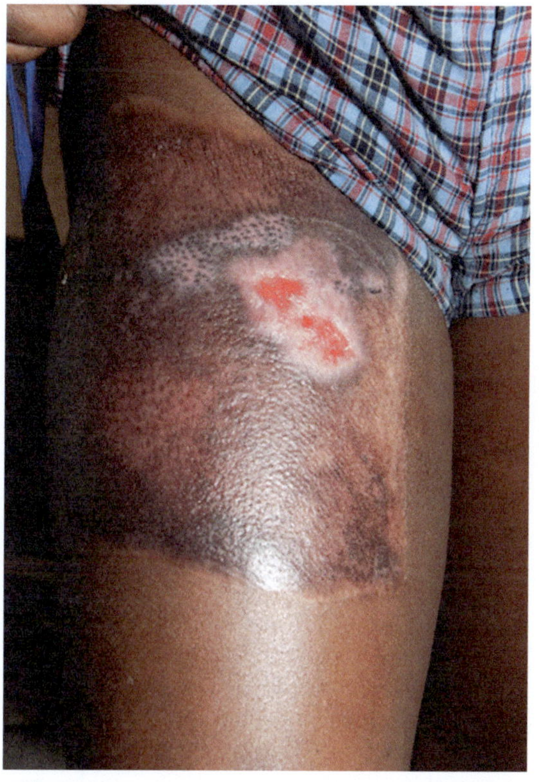

Fig. 8.16 Re-pigmentation tends to lag behind re-epithelialization. At the hair follicles and other skin adnexa, melanocytes differentiate to produce pigmented dots that eventually coalesce to re-pigment the wound. Deeper wounds (such as around the open area) tend to pigment later than more superficial areas

wounds and then differentiate into mature melanocytes to produce melanin. Since hair pigmentation is regulated in a somewhat different fashion than skin pigmentation, the "hair melanocytes" might have to change their phenotype into skin pigment-producing cells. More superficial wounds re-pigment faster than deeper burns. Deeper burns may never re-pigment. It will often take a year for a wound to regain its original pigmentation. Unfortunately, we have very little control over how much a wound pigments. We always tell patients that they should avoid sun so that the wounds will not "over-pigment," but color differences may persist. There are some medications that may help with pigmentation changes, but they are very difficult to regulate. We certainly could use more research about the regulation of pigmentation.

Factors That Inhibit Wound Healing

Most healthy people heal without much trouble. There are, however, people with problems that significantly impair tissue repair. It is important for caregivers to know which patients are at risk for these impairments. Healing is altered in those patients who are very old, malnourished, have infections, diabetes mellitus, and impaired oxygenation and systemic illnesses; or receive agents that impair rapid cellular growth—steroids, chemotherapy agents, or radiation. This section will briefly comment on these impairments, but the effects of these problems are reviewed in greater detail in excellent reviews [31–33].

There are well-known changes to the skin that occur as one ages [34–38]. There are *intrinsic* changes that include thinning, stretching, sagging, wrinkling, pigment changes, and loss of skin adnexa. These normal changes of aging can be accelerated to produce *extrinsic* changes. Exposure to sunlight is the most well-known extrinsic factor that accelerates aging of skin. Loss of skin adnexa, especially hair follicles, can predispose the elderly to a wound that fails to re-epithelialize. Even a very superficial partial-thickness burn will fail to heal if there are no skin adnexa. Caregivers may suggest that the wound "converted" to full-thickness, but, in reality, without skin adnexa the wound has no chance to re-epithelialize. The thinning of the dermis also makes skin grafting more risky since harvesting split-thickness skin may lead to a donor site that fails to heal. A benefit of loose skin, however, is that smaller wounds can contract with lower chance of contracture. As the population ages, these issues will become more important in the management of our aging population. Fortunately, the outcomes for older patients with burns are improving.

It has been known for almost a century that malnutrition impairs tissue repair [39–41]. If nutritional intake is impaired at the time of wounding, tensile strength of an incision will decrease in proportion to the deficit. Restricting both total calories and protein, or simply protein by itself will impair tissue repair. This fact is even more important for the hypermetabolic burn patient. Failure to provide adequate nutrition will impair the healing of the wounds. Deficiencies in individual nutrients, including arginine, zinc, copper, vitamins A, and C, will all impair tissue repair. It is important to remember that failure to heal a wound may ultimately lead to sepsis and multiple organ dysfunction syndrome that lead to the death of the patient.

The role of infection is not as clear as one would expect [42–46]. Minor infections may stimulate the inflammatory response and improve healing. Traditionally, when bacteria increase in number to reach greater than 10^5/g tissue, healing is impaired and skin grafts are unlikely to take [46, 47]. Some infections can have profound effects on healing. *Pseudomonas aeruginosa* is a common contaminant in the wound that often leads to a yellow exudate. The exudate is not a problem, but on occasion, *Pseudomonas* invades tissue to create purple/gray punched out lesions that destroy large areas of skin (Fig. 8.17). These infections are often fatal unless aggressively treated.

Diabetes mellitus is a well-known cause of impaired tissue repair [48–52]. There are three major reasons why diabetes is a detriment to wound healing. First, there is a vascular component where diabetics are predisposed to atherosclerosis and thus have macrovascular disease. In addition, there are microvascular changes, including capillary basement membrane thickening, that inhibit flow of nutrients to the site of

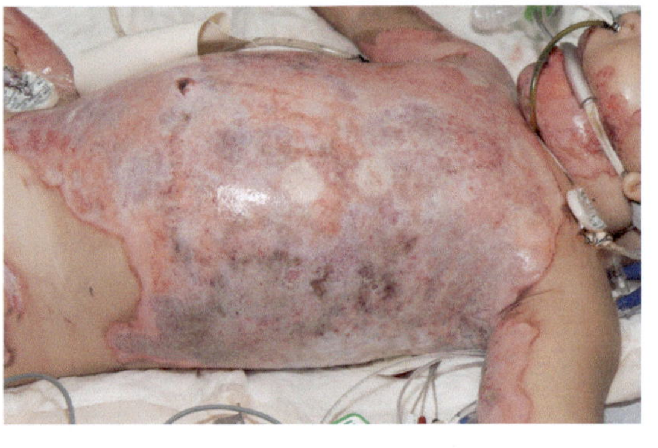

Fig. 8.17 This is an example of a superficial scald burn that was invaded by *Pseudomonas aeruginosa*. The child became profoundly unstable, and despite aggressive excision of the wound, she ultimately died of sepsis

healing. Second, people with diabetes frequently develop peripheral neuropathy leading to insensate feet. Therefore, people do not notice when their feet are being injured, so they develop deep injuries. We have treated many diabetics who have walked out on hot surfaces, or have tried to warm their feet in hot water or near heaters, who have developed full-thickness burns [53]. These burns lead to a need for prolonged care and frequently amputations. Loss of the normal reflexes to maintain the arch of the foot leads to pressure points on the first or second metatarsal heads, which leads to the typical plantar ulcers at these points. In addition, loss of sympathetic nerves leads to loss of sweating that leads to dry, cracking feet. These areas are prone to infection. The third problem with diabetes is that there is an impaired ability to deal with infections that is at least somewhat related to hyperglycemia. It is not uncommon for major infections to develop in small wounds, which ultimately leads to extensive tissue destruction. People with diabetes have the highest nontraumatic amputation rate of all groups. Studies reveal that once a wound develops in a diabetic patient, they have a very high chance of never healing that wound [54].

Oxygen is essential to the healing process and one of the major reasons for a wound not to heal is a poor blood supply [55]. One of the primary reasons for performing vascular surgery to the extremities is because a limb has a wound that does not heal. One must consider the perfusion of a limb when trying to get a burn to heal or to determine whether a graft will take. Many systemic diseases inhibit the healing process. Uremia, for instance, is a cause for impaired healing [51]. Any process that increases tissue edema also inhibits delivery of nutrients to the wound and is a detriment to tissue repair. One must consider any process that increases the metabolic demand on the body "takes away" nutrients from the wound. Since the metabolic demand of major burns is so extensive, wounds tend to take longer to heal in the massively burned patients. Finally, since wound healing demands the rapid migration and proliferation of cells at the site of injury, any drugs or treatments that inhibit cell growth or migration inhibit the healing process. Steroids have been known to inhibit tissue repair for years [56, 57], probably because of their anti-inflammatory activities. The goal of chemotherapy agents [58–61] and radiation [62–64] therapy are to kill rapidly proliferating cancer cells while allowing the quiescent cells to survive. For healing to occur, however, rapid proliferation of cells is required. Therefore, people being treated for malignancies or for major autoimmune diseases tend to have more healing difficulties. All of these factors must be considered when treating burn patients.

Topical Agents for Burn Wound Healing

Topical agents have been used to treat burns for centuries. Topical agents have been designed to provide a moist environment to optimize re-epithelialization and to provide antimicrobials to retard microbial growth. There are some misconceptions about burn topicals that need to be clarified. Some people believe that the topical agents "heal the wound," but they do not; people heal their own wounds, but topicals can optimize healing. Other people believe that topical agents can "accelerate" healing, but in reality, it is extremely difficult to accelerate healing in healthy people. Studies with growth factors from the past suggested that healing in healthy people could be accelerated by a half day [31]. This result was statistically significant but clinically irrelevant. No one would pay thousands of dollars for a wound to heal a half-day faster. The use of growth factors to improve impaired healing is of value and might prevent scar formation [33, 65, 66]. Since growth factors either from genetically engineered proteins or from cultured cells are extremely expensive, so one must balance the cost versus benefit. The other misconception is that topical antimicrobials eliminate bacteria. They suppress growth but they do not kill all microorganisms. Most topical agents will kill specific bacteria, but do not cover other potential pathogens so that other potentially more resistant organisms may grow. For instance, mafenide acetate kills many bacteria, but does not cover yeast. These wounds tend to colonize yeast and not bacteria. As a matter of fact, topical agents may contribute to resistant organisms that are quite prevalent in the burn unit. A significant question is whether any antimicrobial agent is helpful or not. Maybe, leaving the normal flora would be better for the wound. This section will briefly cover many of the typical topical agents used for burns [67–70]. The goal should always be to have an agent that minimizes infection, optimizes healing, and is not toxic to the cells healing the wound.

Bacitracin and Other Antimicrobial Ointments

There are many antimicrobial ointments that are inexpensive and effective for the treatment of small, superficial burns. Ointments help maintain the moist environment to optimize the migration of keratinocytes, the antimicrobials minimize infection, and they are fairly inexpensive. One of the most commonly used ointments is *bacitracin*. Bacitracin is effective against gram-positive organisms, which are the predominant early organisms in a wound. It has little efficacy against gram negatives or yeast, so one must watch for the appearance of these organisms. The ointment is usually applied with a nonsticky dressing and has to be changed twice per day. It is also applied to faces without any other dressing two to three times per day. The positive aspects of bacitracin are that it is inexpensive and easy to use for small burns. The down side is that the dressings have to be removed and changed, which is quite painful. After a week or so, bacitracin will almost always lead to a maculo-papular rash that may be an overgrowth of yeast or just a contact dermatitis. Patients just need to stop using bacitracin and it will go away. There are other topical ointments that are also used such as neomycin or Neosporin (Johnson & Johnson, Inc., New Brunswick, NJ) that are effective. On occasion, especially when a rash from bacitracin occurs, we will often use an ointment lacking any antimicrobials to cover the wound. These untreated ointments may be just as effective as those that have antimicrobials for small superficial wounds.

Silver Sulfadiazine

Silver sulfadiazine has been the prototypical burn cream used for decades. It was originally named "Silvadine," although the product with that name is no longer made. The cream has efficacy against gram positive and negative organisms, along with some yeast. It is very soothing and has been a standard antimicrobial that has been used for decades. It is a "sulfa drug" that is combined with silver, which both have antimicrobial effects. The typical leukopenia observed the first few days after burn injury has been attributed to silver sulfadiazine, but it is more likely due to margination of the inflammatory cells into the wound. There are now multiple studies that suggest that re-epithelialization is impaired with its use compared to other dressings, so it is not the optimal agent for partial-thickness burns [71, 72]. We usually use it for deep burns prior to performing excision and grafting. One product combines silver sulfadiazine with cerium nitrate to add extra antimicrobial effects [73, 74]. Since the philosophy for many centers is to treat deep burns aggressively with early excision and grafting, these topical agents are not as frequently used as in the past.

Bismuth Dressing (Xeroform)

Another dressing that has been around for decades is Xeroform (DeRoyal Industries, Powell, TN), which is a bismuth-containing ointment placed on a fine mesh gauze. Another variation of this type of dressing is called "Scarlet Red" due to its red color. Scarlet red is no longer manufactured. These agents retain some moisture on the wound surface and have some antimicrobial effects. They may stick to the wound, however. We tend to use Xeroform on smaller open wounds as they approach their final closure. They are very easy to apply and are easy for the patient or their families to learn to use.

Mafenide Acetate

Mafenide acetate (Sulfamylon, Mylan Pharmaceuticals, Hertoferdoshire, UK) was developed decades ago with the specific purpose of reducing *Pseudomonas aeruginosa* infections [75, 76]. In the past, the typical treatment of burns was to allow for the eschar to "separate" spontaneously and then graft the underlying granulation tissue. One problem with this approach was that, on occasion, *Pseudomonas aeruginosa* would become "invasive" leading to a profound sepsis that was often rapidly fatal even when aggressively excising the wound (Fig. 8.17). Mafenide acetate is highly effective against the bacteria and reduced these devastating infections. Mafenide acetate is a "sulfa drug" that exists as a cream or can be made as a solution. It penetrates into eschar better than any other antimicrobial agent, so it is a good choice for treating deep ear burns to reduce the chance of developing chondritis—an infection of the cartilage that is highly destructive. It is occasionally irritating to the wound and should be stopped when it causes pain. As a solution, it has often been used as an irrigant to reduce infections in skin grafts. Mafenide acetate has no efficacy against yeast or fungus, so many people add nystatin or miconozole to the solution. If not, yeast overgrowth will often occur. Mafenide acetate is a carbonic anhydrase inhibitor, so it may cause a metabolic acidosis that can be treated with sodium bicarbonate.

Bleach Products

An old product to treat wounds has been "Dakins solution" (sodium hypochlorite), which is a dilute concentration of bleach. Bleach kills all forms of antimicrobials, but can, at high concentrations, be toxic to normal cells. We tend to use this product when wounds become invaded with fungi.

Acetic Acid

Another older treatment that has re-emerged in recent years has been acetic acid that has some efficacy in treating chronically open wounds.

Silver Products

Silver, by itself, has antimicrobial effects [67, 77]. An old but effective silver product is silver nitrate solution. It covers most bacteria and yeast or fungus. The silver ion precipitates when it combines with chloride. The silver chloride precipitate will stain all other tissues and all other items with a dark brown color. This stain is very difficult to remove from floors, walls, and clothing. In addition, when the silver precipitates, it exposes tissue to water so that patients can develop hyponatremia.

Many dressings now come with silver adhered to the material. Some have nanocrystalline silver and others have other forms of the element. The idea is to add an antimicrobial to a dressing that is designed to optimize the healing environment. Some microorganisms, however, develop resistance to silver ions through mechanisms that include the excretion of the ion.

Biologic Dressings

Since the goal is to maintain a moist environment on the surface of the wound that allows for rapid epithelial migration, many dressings have been designed to carry out this goal [78, 79]. "Biologic dressings" are a class of dressings that are designed for this purpose. One of the earliest types of dressing to be developed was a polyurethane dressing that would adhere to the surrounding normal skin. Two of the very common products are OpSite (Smith & Nephew, London, UK) and Tegaderm (3M, St. Paul, MN). These dressings allow for some evaporation of water through the dressing to reduce pooling of serum, but not enough to allow desiccation. They are superb for small superficial wounds and small split-thickness donor sites. They do tend to collect fluid beneath them that often will leak if not aspirated with a needle. The underlying fluid may become contaminated with bacteria, which can lead to a wound infection. It is often very difficult to have the dressing adhere to larger donor sites or wounds so that the dressing may slip off the wound.

Another well-known dressing that has been around for decades is Biobrane (Smith & Nephew, London, UK), which has type I collagen attached to a nylon/silicone sheet. The collagen sticks to the wound and the silicone acts as a barrier to prevent drying. The wound re-epithelializes underneath the dressing and falls off when completely a new epithelium is generated. This dressing works very well for superficial wounds, split-thickness donor sites, and for people with toxic epidermal necrolysis syndrome (or Stevens-Johnson Syndrome). One must monitor the wound for the collection of pus beneath the dressing. If it does get infected, the pus trapped under the silicone has the potential for invading the wound. Some companies have attached cultured fibroblasts to Biobrane to release growth factors that may enhance wound closure. The added cells may accelerate healing by a day or so, but their costs are prohibited for most wounds—costing more than a thousand dollars for a small sheet. Other allogeneic skin substitutes have been developed, but they have the same issues as the cells combined with Biobrane.

Currently, there are several products that adhere to the wound and optimize healing of partial-thickness wounds. These products such as MepilexAG (Molnlycke Health Care, Norcross, GA), AquacellAG (ConvaTec, Inc., Bridgewater, NJ), and others have changed the practice of treating small, superficial wounds. In the past, many patients were admitted to burn centers to apply twice a day dressings. The wounds would need to be washed and dressed with an ointment and some other form of dressing. The patients required inpatient treatment because of the pain and the time required to learn how to dress the wounds. Now most burn centers treat these wounds as outpatients. The wound is cleaned and then covered with a biologic dressing that requires changing every 4–7 days. The patient can be sent home without a need for dressing changes until those outpatient visits. This change in philosophy has been popular for the medical staff as well as for the patients and their families. This change in philosophy has also significantly reduced the numbers of admissions.

Summary

The basic principles of wound healing apply to all types of injuries and tissues. The wound must re-create the strength of the wound to match the dermis by creating a less than perfect scar. The same cells, fibroblasts, which create the scar, are involved in contracting a wound. The epithelium must be re-form to create the barrier to water loss and microbial infection. Most healing proceeds with little difficulty, but certain abnormalities such as malnutrition, infection, diabetes mellitus, poor blood supply, and drugs that impair growth—steroids, chemotherapy agents, and radiation—impair the healing process. One must remember these inhibitors of tissue repair to optimize healing. It is clear that recreating the barrier, the epithelium, within 2 weeks or so is essential to minimize scarring. The factors that influence scarring will be covered in Chap. 20. Topical agents are designed to optimize the re-epithelialization process and inhibit (but not stop) microbial growth. The strategies to cover the deeper and more extensive wounds will be covered in the next chapter.

References

1. Deitch EA, Wheelahan TM, Rose MP, Clothier J, Cotter J. Hypertrophic burn scars: analysis of variables. J Trauma. 1983;23(10):895–8.
2. Chung WH, Hung SI. Recent advances in the genetics and immunology of Stevens-Johnson syndrome and toxic epidermal necrosis. J Dermatol Sci. 2012;66(3): 190–6.
3. Downey A, Jackson C, Harun N, Cooper A. Toxic epidermal necrolysis: review of pathogenesis and management. J Am Acad Dermatol. 2012;66(6): 995–1003.
4. Nishifuji K, Shimizu A, Ishiko A, Iwasaki T, Amagai M. Removal of amino-terminal extracellular domains of desmoglein 1 by staphylococcal exfoliative toxin is sufficient to initiate epidermal blister formation. J Dermatol Sci. 2010;59(3):184–91.
5. Nishifuji K, Sugai M, Amagai M. Staphylococcal exfoliative toxins: "molecular scissors" of bacteria that attack the cutaneous defense barrier in mammals. J Dermatol Sci. 2008;49(1):21–31.
6. Coulombe PA, Kerns ML, Fuchs E. Epidermolysis bullosa simplex: a paradigm for disorders of tissue fragility. J Clin Invest. 2009;119(7):1784–93.
7. Varkey M, Ding J, Tredget EE. Differential collagen-glycosaminoglycan matrix remodeling by superficial and deep dermal fibroblasts: potential therapeutic targets for hypertrophic scar. Biomaterials. 2011;32(30): 7581–91.
8. Driskell RR, Lichtenberger BM, Hoste E, et al. Distinct fibroblast lineages determine dermal architecture in skin development and repair. Nature. 2013;504(7479):277–81.
9. Medzhitov R. Origin and physiological roles of inflammation. Nature. 2008;454(7203):428–35.

10. Simpson DM, Ross R. The neutrophilic leukocyte in wound repair a study with antineutrophil serum. J Clin Invest. 1972;51(8):2009–23.
11. Leibovich SJ, Ross R. The role of the macrophage in wound repair. A study with hydrocortisone and antimacrophage serum. Am J Pathol. 1975;78(1):71–100.
12. Carmeliet P, Jain RK. Molecular mechanisms and clinical applications of angiogenesis. Nature. 2011;473(7347):298–307.
13. Herbert SP, Stainier DY. Molecular control of endothelial cell behaviour during blood vessel morphogenesis. Nat Rev Mol Cell Biol. 2011;12(9):551–64.
14. Hong WX, Hu MS, Esquivel M, et al. The role of hypoxia-inducible factor in wound healing. Adv Wound Care. 2014;3(5):390–9.
15. Nauta TD, van Hinsbergh VW, Koolwijk P. Hypoxic signaling during tissue repair and regenerative medicine. Int J Mol Sci. 2014;15(11):19791–815.
16. Brown DL, Kao WW, Greenhalgh DG. Apoptosis down-regulates inflammation under the advancing epithelial wound edge: delayed patterns in diabetes and improvement with topical growth factors. Surgery. 1997;121(4):372–80.
17. Greenhalgh DG. The role of apoptosis in wound healing. Int J Biochem Cell Biol. 1998;30(9):1019–30.
18. Garbin S, Pittet B, Montandon D, Gabbiani G, Desmouliere A. Covering by a flap induces apoptosis of granulation tissue myofibroblasts and vascular cells. Wound Repair Regen. 1996;4(2):244–51.
19. Darby IA, Bisucci T, Pittet B, Garbin S, Gabbiani G, Desmouliere A. Skin flap-induced regression of granulation tissue correlates with reduced growth factor and increased metalloproteinase expression. J Pathol. 2002;197(1):117–27.
20. Suarez E, Syed F, Rasgado TA, Walmsley A, Mandal P, Bayat A. Skin equivalent tensional force alters keloid fibroblast behavior and phenotype. Wound Repair Regen. 2014;22(5):557–68.
21. Ogawa R. Mechanobiology of scarring. Wound Repair Regen. 2011;19 Suppl 1:s2–9.
22. Ogawa R, Okai K, Tokumura F, et al. The relationship between skin stretching/contraction and pathologic scarring: the important role of mechanical forces in keloid generation. Wound Repair Regen. 2012;20(2):149–57.
23. Greenhalgh DG, Palmieri TL. Zigzag seams for the prevention of scar bands after sheet split-thickness skin grafting. Surgery. 2003;133(5):586–7.
24. Woodley DT, O'Keefe EJ, Prunieras M. Cutaneous wound healing: a model for cell-matrix interactions. J Am Acad Dermatol. 1985;12(2 Pt 2):420–33.
25. Woodley DT, Wynn KC, O'Keefe EJ. Type IV collagen and fibronectin enhance human keratinocyte thymidine incorporation and spreading in the absence of soluble growth factors. J Invest Dermatol. 1990;94(1):139–43.
26. Cheng CF, Fan J, Bandyopahdhay B, et al. Profiling motility signal-specific genes in primary human keratinocytes. J Invest Dermatol. 2008;128(8):1981–90.
27. Li W, Henry G, Fan J, et al. Signals that initiate, augment, and provide directionality for human keratinocyte motility. J Invest Dermatol. 2004;123(4):622–33.
28. Junker JP, Kamel RA, Caterson EJ, Eriksson E. Clinical impact upon wound healing and inflammation in moist, wet, and dry environments. Adv Wound Care. 2013;2(7):348–56.
29. Lin JY, Fisher DE. Melanocyte biology and skin pigmentation. Nature. 2007;445(7130):843–50.
30. Greenhalgh DG. A primer on pigmentation. J Burn Care Res. 2015;36(2):247–57.
31. Greenhalgh DG. The role of growth factors in wound healing. J Trauma. 1996;41(1):159–67.
32. Anderson K, Hamm RL. Factors that impair wound healing. J Am Coll Clin Wound Specialists. 2012;4(4):84–91.
33. Barrientos S, Brem H, Stojadinovic O, Tomic-Canic M. Clinical application of growth factors and cytokines in wound healing. Wound Repair Regen. 2014;22(5):569–78.
34. Greenhalgh DG. Management of the skin and soft tissue in the geriatric surgical patient. Surg Clin North Am. 2015;95(1):103–14.
35. Archer SB, Henke A, Greenhalgh DG, Warden GD. The use of sheet autografts to cover extensive burns in patients. J Burn Care Rehabil. 1998;19(1 Pt 1):33–8.
36. Gould L, Abadir P, Brem H, et al. Chronic wound repair and healing in older adults: current status and future research. J Am Geriatr Soc. 2015;63(3):427–38.
37. Birch MP, Messenger JF, Messenger AG. Hair density, hair diameter and the prevalence of female pattern hair loss. Br J Dermatol. 2001;144(2):297–304.
38. Zouboulis CC, Makrantonaki E. Clinical aspects and molecular diagnostics of skin aging. Clin Dermatol. 2011;29(1):3–14.
39. Kavalukas SL, Barbul A. Nutrition and wound healing: an update. Plast Reconstr Surg. 2011;127 Suppl 1:38s–43.
40. Nordlund MJ, Pham TN, Gibran NS. Micronutrients after burn injury: a review. J Burn Care Res. 2014;35(2):121–33.
41. Abdullahi A, Jeschke MG. Nutrition and anabolic pharmacotherapies in the care of burn patients. Nutr Clin Pract. 2014;29(5):621–30.
42. Levenson SM, Kan-Gruber D, Gruber C, Molnar J, Seifter E. Wound healing accelerated by Staphylococcus aureus. Arch Surg. 1983;118(3):310–20.
43. Tenorio A, Jindrak K, Weiner M, Bella E, Enquist IF. Accelerated healing in infected wounds. Surg Gynecol Obstet. 1976;142(4):537–43.
44. Irvin TT. Collagen metabolism in infected colonic anastomoses. Surg Gynecol Obstet. 1976;143(2):220–4.
45. Bucknall TE. The effect of local infection upon wound healing: an experimental study. Br J Surg. 1980;67(12):851–5.
46. Smith M, Enquist IF. A quantitative study of impaired healing resulting from infection. Surg Gynecol Obstet. 1967;125(5):965–73.

47. Krizek TJ, Robson MC. Evolution of quantitative bacteriology in wound management. Am J Surg. 1975; 130(5):579–84.
48. Greenhalgh DG. Wound healing and diabetes mellitus. Clin Plast Surg. 2003;30(1):37–45.
49. Baltzis D, Eleftheriadou I, Veves A. Pathogenesis and treatment of impaired wound healing in diabetes mellitus: new insights. Adv Ther. 2014;31(8):817–36.
50. Malay DS, Margolis DJ, Hoffstad OJ, Bellamy S. The incidence and risks of failure to heal after lower extremity amputation for the treatment of diabetic neuropathic foot ulcer. J Foot Ankle Surg. 2006; 45(6):366–74.
51. Yue DK, McLennan S, Marsh M, et al. Effects of experimental diabetes, uremia, and malnutrition on wound healing. Diabetes. 1987;36(3):295–9.
52. Christman AL, Selvin E, Margolis DJ, Lazarus GS, Garza LA. Hemoglobin A1c predicts healing rate in diabetic wounds. J Invest Dermatol. 2011;131(10): 2121–7.
53. Barsun A, Sen S, Palmieri TL, Greenhalgh DG. A ten-year review of lower extremity burns in diabetics: small burns that lead to major problems. J Burn Care Res. 2013;34(2):255–60.
54. Margolis DJ, Kantor J, Berlin JA. Healing of diabetic neuropathic foot ulcers receiving standard treatment. A meta-analysis. Diabetes Care. 1999;22(5):692–5.
55. Sen CK. Wound healing essentials: let there be oxygen. Wound Repair Regen. 2009;17(1):1–18.
56. Dostal GH, Gamelli RL. The differential effect of corticosteroids on wound disruption strength in mice. Arch Surg. 1990;125(5):636–40.
57. Howes EL, Plotz CM, Blunt JW, Ragan C. Retardation of wound healing by cortisone. Surgery. 1950;28(2): 177–81.
58. Curtsinger LJ, Pietsch JD, Brown GL, et al. Reversal of Adriamycin-impaired wound healing by transforming growth factor-beta. Surg Gynecol Obstet. 1989;168(6):517–22.
59. Falcone RE, Nappi JF. Chemotherapy and wound healing. Surg Clin North Am. 1984;64(4):779–94.
60. Ferguson MK. The effect of antineoplastic agents on wound healing. Surg Gynecol Obstet. 1982;154(3): 421–9.
61. Shamberger RC, Devereux DF, Brennan MF. The effect of chemotherapeutic agents on wound healing. Int Adv Surg Oncol. 1981;4:15–58.
62. Luce EA. The irradiated wound. Surg Clin North Am. 1984;64(4):821–9.
63. Waghmare CM. Radiation burn – from mechanism to management. Burns. 2013;39(2):212–9.
64. Bui E, Joseph B, Rhee P, Diven C, Pandit V, Brown CV. Contemporary management of radiation exposure and injury. J Trauma Acute Care Surg. 2014;77(3): 495–500.
65. Pierce GF, Mustoe TA, Lingelbach J, Masakowski VR, Gramates P, Deuel TF. Transforming growth factor beta reverses the glucocorticoid-induced wound-healing deficit in rats: possible regulation in macrophages by platelet-derived growth factor. Proc Natl Acad Sci U S A. 1989;86(7):2229–33.
66. Suh DY, Hunt TK, Spencer EM. Insulin-like growth factor-I reverses the impairment of wound healing induced by corticosteroids in rats. Endocrinology. 1992;131(5):2399–403.
67. Greenhalgh DG. Topical antimicrobial agents for burn wounds. Clin Plast Surg. 2009;36(4):597–606.
68. Brown RL, Greenhalgh DG. Mouse models to study wound closure and topical treatment of infected wounds in healing-impaired and normal healing hosts. Wound Repair Regen. 1997;5(2):198–204.
69. Neely AN, Gardner J, Durkee P, et al. Are topical antimicrobials effective against bacteria that are highly resistant to systemic antibiotics? J Burn Care Res. 2009;30(1):19–29.
70. Erfurt-Berge C, Renner R. Recent developments in topical wound therapy: impact of antimicrobiological changes and rebalancing the wound milieu. BioMed Res Int. 2014;2014:819525.
71. Genuino GA, Baluyut-Angeles KV, Espiritu AP, Lapitan MC, Buckley BS. Topical petrolatum gel alone versus topical silver sulfadiazine with standard gauze dressings for the treatment of superficial partial thickness burns in adults: a randomized controlled trial. Burns. 2014;40(7):1267–73.
72. Rashaan ZM, Krijnen P, Klamer RR, Schipper IB, Dekkers OM, Breederveld RS. Nonsilver treatment vs. silver sulfadiazine in treatment of partial-thickness burn wounds in children: a systematic review and meta-analysis. Wound Repair Regen. 2014;22(4): 473–82.
73. Garner JP, Heppell PS. Cerium nitrate in the management of burns. Burns. 2005;31(5):539–47.
74. Oen IM, van Baar ME, Middelkoop E, Nieuwenhuis MK. Effectiveness of cerium nitrate-silver sulfadiazine in the treatment of facial burns: a multicenter, randomized, controlled trial. Plast Reconstr Surg. 2012;130(2):274e–83.
75. Maggi SP, Soler PM, Smith PD, Hill DP, Ko F, Robson MC. The efficacy of 5% Sulfamylon solution for the treatment of contaminated explanted human meshed skin grafts. Burns. 1999;25(3):237–41.
76. Heinle EC, Dougherty WR, Garner WL, Reilly DA. The use of 5% mafenide acetate solution in the postgraft treatment of necrotizing fasciitis. J Burn Care Rehabil. 2001;22(1):35–40.
77. Klasen HJ. A historical review of the use of silver in the treatment of burns. II. Renewed interest for silver. Burns. 2000;26(2):131–8.
78. Sood A, Granick MS, Tomaselli NL. Wound dressings and comparative effectiveness data. Adv Wound Care. 2014;3(8):511–29.
79. Wasiak J, Cleland H. Burns: dressings. BMJ Clin Evid. 2015:pii1903.

Operative Management of Burns

9

David G. Greenhalgh

Introduction

Burns that take longer than 2–3 weeks to re-epithelialize will develop hypertrophic scarring. In addition, any burn that is of full-thickness will heal by scar formation and contraction. Therefore, to minimize scarring, surgery is the best option for most of these patients. The goal for any treatment of burns is to optimize the functional and cosmetic outcomes of burns. The objective of this chapter is to provide surgical strategies for obtaining the best outcomes possible for burn wounds. It is important to remember that there are different options for different types of burns. The size of the burn may limit the operative options. In addition, it is important to understand that the severity of injury also dictates the choice of procedures that are possible for that patient. For instance, one should have an excellent outcome in an isolated hand burn that is barely full-thickness. The same outcome would not be expected for a fourth-degree hand burn in a patient with 90 % total body surface area (TBSA) burn. The principles of operative management of burns will be covered in this chapter.

D.G. Greenhalgh, M.D. (✉)
Shriners Hospitals for Children Northern California, University of California, Davis Medical Center, 2425 Stockton Boulevard, Sacramento, CA 95817, USA
e-mail: dggreenhalgh@ucdavis.edu

Deciding to Graft or Not

The basic tenet is that *grafting should reduce the ultimate scarring of the burn wound.* Small full-thickness burns that are localized in areas without functional importance and with surrounding loose skin can contract without major problems. Burns on the lower abdomen or buttocks can contract to leave small and hidden scars. One must also consider that small skin grafts in the middle of a large surface area may look worse than allowing the wound to contract. A common problem is the child with a chest and abdominal scald with all areas, but one small area healing in 2 weeks. Should that remaining open area be grafted or allowed to heal with the potential for hypertrophic scarring? A small graft in the middle of the upper chest is quite unsightly, so allowing it to heal and dealing with a small hypertrophic scar may be the better option.

The timing of skin grafting is another decision that must be made. If the burn is clearly superficial, then allowing it to heal is the best option. While many surgeons will debride superficial burns, I do not believe that superficial burns require any operative debridement to improve re-epithelialization. Usually, the wound may be washed and loose blisters wiped away and the dressing (preferably a biologic dressing) should be applied. If the burn is clearly full-thickness then there is no need to delay, so excision and grafting should proceed as soon as the operating

D.G. Greenhalgh (ed.), *Burn Care for General Surgeons and General Practitioners*,
DOI 10.1007/978-3-319-29161-1_9

room schedule allows. The real difficulty occurs in those burn wounds that are considered to be of "indeterminant" depth. The simplest solution is to wait 2 weeks and then graft if the wound has not healed. The problem with waiting is that one is often left with a wound that is half-healed—so do you allow it to re-epithelialize or just graft the open area? Unfortunately, I have observed several nicely healed grafts surrounded by hypertrophic scarring (of the area that had just healed around 2 weeks). There are many devices that can determine local blood flow (laser Doppler devices, infra-red spectrometers, and other devices) that may help. It is not clear, however, whether the information they provide is better than that of an experienced clinician. The other problem with these instruments is that they are less helpful with larger surface area burns. If one tries to measure local blood flow over an entire arm, there may be areas that have good blood flow and other areas that have poor perfusion. Since the depth of the burn may not be uniform, it is difficult to make a decision of whether to graft part or the entire arm. *Whether to perform excision and grafting or not is one of the most difficult decisions in burn surgery.*

Principles of Skin Grafting

There are several important principles about grafting that guide the surgeon. Like other forms of tissue repair, there are *three phases of skin graft healing*. The first phase of skin graft healing is the *Phase of Imbibition*. Immediately after the graft is placed, it survives by diffusion of nutrients from the wound bed to the graft. Thus, the skin graft "imbibes" nutrients from the wound bed. Any barrier between the wound bed and graft leads to the graft's death. Therefore, any hematoma, seroma, foreign body, inadequate excision (nonviable wound bed), and exposed ungraftable tissue (tendon, bone) will lead to graft loss. Since the epidermis must survive, even a graft that is too thick may lead to epidermolysis and ultimately graft loss. After 2–4 days, the second phase, called the *Phase of Vascularization*, is noted by the graft developing the red color of the invading blood supply. During this phase, capillaries invade the graft through the process of angiogenesis and a process called "inosculation". During inosculation, exposed capillaries of the wound bed "hook up" with open capillaries of the graft. During this phase, it is important to prevent sheering of the graft or else the disrupted capillaries form hematomas that lead to graft loss. The final phase, the *Phase of Maturation*, starts as collagen molecules from the wound bed "attach" the graft to the body. This process, like all maturing wounds, lasts up to 2 years until the graft is no longer red. It is typical that all grafts get thicker and redder for 3–4 months and then the vascularity gradually fades and the graft thins. During this phase, if the balance of collagen synthesis and collagen breakdown is "tipped" towards excessive collagen production, a hypertrophic scar results. Studies suggest, however, that skin grafts tend to induce apoptosis of the inflammatory cells and fibroblasts to reduce scar formation [1–3]. More information about scar management is described in Chap. 20 about managing scars.

Another important principle is that *the thicker the skin graft, the less it tends to shrink* over time. Therefore, the goal for the best outcome is to get the thickest graft possible. The balance, however, is that the donor site is another wound that needs to heal with minimal scarring. There are two types of skin grafts that differ based on the donor—split-thickness and full-thickness skin grafts. Split-thickness skin grafts are harvested through the middle of the dermis and thus "split" the dermis of the donor site. Since the dermis and its skin appendages remain, the donor site must re-epithelialize to heal. One should consider the donor site healing as being similar to that of a partial-thickness burn. As described in the chapter on wound healing (Chap. 8), the goal is to have the harvest site heal within 2–3 weeks to minimize the chances of donor site scarring. Thus, there is always a balance between harvesting the thickest skin possible while minimizing the donor site morbidity when performing split-thickness skin grafts. Since there is often a large surface area of available donor site, split-thickness skin grafts are used to cover larger defects.

Full-thickness skin grafts, by definition, are harvested completely to the subcutaneous fat. These are the thickest possible grafts, but the surface area that can be utilized is limited since there is always a full-thickness defect that remains. Typically, the donor site wounds are closed primarily (with stitches), but it is possible to harvest larger full-thickness grafts and then apply split-thickness grafts over the full-thickness wound. Full-thickness grafts are usually used for small grafts on the hand or face. Any area with loose skin can be used for skin harvest since trying to close the donor site in tighter areas will lead to contractures. The inguinal region and the lower abdomen are good sites for harvest for all places except the face. For instance, the groin can be used to cover a large portion of the palm. One must be careful when harvesting skin from obese people since their dermis often becomes quite thick. Thicker dermis tends to interfere with absorption of the nutrients from the wound bed (phase of imbibition) and the epidermis may die. Any fat must be removed with scissors and I often remove dermis in the thicker grafts at the same time. I will also try to remove hair follicles that protrude into the fat to minimize the transfer of hair. Due to differences in color, skin should be harvested from behind the ears or at the lower neck for full-thickness skin grafts of the face.

Preparation for Skin Grafting

As for any surgery, preparation is important for patients undergoing skin grafts. While small grafts are not as difficult to prepare for, large grafts do require significant preparation, which is greatly helped by having an experienced operative team. Once the decision for grafting is made, one must choose the patient position that allows for the best access to both the donor site and the graft. If the back is needed as a donor site, one can roll the patient on his/her side, prep the back, place drapes, and then prep the rest of the patient. When it is time for harvest, the patient can be rolled to obtain the skin. It is quite common for large amounts of the body to be exposed during the procedure. Since thermoregulation of the skin is destroyed with the burn, large areas of exposure can cause the patient to lose a large amount of heat. It is routine to raise the temperature in the operating room to 85–90° Fahrenheit (29.4–32.2 °C) for patients with large burns. Small children may need the operating room to be even warmer. Monitoring the patient is also a challenge since many of the typical sites for attaching devices are burned or required for donor site harvest. EKG pads may be stapled to parts of the trunk to improve adherence to the skin. Pulse oximeters may have to be attached to ears or other unusual sites (nose, tongue, others). Since bilateral extremities are often involved, blood pressure monitoring may be difficult without an arterial line (often placed in the femoral artery).

One of the most important perioperative considerations is to be prepared for significant blood loss. One may forget that burn excision exposes large surfaces to bleeding that can quickly overwhelm anesthesiologists. In the current era of massive excisions, no large burn case should be performed without having typed and crossed blood available. Housinger, et al, published that a patient loses around 2 % of a blood volume per percent burn excision [4]. If one excises both arms, hands, and legs (around 54 % total body surface area [TBSA]), then one would expect to lose an entire blood volume during the excision. If no blood were available, then the patient would not survive the excision. As for any massive transfusion, fresh frozen plasma and platelets should also be available. The actual ratio of blood cells to specific clotting factors still needs to be worked out. There are many techniques that can reduce blood loss. For distal limb excisions, we always use tourniquets, but bleeding still occurs after the tourniquet is removed. Tourniquet excisions require more skill to judge the depth of excision since the typical practice of excising to bleeding tissue is not possible. The use of epinephrine in saline soaks is nearly universal as a hemostatic adjunct. In addition, injection of a solution containing epinephrine (tumescence) reduces bleeding from excision and donor sites. The solution for injection that we use contains 2 mg (2 ml 1:1000) epinephrine per liter of lactated Ringers solution. The most efficient method

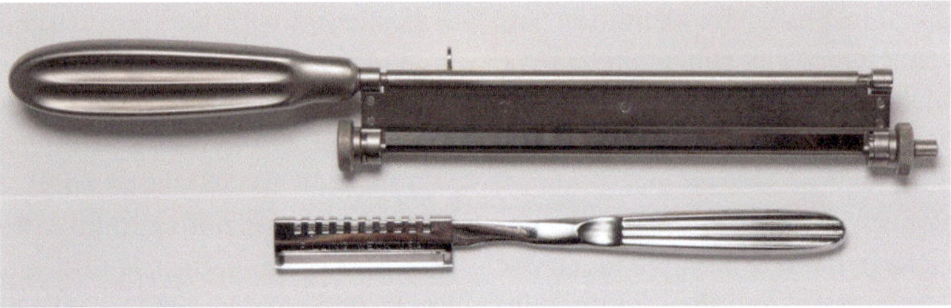

Fig. 9.1 *Goulian knife (smaller) and Watson knife*. The Goulian knife is essentially a small blade with a pre-set guard. The depth of the cut depends on many factors other than the guard thickness such as how pressure and traction is applied to the excised tissue. The Watson knife has a larger blade and an adjustable guard. It is used to excise large surface areas

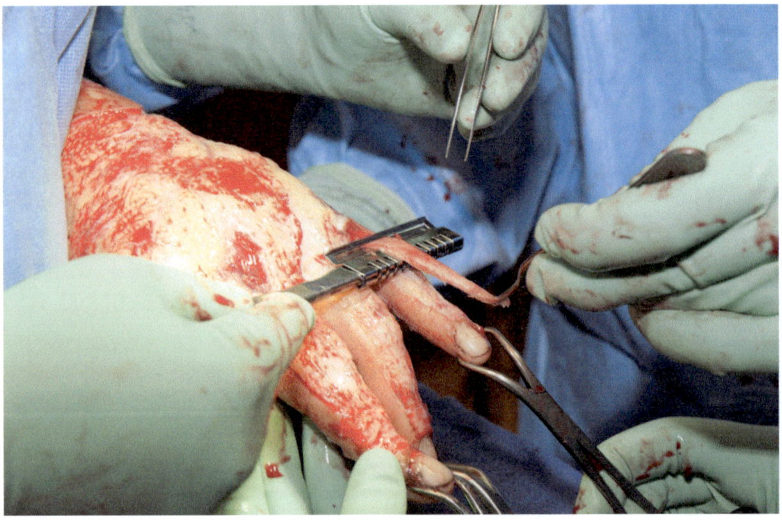

Fig. 9.2 The Goulian knife being used to excise a finger burn. Applying traction to the eschar as it is being excised helps to regulate the depth of excision. The remaining fat is pale and glistening—a depth that will accept a skin graft

of delivery is to use roller pumps with 18-gauge spinal needles to inject large amounts of fluid. While there are theoretic concerns about the dose of epinephrine, we do not have problems with large amounts of fluid even in children. We also use topical thrombin spray, which may shorten the time until hemostasis. Fibrin sealants may also aid with hemostasis and assist with adhering the grafts to the wound bed. The use of tranexamic acid, an inhibitor of fibrinolysis, may also help.

The main instruments used for burn excisions are relatively basic in this age of robotic surgery. In essence, most excisions are performed with blades with some form of "guard" that limits the depth of excision. The Goulian knife is a blade that has variable guards that have numeric labels that are supposed to indicate the thousandth of an inch from the blade (Figs. 9.1 and 9.2). These guards are often bent and one must be careful to not rely on those numbers to determine the depth of the excision. The larger knives include Watson and Humby knifes (Fig. 9.3). We use the Watson knife for excising larger burned areas. There is a device, called the VersaJet (Smith & Nephew, Hull, United Kingdom), which uses a water jet to excise tissue, but I find that it is too slow for excisions of larger areas of burn. For full-thickness skin grafts, a simple scalpel blade is used. To harvest split-thickness skin grafts, most people use a powered dermatome. There are several manufac-

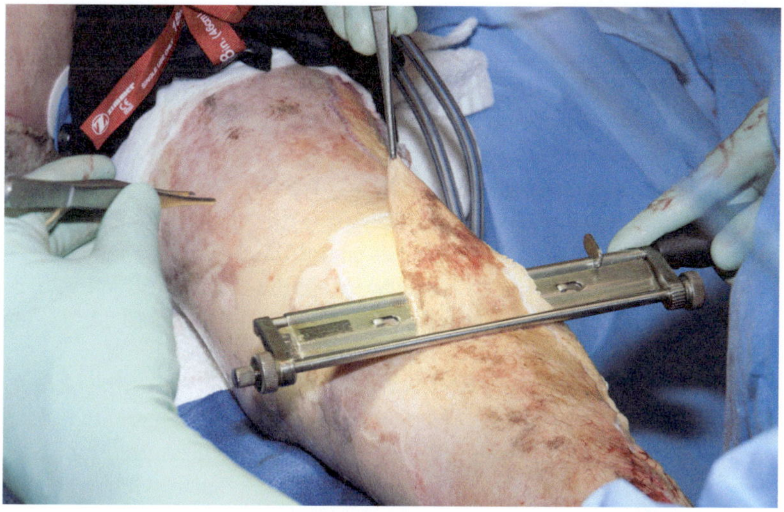

Fig. 9.3 The Watson knife is being used to excise a large area of eschar from the arm. The traction helps with the excision

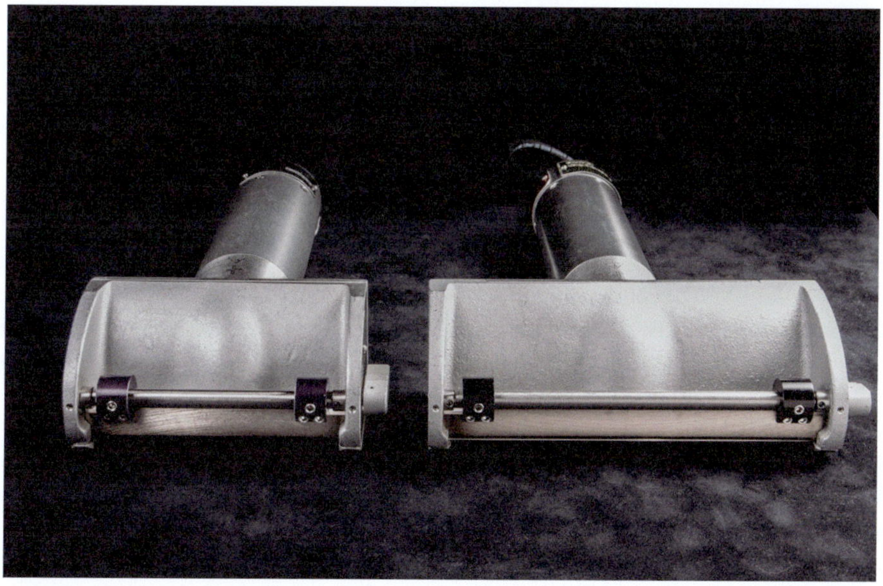

Fig. 9.4 The Padgett 4 and 6 in. dermatomes. The 6 in. dermatome is more difficult to use, but can produce wide pieces of skin that can reduce seams in the graft

turers of dermatomes and which one is used is dependent on the preferences of the surgeon. We use the Padgett Dermatome (Integra LifeSciences Corp., Cincinnati, OH), which has both a four- and six-inch wide blade (Fig. 9.4). The 6-in. dermatome is a little more difficult to use, but allows for very large pieces of skin that can minimize the seams between grafts.

Anesthesia

It is not possible to cover all of the essential components of anesthesia in this chapter, but instead, the key principles will be covered. Excellent reviews on anesthesia for burn patients are available for more in-depth guidance [5–8]. The first issue is dealing with the difficult airway. There may be edema that obscures the airway during the resuscitation period. Scarring may limit the ability for neck extension or mouth opening. These issues are covered in detail in Chap. 3. The second issue is securing the airway, which is often difficult but is also covered in Chap. 3. It is often common to have disagreements about the timing of feedings prior to surgery. Stopping feedings at midnight the day before surgery in a large burn patient who requires frequent surgical procedures leads to a significant deficit in nutrition. Many burn centers place post-pyloric feeding tubes that allow for feedings up to, and in some centers, throughout surgery. Monitoring the patient is another challenge that is covered above. We will place monitors, including EKG leads and pulse oximeters on any available site. Arterial lines are also very helpful for major burn excisions. Monitoring the temperature is also essential as the patient may become quite cold over time. The burn operating room is renowned for being very warm. As stated above, adequate blood products must be available prior to major excisions.

There are many pharmacologic considerations for the anesthesiologist. The pharmacokinetics and pharmacodynamics of burn patients are significantly changed. During the first 48 h, the so-called "ebb" phase of the initial burn resuscitation, the cardiac output is decreased. Therefore, there is decreased hepatic and renal blood flow, which may decrease elimination of some drugs. After 48 h, there is a marked hyperdynamic phase that results in the most severe hypermetabolic response of any injury or disease. The cardiac output is increased in association with a marked decrease in systemic vascular resistance. The calorie requirements approach twice normal compared to normal people. There is an increase in renal and hepatic blood flow that often increases the clearance of drugs. Increased hepatic clearance, exemplified by drugs such as propofol and fentanyl, reduces their duration of action. Another important factor is that two major drug-binding proteins, albumin and alpha$_2$-acid glycoprotein (AAG), are changed in opposite ways. Albumin levels typically drop to very low levels, and despite replacements, typically remain almost half normal. Albumin binds mainly acidic and neutral drugs, such as benzodiazepines, and since albumin levels are lower, there is decreased binding, increased free drug, and increased volume of distribution. AAG, being an acute phase reactant, is increased after a burn. AAG binds to cationic drugs, such as lidocaine, propranolol, muscle relaxants, and some opioids. Increased AAG leads to decreased free drug availability.

Choosing which paralytic agents to use in burn patients is very important. The initial muscle contractions caused by the depolarizing agent succinylcholine may lead to excessive potassium release which may lead to a hyperkalemia and cardiac arrest. It is stated that this effect does not occur for 48 h, so it is recommended to avoid succinylcholine after 2 days post-burn. On the other hand, there is a decreased sensitivity to nondepolarizing paralytic drugs [9]. Therefore, the dose of a nondepolarizing paralytic agent needs to be increased, and at the same time, there is a delay in its onset of activity. Burn patients have significant amounts of pain, so they are given more narcotics and other sedatives than most patients. They often develop tolerance so that during induction and upon emergence much higher doses are required than usual. Ketamine is a useful drug that is used both for anesthesia and moderate sedation. This drug increases secretions, but is safer for maintaining the airway. We have used both intravenous and intramuscular ketamine for years with minimal complications [10]. Like narcotics, ketamine tolerance is increased with time and higher doses are required with time. In addition, low-dose ketamine, by binding to *N*-Methyl-D-aspartate (NMDA) receptors, acts synergistically with narcotics to improve pain while lowering the latter drug's dose requirements.

It is very helpful to have free communication between the surgeon and anesthesiologists throughout the case. The amount of blood loss can be excessive over a short period of time, so the surgeon should let the anesthesiologist know when rapid blood loss is about to occur. Along the same vein, the anesthesiologist should feel free to tell the surgeon to slow down or stop when hypotension is threatening the patient. Another period of patient stress occurs when tourniquets are released since the patient often is exposed to the "reperfused" blood from the extremity. The released blood also contains increased acid and other cell byproducts that produce a mild to moderate "ischemia-reperfusion" response, which also can lower blood pressure. Clearly, free and ample communication between the two teams leads to better outcomes.

Burn Excision

The most important principle of burn excision is to excise deep enough to expose a viable wound bed that will allow the skin graft to "imbibe" nutrients from the wound bed and thus survive until a vascular supply is created. In other words, the wound bed must have viable tissue that is not infected. The excision can be taken down to bleeding dermis, fat, fascia, or muscle. Grafts will not take on bone, tendon, or foreign bodies (hardware). Tangential excision is the most common method performed. Goulian or Watson knives are typically used to remove layers of burn, traditionally until bleeding is observed. Other instruments, such as the VersiJet™, scissors, or free blades, are also utilized. As described above, bleeding can be quite extensive with an open wound. The bleeding can obscure the view of the wound bed, so sweeping the knife, blade down and backwards will clear the site for better visualization. Injection of epinephrine-containing solutions (2 mg epinephrine/l lactated Ringer's) will greatly reduce the bleeding. For extremities, tourniquets eliminate bleeding but one can no longer rely on bleeding for adequacy of excision. The dermis must have a glistening appearance and fat must have a "normal" yellow color (Fig. 9.2). One misconception is that one cannot graft on a bed of fat, but we have excellent success with grafting on fat. Some feel that the bed must be "conditioned" with allograft skin prior to obtaining take, but that is also not necessary. If one is planning to place sheet grafts (skin with no meshing), then all of the dermis, with all of its adnexa, must be removed from the recipient site. Otherwise, any remnant hair follicles or other glands will continue to produce their product or slough cells and an inclusion cyst will result. Large numbers of remnant glands will lead to multiple skin bridges and cysts that have been called "sponge skin" [11].

Fascial excision is a technique where all of the tissue is excised as a unit down to the fascia. This method may reduce bleeding since the cautery can be used to remove the burn and fat, and there are only perforating vessels that must be controlled. The technique does permanently remove all fat, so the fat never develops below the skin graft. Thus, the skin is stuck to the fascia/muscle and has no mobility. In addition, the extremities lose their normal contours and have a "spindly" appearance. At the borders of the excision, where fascial excision is next to fat-containing tissue, is a sharp step-off that is quite noticeable. In addition, when fascial excisions are performed circumferentially on legs, the graft tends to contract and limit venous and lymphatic return, so there is an increased incidence of distal edema. Cellulitis, which is associated with decreased lymphatic and venous return, may also occur and be difficult to treat. Some of my colleagues feel that fascial excisions are the best options for the elderly or obese patient because of the belief that grafts do not take as well on fat, especially in the elderly. Except when the depth of the burn is down to fascia, I never perform fascial excisions because of the cosmetic and functional issue. Our results in the elderly and obese patients are fine with grafting on fat.

Full-Thickness Skin Grafts

Since thicker grafts shrink the least of any graft, full-thickness grafts are preferred for small and functionally important areas such as the face or hand. They are obviously limited by the fact that donor site must be closed primarily or covered with a split-thickness skin graft (which is rarely performed). Most of the time, the site of harvest is chosen for its ease of closure combined with the ability to hide the incisional scar. The color of the skin is another important consideration since skin harvested from below the clavicle is usually a different color than that of the face or neck. Therefore, full-thickness grafts for the face should be harvested above the clavicle.

My preferred donor site for full-thickness grafts below the clavicle is from the inguinal region. An ellipse of skin can be harvested that covers an entire palm with little difficulty closing the incision. Local anesthetic containing epinephrine is injected into the area and a full-thickness piece of skin is harvested down to fat. The harvest can be performed right on the dermis or a little fat can be left on the skin for later removal. The donor site is closed with buried dissolvable stitches. The ultimate scar is rarely noticed since it is at the crease of the leg. An alternative is the lower abdomen where skin can be harvested as for an abdominoplasty. One must be careful when using lower abdominal skin from obese patients since the dermis is often quite thick due to the weight of pannus. Any other site can be used, including the upper, inner arm, gluteal crease, or others. For the face, skin can be harvested from the supraclavicular region or from behind the ear. When using the posterior auricular region, skin is harvested in equal amounts from the head and posterior ear; then the skin edges are sewn to each other (removing space from behind the ear).

Once the full-thickness skin is harvested, it must be prepared for grafting by cutting away any fat from the dermis. One may grasp both ends of the ellipse with hemostats and then use scissors to trim the fat. One must also look for hair follicles, which for inguinal or abdominal skin project beneath the dermis. The hair follicle bulbs should be trimmed to minimize the transfer of hair. If the dermis is thicker than desired, it should be thinned with scissors until the desired thickness is obtained. The excessively thick dermis of heavyset people acts as a barrier to diffusion of nutrients that may lead to epidermolysis. If the epidermis is lost, then the graft will ultimate fail unless regrafted with a thinner (split-thickness) graft.

A benefit of full-thickness skin grafts is that they have minimal discomfort when compared to split-thickness grafts. Closing the donor site eliminates the exposed wounds of split-thickness grafts. The improved comfort makes it quite easy to perform full-thickness grafts as outpatient procedures. Full-thickness skin grafts also have the benefit of contracting less than thinner grafts, so they are very useful for small hand or face defects.

Split-Thickness Skin Grafts

Split-thickness skin grafts are required to cover any sizeable surface area of the body. The term "split-thickness" is derived from the fact that the dermis is "split" so that a portion of dermis that carries the epidermis is transferred while the remaining dermis heals by re-epithelialization. The surgeon can vary the thickness of the donor skin. The same principle of minimizing scarring applies—that thicker skin contracts less than thinner skin, but one must consider the healing of the donor site. As stated in the chapter on wound healing (Chap. 8), if the donor site takes longer than 2–3 weeks to re-epithelialize, then there is a likelihood that the donor site will develop hypertrophic scarring. If one takes a thick split-thickness skin graft, then it is at the expense of a higher risk for delayed donor site healing and hypertrophic scarring. The surgeon must balance the risks of donor site scarring with optimizing the functional and cosmetic outcomes of the graft. There are strategies for optimizing both outcomes. When possible, the donor site should be chosen in an area that tends to be hidden. Classically, harvesting skin from the lateral thigh from the hip to the knee has been the donor site of choice. If that area develops hypertrophic scarring, then the lower, lateral thigh will be exposed when wearing shorts. If, on the other hand, the skin is harvested from the upper lateral thigh and then coursing anteriorly and medially in a circumferential fashion, then that donor site is easily covered with shorts (Fig. 9.5). The back is a particularly forgiving site for harvest, with scarring being less common than the thigh (Fig. 9.6) [12]. The back is easier to approach in a child than an overweight adult, however. The lower

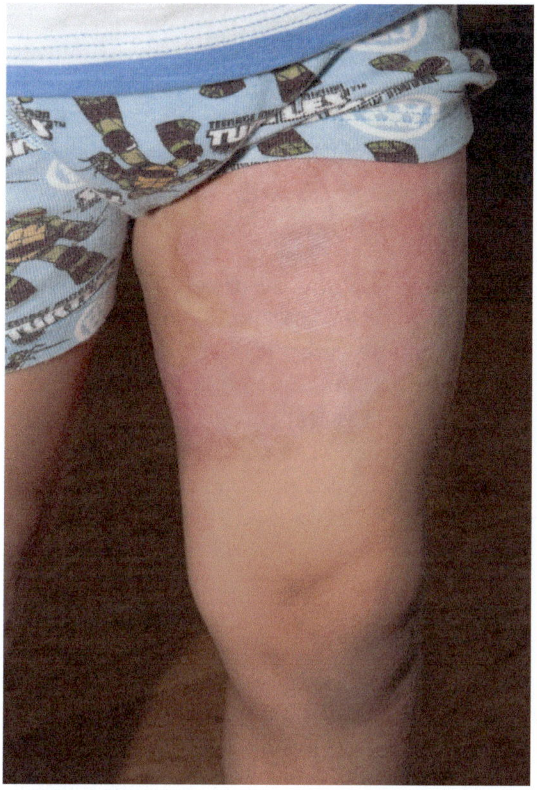

Fig. 9.5 This circumferential thigh donor site is easily covered with shorts

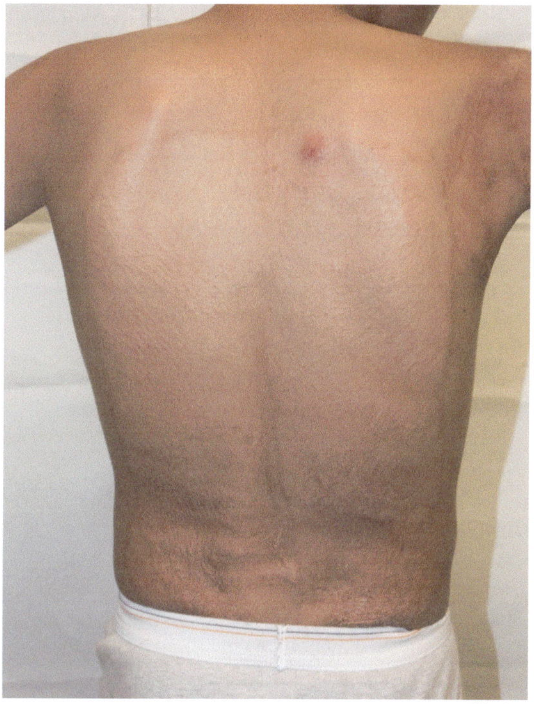

Fig. 9.6 The ultimate result of a back donor site is quite acceptable. Back donor sites tend to do well because the skin is thicker than other parts of the body

back is preferred since that area may also be covered with shorts. The upper back should be avoided, especially in young women who might want to wear clothing exposing the upper back. For patients with massive (>80 % TBSA) burns, any available skin is fair game. I have harvested from all areas (including the genitalia and hands) except for the face.

There are several "principles and tricks" (Table 9.1) that can be used to optimize harvesting split-thickness skin grafts. While hand-held instruments, such as Goulian and Watson knives, can be used to harvest skin, they are less reliable and rarely used at least in developed countries. There are several powered dermatomes that are available and it probably does not really matter which one is used, but it is best to become familiar with one and use it consistently. For a small and less important harvest, preparation of the donor site is not necessary. The lateral thigh works well, but the donor site will have considerable oozing of blood. For important grafts, or if one needs to harvest large areas of split-thickness skin grafts, preparation of the harvest site is important. Injection of an epinephrine-containing solution ("Pitken" solution containing 2 mg epinephrine per liter lactated Ringer's solution) has two advantages; it minimizes donor site bleeding and provides a uniform, firm surface for a reliably consistent skin graft. If one needs to harvest from a surface that has bony prominences (back), has a soft consistency (abdomen), or is not flat enough for a wide harvest (scalp), injection of a "Pitken" solution is very helpful. One can inject epinephrine-containing solutions by hand-held syringes, but it requires time and patience. People have also used pressure devices placed around intravenous bags, but we prefer to use a roller-pump to push the fluid into the subcutaneous space. We have injected many liters into large surface areas to allow for extensive harvests.

One must then set the thickness of the dermatome to harvest the desired thickness of skin. The

Table 9.1 Tricks to improve split-thickness skin graft harvest

Choosing a harvest site
Choose a site that optimizes the thickness of the donor while minimizes scarring (such as the back)
Choose a site that is hidden if it scars (lower back, circumferential upper thigh)
Avoid cosmetically important areas (upper chest or back, face, hands)
Avoid areas that are prone to scarring (lower legs)
Match donor color to recipient color (skin above clavicle for face)
Always harvest 20 % more than anticipated (donors shrink)
Prep and drape more donor site areas than expected (more than expected may be needed)
Harvest "tricks"
Inject the donor site with epinephrine-containing solution to create a uniformly firm surface
Harvesting from firmer surfaces (scalp, lower legs) produces thicker skin (dermatome can be set thinner)
Harvesting from softer surfaces (abdomen, buttocks) produces thinner skin (dermatome should be set thicker)
Check donor skin thickness as you harvest by looking at the dermal side
Adjust dermatome thickness as you harvest to obtain the appropriate thickness (especially when traveling from firm to soft surface such as outer thigh to inner thigh)
The first harvest is always thicker
If the harvest becomes too thin or tears, obtain new blade

typical thickness used for most grafts is between 10 and 12 thousands of an inch. Thicker grafts are used for more functional areas such as the hands or face (15–18/1000 in.). Many surgical residents have been taught to check the thickness of the dermatome by placing a scalpel blade between the dermatome blade and its surface. This is a practice that should be avoided because it is inaccurate and may dull the dermatome blade. It turns out that the numbers on the dermatome may determine the gap between blade and dermatome surface, but they do not determine the thickness of the harvested skin. Another "principle" is that the donor skin is thicker when harvested from a firm surface. Thus, when harvesting skin from a lower leg or scalp, the dermatome should be set on the thinner side (8–10/1000 in.) to obtain skin at 12/1000 in.. When harvesting from a soft surface, especially the abdomen, the dermatome may have to be set at 20–25/1000 in. to obtain a piece of skin that is 12/1000 in. thick. Another "trick" is that one should check the thickness of the skin as it exits the dermatome to check for its thickness. I usually examine the dermal side to obtain the best feedback. A skilled burn surgeon uses the "trick" to adjust the dermatome thickness as the skin is being harvested to maintain the desired thickness for the entire graft. For instance, when harvesting a circumferential upper thigh donor site, the dermatome may be set at 12/1000 in. to start, but as the softer medial thigh is approached, the dermatome thickness usually needs to be increased to 18–20/1000 in.

The angle of dermatome as it harvests skin is important for obtaining consistent skin. Usually, the dermatome is maintained at a 45° angle as it contacts the skin. The same angle must be maintained as one harvests the skin. When obtaining skin from a circular surface, such as the upper thigh or scalp, one must remember to maintain that 45° angle throughout the harvest. I tend to think of maintaining a constant tangent of a circle as I move around the circular surface (Fig. 9.7). Another "trick" for harvesting multiple pieces of skin is that the first piece tends to be the thickest, while subsequent harvests tend to be thinner. If the harvest skips or becomes inconsistent, then the blade is becoming dull and a new blade will help with a more consistent subsequent harvest.

The next decision is whether to mesh the skin or leave it as an intact sheet of skin. There are several types of skin meshers that will expand the skin from a size of 1:1 to 6:1. It is important to remember that the size of the harvested skin ends up being smaller than the original donor site since it shrinks in size. If one places a large volume of subcutaneous "Pitken" solution, the donor skin is stretched due to the tension. Therefore, if the skin is stretched, then the donor site shrinks even more. As a "principle," donor skin should always be harvested 20 % larger than one expects to need for covering the excised area. One must be cautious when harvesting skin that exactly matches a template of the recipient site. This principle also explains the naming of a 1:1 mesher; its expansion returns the skin to roughly the original size of the harvest. The number of the expansion indicates a rough degree of expansion so that a 4:1 meshed autograft is four times it original size. The

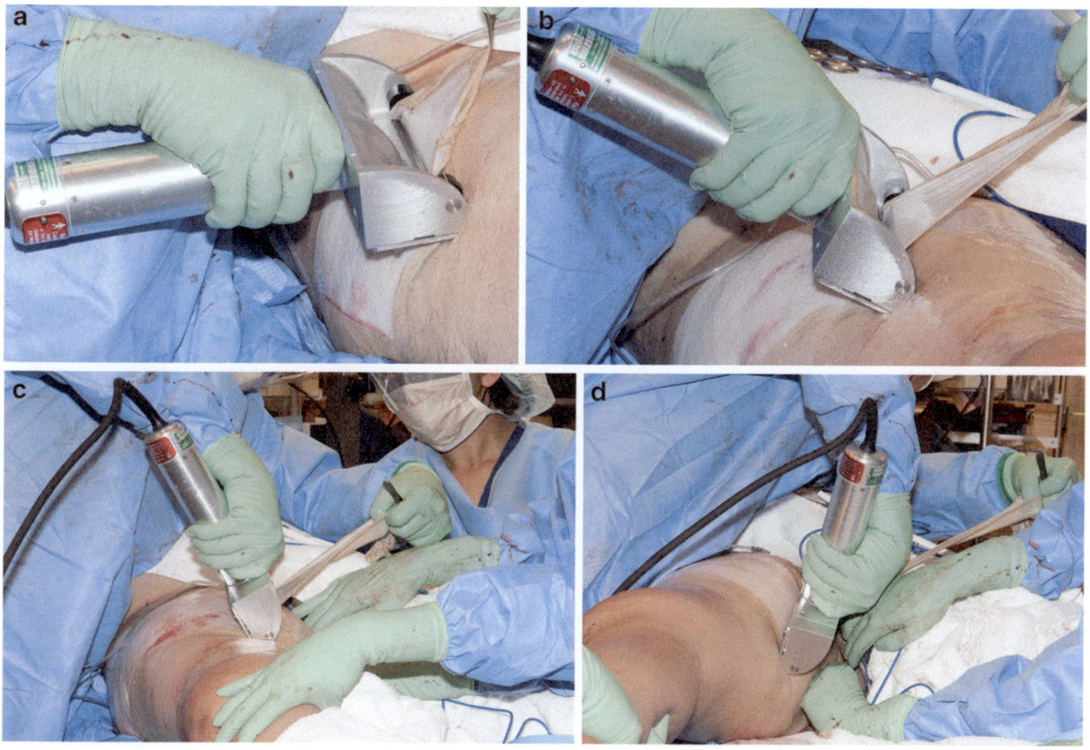

Fig. 9.7 (**a–d**) When harvesting skin around a circumferential donor site, the 45° angle on the skin must be maintained throughout the harvest

largest expansion that I use is 4:1 mesh since the 6:1 expansion tends to be difficult to handle. There is another strategy, called the "Meeks" technique, which allows for even greater expansion. This technique is a modification of the "postage stamp" grafting technique where tiny stamp-sized pieces of skin are distributed throughout the recipient site. For the "Meeks" technique, a piece of skin is placed shiny side up on a stretchy cloth and then blades are run perpendicular to each other to create small squares of skin. The cloth is then stretched to spread the squares over a large area and inverted to place the skin on the bed. Impressive expansion of skin is accomplished with this technique.

Meshed grafts are the easier method for covering a wound. They also have the advantage of making it easier to prevent blood and serum from collecting beneath the graft and interfere with take (especially for wider meshed skin). Another advantage is that meshing will reduce the amount of donor site that is available. Meshed skin is not without its problems. The main issue is that the meshed pattern will last for life. Healing of a meshed graft involves graft adherence, but for the interstices, scar formation, re-epithelialization, and contraction also occur to leave the pattern for life. If the interstices take longer than 2–3 weeks to re-epithelialize, the scarring can be significant (Fig. 9.8). Because of these problems, I prefer to utilize sheet split-thickness skin grafts when practical. Sheet grafts require more work since hemostasis must be meticulous and more donor sites are required. One must also pay more attention to the seams between sheet grafts since, like any incision, a straight line tends to create more tension and thus more hypertrophic scarring. One can create seams that are in a zigzag pattern to minimize these issues [13]. For larger sheet grafts, the goal is to obtain the widest and most consistent skin available. The 6-in. wide dermatome (Padgett, Integra LifeSciences, Inc.,

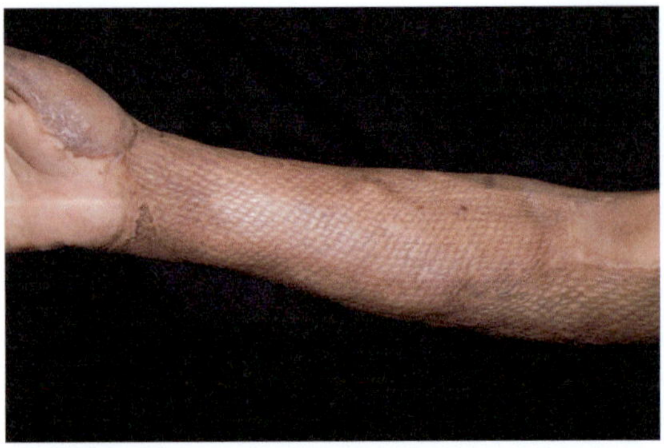

Fig. 9.8 This is the typical meshed pattern of an arm grafted with 2:1 mesh. While the graft is supple and mobile, the meshed pattern will persist for life. The thumb has a sheet graft for comparison

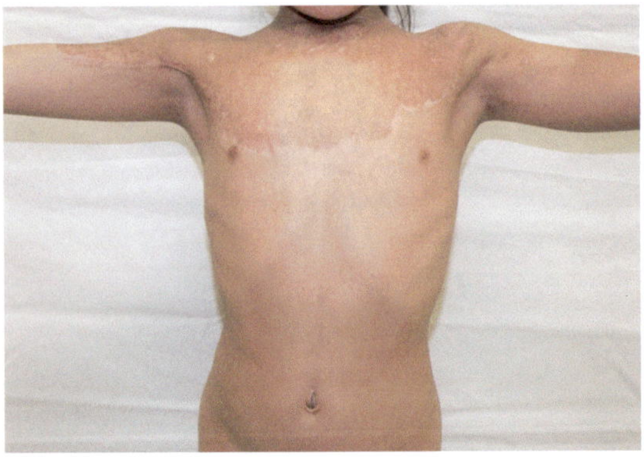

Fig. 9.9 This child has one 6 in. wide sheet graft that covers her entire upper chest and right arm. The cosmetic outcome is excellent

Cincinnati, OH), while more difficult to use, leads to the ability to cover all or most of a dorsal hand. The postoperative care is a little more involved with sheet grafts. We always check the grafts on postoperative day 1 to check for hematomas or seromas. If fluid is found beneath the graft, the skin may be nicked with a blade to remove any hematoma or seroma. On occasion, large hematomas develop, but at day one the graft can be partially removed, the blood evacuated, and the graft replaced with satisfactory results. The extra effort for placing sheet grafts is worthwhile since the ultimate graft is much better cosmetically and functionally (Fig. 9.9).

Postoperatively, the grafts are usually covered with fine mesh gauze soaked in a topical solution. For mesh grafts, a moist environment is desired to improve on the rate of re-epithelialization. Sheet grafts can be covered with same dressing or they can be left open to air with good results. Areas such as the chest are often left open so that hematomas can be removed. Some surgeons advocate the use of negative pressure devices to improve graft take, but I have not found that technique necessary.

Management of Hand Burns

Hand burns are very common since they are often exposed to the heat source or they are involved in the inciting event or are used to stop the burning process. For instance, a very common injury occurs when someone tries to carry out a frying pan of burning grease. As the pan is carried, the air movement pushes the flames over the thumb, index finger, and dorsal hand. The hands are also used to protect the face when escaping a room engulfed in flames. Toddlers explore their environment with their hands and, unlike adults, they freeze when they contact a hot surface—leading to deep palmar burns. Because hands are exposed to the public and are essential for normal activities, one must ensure that hand burns have the best outcome possible. As for any burn, if they heal within 2 weeks then they do well. If healing takes longer than 2 weeks, then hypertrophic scarring can interfere with normal range of motion. Therefore, one should have a low threshold to graft a deep burn of the hand. Some people advocate that the hand should be covered with a dermal substitute in order to have an improved outcome, but I have had excellent results with immediate sheet autografts.

Full-thickness *palmar burns* that are typically observed in toddlers are usually treated as outpatient procedures. Tourniquets are used to make visualization of the burn easier. The burn is excised to fat with a Goulian knife and a full-thickness skin is harvested from the inguinal region. The full-thickness graft is then sutured in place with a chromic suture, left long to use a tie-over bolster. A nonsticky dressing is applied over the graft and covered with cotton soaked in

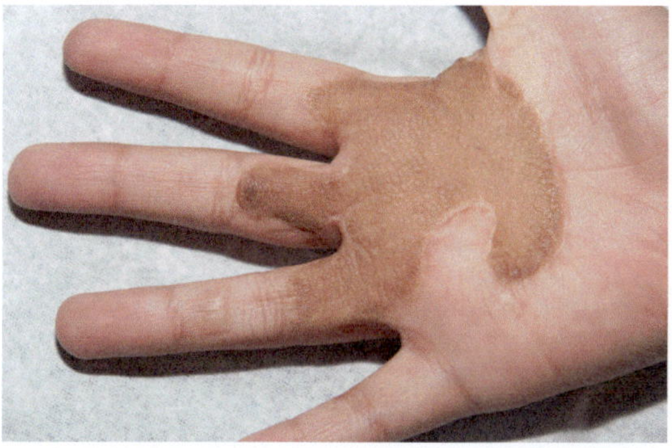

Fig. 9.10 This palm burn was covered with a full-thickness skin graft. The mobility is excellent but there is obvious hyperpigmentation

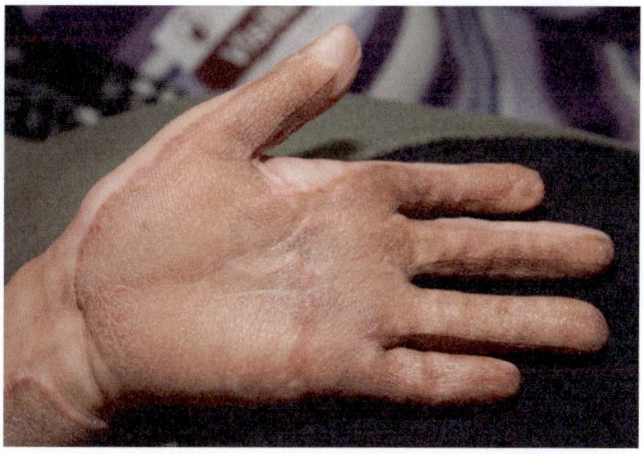

Fig. 9.11 When grafting the entire palmar surface of hand, there is not enough skin available to graft the area without a seam, so a thick split-thickness graft using the 6-in. dermatome was used to create a single graft

saline and tied into place. The rest of the hand is wrapped in cotton, and ultimately, CoBan™ Self-Adherent Dressing (3M, St. Paul, MN) is used to cover the entire package. So far, I have never had a patient get out of this self-adherent dressing. The dressing is left untouched for a week and then the dressing is removed and hand therapy is started. There are two problems with this technique—increased pigmentation and transfer of hair. Since the palm lacks pigment, grafts tend to be darker than the rest of the hand. The alternative is to harvest skin from the plantar aspect of the foot, but this skin is very rigid and due to the thickness of the epithelium is difficult to handle. The other problem is that some hair may be transferred, but it can be removed with laser treatment. Other than these two problems, the results are excellent (Fig. 9.10) [14–16]. If the entire palmar surface needs covering, then a thick split-thickness skin graft can be used (Fig. 9.11).

Dorsal hand burns are also quite common. The results from hand grafts can be excellent. Tourniquets make the excision much easier than if bleeding is allowed. Excising the dorsal fingers requires skill to ensure that deeper structures remain uninjured. Traction can be maintained by grasping the pads of the fingers with penetrating towel clips. After excising the burn, the towel clips are used to suspend the hand from a hand holder that makes placement much easier. Since sheet grafts should be used, the burn is then excised down to fat to prevent any inclusion cysts. Meshed hand grafts should only be used when donor sites are limited in massive burns. Even burns in patients with 60–70 % TBSA sheet grafts are preferred and the rest of the arm can be covered with a mesh graft. The goal for the graft is to minimize any seams, so the 6-in. dermatome provides enough width to cover all or most of the hand. Thicker skin should be used to reduce contractures, so I use 15–16/1000th in. skin. If the surgeon needs to cover the entire arm and hand, then the thickest skin should be used on the hand and the thinner skin is used on the more proximal arm.

A good strategy is to apply the sheet skin to the fifth finger and then spread it over the other fingers. The skin is then cut between the fingers as one proceeds toward the index finger. To cover the thumb, the skin can be curved up towards the thumb and attached. Another strategy is to harvest skin in the shape of an "L" to fit the shape of the skin. The graft may be sutured, but it is much more expeditious to staple the graft in place. The hand is then wrapped in a fist position to stretch the graft over the dorsal fingers. We usually check the graft on postoperative day 1 to check for any hematoma and the staples are removed on postoperative day 5. Range of motion is started on this day. The outcomes are quite good (Fig. 9.12).

Burns that involve *both the dorsal and volar side of the hand* are more challenging. The excision is carried out in the same manner as before. The challenge is covering the circumferential

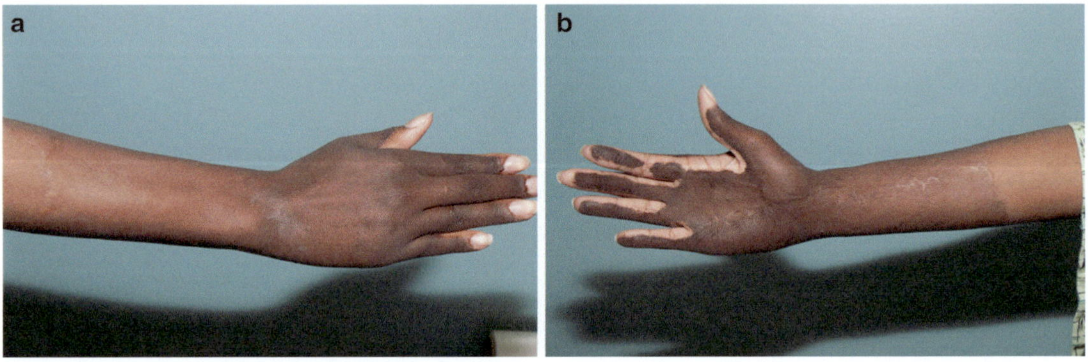

Fig. 9.12 (**a**–**b**) This is an example of a 6-in. wide sheet graft that covered the entire dorsal hand (**a**). The seam on the volar side has a zigzag pattern to minimize contraction. The palm was covered with a full-thickness graft. This picture was taken several years after grafting

finger burns. Usually, two sheets of skin are used—one for the dorsal side and one for the palmar side. The best strategy is to wrap each finger circumferentially so that the seams are between the fifth and ring fingers; and between the middle and index fingers. The seam of the thumb should be on the ulnar side. The graft should be positioned in neutral and the aftercare is the same as before.

Deeper (fourth-degree) burns to the hand are not uncommon, especially in young children. The saving grace for the very young child is that their fingers have fat that offers some protection. We rarely amputate any digits during the first excision, but will cover the area with autograft or allograft. When the depth is not clear, autografting may cover more than anticipated (especially when there is plenty of donor site availability). The principle for amputations is to preserve as much length as possible. The most common defect is exposure of the dorsal proximal interphalangeal (PIP) joint. When this is the only exposed area of a hand graft, simple immobilization is possible by using Kirschner wires to immobilize the joint. The defect will usually fill in on its own. More extensive exposure requires flap coverage, which will not be covered here.

Management of Face Burns

Optimal healing of face burns is extremely important since, for obvious reasons, the face is what is presented to the public. Even mild scarring is difficult to hide, so the burn surgeon must optimize healing and minimize scarring. Fortunately, the face is more resistant to severe burns. There are several reasons; first the face tends to be protected with hands or in other ways when exposed to heat. In addition, it is very vascular and its vascularity diffuses heat to decrease the depth of injury. Therefore, in facial burns of indeterminate depth, it is worth waiting to determine whether healing occurs within 2 weeks. If the burn is obviously deep or if it has not healed within 2 weeks, then grafting is usually needed.

There are several important principles that need to be remembered when excising and grafting a face. First, one must be prepared for a significant amount of blood loss since the face has been documented to lose approximately 4.5 % of a blood volume per percent excision [4]. If one excises an adult face covering 5 % TBSA, then one would expect to lose just below a quarter of a blood volume. In a young child, with the head and face covering a larger relative surface area, a 10 % excision would lead to nearly the loss of nearly half of a blood volume. Second, the skin color of the face is different than any skin harvested below the clavicle. If one places a small graft from the thigh on a face, the ultimate color will be noticeably yellower than the rest of the face. Even a perfect graft would still be very noticeable (Fig. 9.12). One must also consider where to place any seams between skin grafts. The face is divided into "esthetic units" that

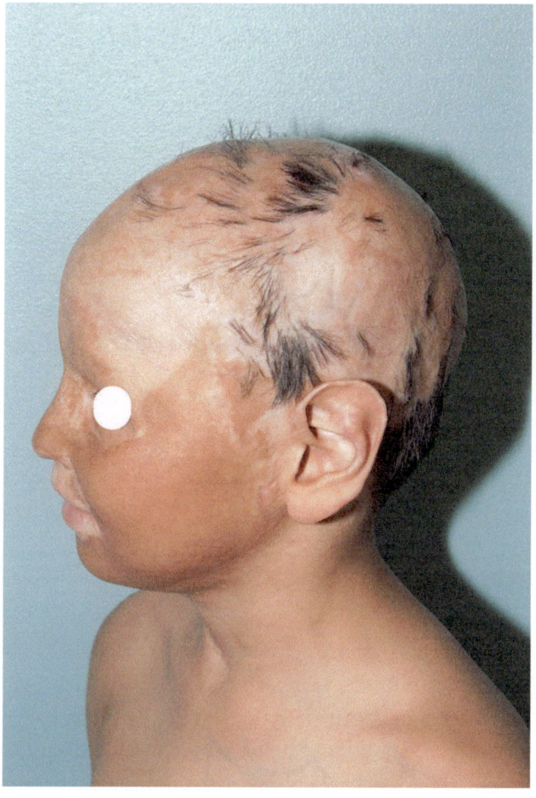

Fig. 9.13 This child did not have viable scalp donor site to cover his lower face burn. A sheet graft was harvested from his back. Despite a graft with minimal scarring there is an obvious color change just above the eye level

should not be violated with seams. No seam should be placed in the middle of the forehead, cheeks, or chin. Any line placed within the unit is easily noticed, but lines placed between esthetic units tend to be less noticed by the human eye. Plastic surgeons always place incisions between esthetic units to "hide" them. Similarly, one should always strive to place skin graft seams between these units—at the level of the eyes, edge of the nose, or bottom of the chin. As described below, if one can minimize the number of seams (down to one), then the cosmetic outcome is even better (Fig. 9.13).

Since excision and grafting of the face is more complex than grafting of any other site, it is best to limit the procedure to just the face. Positioning the patient in slight reverse trendelenberg lowers venous pressure and may reduce bleeding. Injection of solution containing epinephrine (2 mg/l lactated Ringer's) also will reduce bleeding. I tend to start around the eyes and then work towards the periphery. Grasping the eyelid for traction allows for better eyelid excision using the Goulian knife. The medial canthus region is a little more challenging to excise and may require a 15-blade scalpel or scissors. Some prefer to use the VersiJet for these areas. I find that applying traction to the eschar with the first cut will allow for a uniform depth excision that can course from the eyelid, across the medial canthus, and down the lateral nose. The next excision is then carried out using a powered dermatome or Watson knife around the forehead and cheeks. The excision is very bloody, so the anesthesiologists should have blood available or transfusing during the excision. It is also better to complete the excision rapidly before spending a great deal of time with hemostasis since repeated limited excision and cauterization leads to more bleeding than one faster, larger excision followed with more concentrated hemostasis. Once the excision is complete, total hemostasis is required to prevent any hematomas under the graft. Since the face should always be covered with a sheet of skin or skin substitute, any residual bleeding will lead to hematoma formation, so spending a significant amount of time with hemostasis is essential.

Once hemostasis is complete, the surgeon has different options for coverage. Many surgeons prefer to use allograft for temporary coverage as any hematoma will not lead to permanent defects in the skin. Skin substitutes (covered later) are also commonly used. Even with temporary coverage, adherence to placing seams at esthetic units is wise. Placing autograft at the first procedure is an excellent option that will shorten the length of stay. There is a slightly greater chance of hematoma formation, but our experience has shown no difference in outcomes when compared to a two-stage procedure [17]. If there is an isolated area of the face that is being grafted, it is best to harvest skin from the scalp since the color matches the face. Harvesting the scalp is more of a challenge due to the curve of the skull. The hair needs to be shaved with a razor and the scalp must be injected with epinephrine-containing

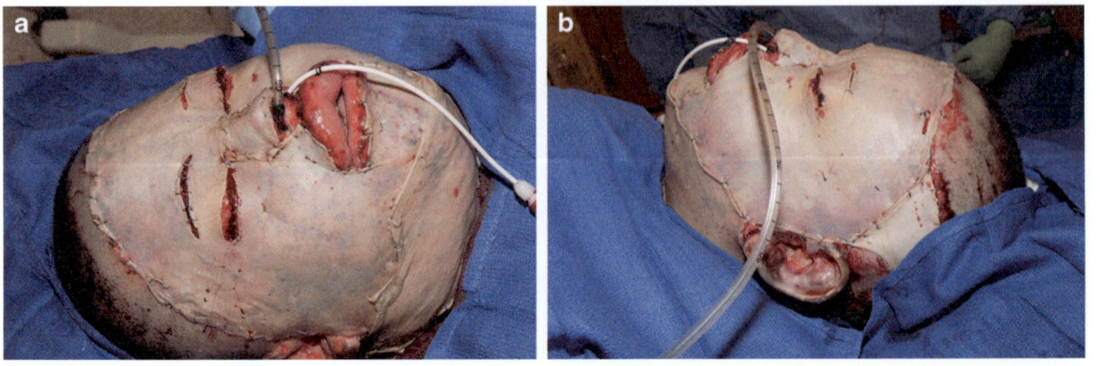

Fig. 9.14 (**a**–**b**) Here are two views of a recently placed graft on a face. Two pieces of skin were harvested in a "U" pattern from the abdomen. One piece of skin was wrapped around the upper face and the other was placed on the lower face and neck

solution. It is best to only partially fill the scalp with fluid so that it remains soft and pliable. If it is filled with fluid until taught, then the curve makes harvesting a wide piece of skin difficult. If it is soft, one can take a flat piece of metal (such as a dermatome guard) and flatten the scalp. The skin is then harvested in a circumferential fashion with the angle of the blade being maintained at around 45°. The dermatome is usually set around 12/1000th inch since the firm scalp leads to thicker harvest than on a softer area. The harvested scalp skin contains small hairs that may be gently scraped away from the dermis on a flat surface with the back of a "pickup" or scalpel handle. The scraping must be performed on the dermal side since the epidermis will be injured otherwise. The graft is then stapled or sutured in place and left open to reveal any hematomas. Postoperatively, hematomas may be drained with rolling (initially) or nicking the skin and draining any fluid.

We have developed a technique that minimizes the seams of the face graft. By harvesting skin in a "U" or circular fashion, one can obtain skin that will wrap around the face. The 6-in. dermatome is especially helpful for these grafts. The entire face is covered with only one seam that is placed at the junction of an esthetic unit. The graft is usually stapled in place except for around the eyelids, which are sutured with a dissolvable suture. The outcomes of these grafts have been very satisfactory (Fig. 9.14).

Strategies for Massive Burns

Excision and grafting of massive burns (>60 % TBSA) requires experience and planning. Decades ago, burn patients were treated conservatively with topical agents until the eschar spontaneously separated and granulation tissue formed. The process of spontaneous eschar separation involves bacterial invasion with the viable tissue developing granulation tissue as a barrier. The enzymes of the bacteria then break the bonds and the nonviable tissue falls away. During this protracted, often many weeks long course, the exposure to bacteria and the nonviable tissue leads to a persistent inflammatory response. In addition, granulation tissue tends to increase scar formation. Recent philosophy dictates that early removal of nonviable tissue and coverage of the open wound should, at least theoretically, reduce the inflammatory response and even mitigate the hypermetabolic response. In the past, it was also taught that patients could only tolerate smaller excisional procedures, limiting burn excisions to 20 % or less. That philosophy has now been disproven by many centers. With an experienced anesthesia and surgical team, massive excisions can be performed within a day of admission.

Our routine is to take the patient the day after admission for tracheostomy and excision of all of the extremities and anterior trunk. We have a team of 4–5 surgeons that makes the procedure

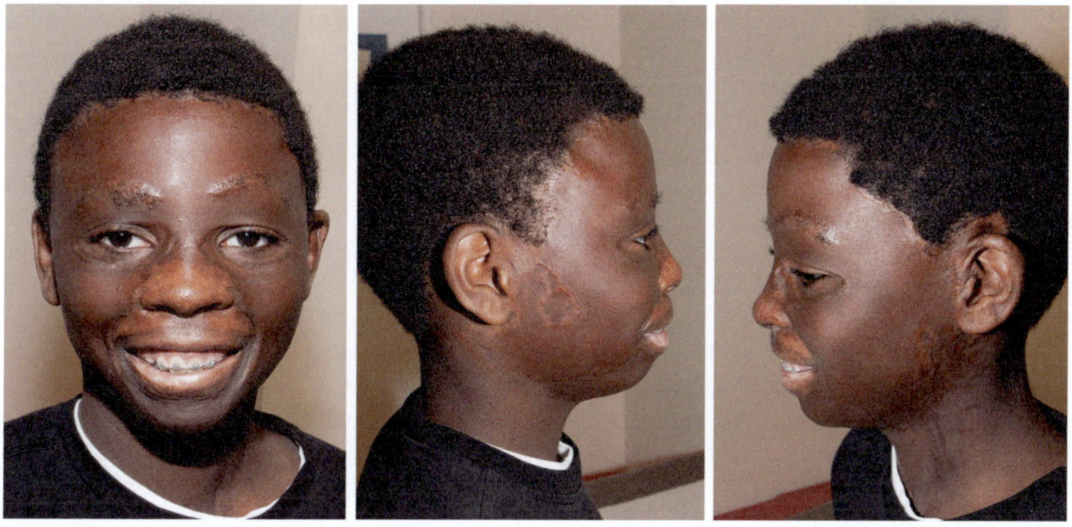

Fig. 9.15 (**a–c**) The result of an entire face graft that is "wrapped around" the face is quite satisfactory 8 years after the grafting

possible for even 90 % TBSA burned patients. All extremities have tourniquets and the anterior trunk is injected with a solution containing epinephrine. Every available donor site is harvested (except for the face and usually the hands). Depending on the size and severity of the burn, the hands may be covered with sheet grafts or a 2:1 meshed graft. If there is questionable viability of the hands, then allograft or 2:1 meshed autograft is used. The rest of the autograft is widely meshed (4:1) and usually used to first cover the arms, and then the feet if available. Some surgeons argue that the back should be covered first, but we cover more functional areas first. The back often has a chance to heal (since it is thicker than other areas), and if not, can be grafted later. When available autograft is exhausted, the remaining areas are covered with either allograft (from a skin bank) or a skin substitute. The widely meshed autograft can be covered with a moist dressing (usually in a topical antimicrobial) or may be covered with allograft (Alexander technique) or xenograft (pig skin). We typically return the next day to excise and cover the back, and then save the face excision and coverage for a third day (since it requires more concentration).

The donor sites should be harvested thinner than for smaller burns since one must wait for donor site healing before it can be reharvested to replace the allograft or dermal substitute. Once the donor site has re-epithelialized, which requires 2–3 weeks, the patient returns for more autografting. During the subsequent phases, matching the donor harvest to the area of excision requires some skill. One technique that helps is to harvest the skin, mesh it, and determine how much can be covered. Then the excision can be performed to match the available skin. This process is repeated multiple times until the patient is totally covered with autograft. In between grafting procedures, one must monitor the patient for infections and sepsis. Fortunately, outcomes for patients with massive burns have improved so that many now survive.

Skin Substitutes

The biggest problem for patients with massive burns is that it requires weeks for donor skin to become available. Therefore, the length of stay of a patient has typically been said to last one day per percent burn. For massive burns, the length of stay is even longer [18]. Investigators and clinicians have been working for decades to shorten the length of stay. Clearly, developing skin substitutes makes the most sense to close the wound faster and thus shorten hospital length of stay. In the future, a patient should be able to have an artificial skin applied over the entire burn soon after the time of injury to allow for rapid closure. While investigations have been ongoing for decades, very little progress has been made to create an adequate cultured skin. The current available skin substitutes are allogeneic and thus rejected. At the current state, the patient's own cells must be grown ex vivo, but the extent of graft take is mediocre at best.

The first strategy to be developed was to regrow the patient's epidermis [19]. In 1984, the Boston group published their experience with covering burns >90 % TBSA with cultured epithelial autografts [20]. To improve graft take, the patients had fascial excisions and then their wounds were covered with cultured epithelial autografts. These patients survived and this technology is still commercially available. One just sends a biopsy, the cells are grown, and weeks later the cells are shipped back to the burn unit. Unfortunately, this technique has problems. First of all, the percentage of "take" of the epithelial cells has been quite low in many centers [21]. The cells have lower resistance to infection, and because they lack a dermis, the skin has lower resistance to shearing [22]. Fascial excision is also disfiguring, so many have attempted to use it on fat where the take is also reduced. Studies have shown that immune-stimulating component of allograft is in the epidermis so the dermis can be retained. The technique of leaving allograft dermis and covering it with cultured epithelial autograft has improved its success [23]. Many centers have had success using a protocol of cultured epithelial autografts and some form of allograft dermis [24–29].

The cultured epithelial autograft studies quickly revealed a need for an artificial dermis. Studies in the 1980s produced dermal substitutes, especially Integra (Integra LifeSciences, Cincinnati, OH) [30] and Alloderm (LifeCell Corporation, Bridgewater, NJ) [31, 32]. Integra is bovine collagen matrix that is covered with a silicone layer (which acts as a pseudo-epithelium). The matrix is placed on the wound bed and a minimum of 2–3 weeks is required for vascular ingrowth. The silicone is removed and a thin autograft is applied to recreate the epithelium. Integra is still being used today, but, unfortunately, it has not had good results with being covered with cultured epithelial autografts. Alloderm, a freeze-dried human dermis, was designed for immediate coverage with autograft, but it is now rarely used for skin grafts. Instead, it is used as an implant for breast augmentations and hernias. Primatrix is a newer dermis made from fetal bovine skin. It is now in its early stages of testing [33, 34].

The ideal goal is to have an autogenous composite skin made of both a dermis and epidermis. There has been a great deal of research in this area, which has produced excellent results [35]. The skin is pliable and has reduced the length of stay of patients with massive burns [36–39]. There are clear problems with pigmentation that should be addressed with the addition of melanocytes. Clearly, the technology to make this type of skin substitute is available, but it appears that its production has not been a priority for many manufacturers or regulators. Burns, while a severe problem for the patient, are not in sufficient numbers to make production of biologic skins a priority for many companies. Allogeneic skins are being produced because they can be used for the more lucrative chronic wound market. Hopefully, in the future, these products will be available to improve the length of stay and outcomes of burn patients with massive wounds.

Summary

There are several basic tenants that can be used to optimize the functional and cosmetic outcomes of burn patients. Clearly, smaller and more superficial burns will do better than those burns that cover large surface areas and are extremely deep. One must strive to optimize re-epithelialization in partial-thickness wounds so that healing occurs within 2 weeks to minimize scarring. If a burn is still open after 2 weeks or if the burn is obviously full-thickness, then skin grafting is usually required. The use of sheet skin graft will minimize the mesh pattern that occurs when meshing skin. Thicker skin does better than thin skin, but the surgeon must balance the thickness of the donor skin with the potential for donor site scarring. For massive burns, the philosophy of early extensive excision with some form of wound coverage appears to have improved survival. While there is extensive experience with skin substitutes, the available products are limited. Hopefully, new and effective products will become available in the future.

References

1. Greenhalgh DG. The role of apoptosis in wound healing. Int J Biochem Cell Biol. 1998;30(9):1019–30.
2. Darby IA, Bisucci T, Pittet B, Garbin S, Gabbiani G, Desmouliere A. Skin flap-induced regression of granulation tissue correlates with reduced growth factor and increased metalloproteinase expression. J Pathol. 2002;197(1):117–27.
3. Garbin S, Pittet B, Montandon D, Gabbiani G, Desmouliere A. Covering by a flap induces apoptosis of granulation tissue myofibroblasts and vascular cells. Wound Repair Regen. 1996;4(2):244–51.
4. Housinger TA, Lang D, Warden GD. A prospective study of blood loss with excisional therapy in pediatric burn patients. J Trauma. 1993;34(2):262–3.
5. Bittner EA, Shank E, Woodson L, Martyn JA. Acute and perioperative care of the burn-injured patient. Anesthesiology. 2015;122(2):448–64.
6. Anderson TA, Fuzaylov G. Perioperative anesthesia management of the burn patient. Surg Clin North Am. 2014;94(4):851–61.
7. Fuzaylov G, Fidkowski CW. Anesthetic considerations for major burn injury in pediatric patients. Paediatr Anaesth. 2009;19(3):202–11.
8. MacLennan N, Heimbach DM, Cullen BF. Anesthesia for major thermal injury. Anesthesiology. 1998;89(3):749–70.
9. Vega-Villa KR, Kaneda K, Yamashita S, Woo S, Han TH. Vecuronium pharmacokinetics in patients with major burns. Br J Anaesth. 2014;112(2):304–10.
10. Owens VFPT, Comroe CM, Conroy JM, Scavone JA, Greenhalgh DG. Ketamine: a safe and effective agent for painful procedures in the pediatric burn patient. J Burn Care Res. 2006;27(2):211–6.
11. Engrav LH, Gottlieb JR, Walkinshaw MD, Heimbach DM, Grube B. The "sponge deformity" after tangential excision and grafting of burns. Plast Reconstr Surg. 1989;83(3):468–70.
12. Greenhalgh DG, Barthel PP, Warden GD. Comparison of back versus thigh donor sites in pediatric patients with burns. J Burn Care Rehabil. 1993;14(1):21–5.
13. Greenhalgh DG, Palmieri TL. Zigzag seams for the prevention of scar bands after sheet split-thickness skin grafting. Surgery. 2003;133(5):586–7.
14. Schwanholt C, Greenhalgh DG, Warden GD. A comparison of full-thickness versus split-thickness autografts for the coverage of deep palm burns in the very young pediatric patient. J Burn Care Rehabil. 1993; 14(1):29–33.
15. Pham TN, Hanley C, Palmieri T, Greenhalgh DG. Results of early excision and full-thickness grafting of deep palm burns in children. J Burn Care Rehabil. 2001;22(1):54–7.
16. Kowalske KJ, Greenhalgh DG, Ward SR. Hand burns. J Burn Care Res. 2007;28(4):607–10.
17. Greenhalgh DG, Hinchcliff K, Sen S, Palmieri TL. A ten-year experience with pediatric face grafts. J Burn Care Res. 2013;34(5):576–84.
18. Taylor SL, Sen S, Greenhalgh DG, Lawless M, Curri T, Palmieri TL. A competing risk analysis for hospital length of stay in patients with burns. JAMA Surg. 2015;150(5):450–6.
19. Burke JF, Yannas IV, Quinby Jr WC, Bondoc CC, Jung WK. Successful use of a physiologically acceptable artificial skin in the treatment of extensive burn injury. Ann Surg. 1981;194(4):413–28.
20. Gallico 3rd GG, O'Connor NE, Compton CC, Kehinde O, Green H. Permanent coverage of large burn wounds with autologous cultured human epithelium. N Engl J Med. 1984;311(7):448–51.
21. Barret JP, Wolf SE, Desai MH, Herndon DN. Cost-efficacy of cultured epidermal autografts in massive pediatric burns. Ann Surg. 2000;231(6):869–76.
22. Desai MH, Mlakar JM, McCauley RL, et al. Lack of long-term durability of cultured keratinocyte burn-wound coverage: a case report. J Burn Care Rehabil. 1991;12(6):540–5.
23. Cuono C, Langdon R, McGuire J. Use of cultured epidermal autografts and dermal allografts as skin replacement after burn injury. Lancet. 1986;1(8490):1123–4.
24. Sood R, Balledux J, Koumanis DJ, et al. Coverage of large pediatric wounds with cultured epithelial autografts in congenital nevi and burns: results and technique. J Burn Care Res. 2009;30(4):576–86.
25. Sood R, Roggy D, Zieger M, et al. Cultured epithelial autografts for coverage of large burn wounds in eighty-eight patients: the Indiana University experience. J Burn Care Res. 2010;31(4):559–68.
26. Atiyeh BS, Costagliola M. Cultured epithelial autograft (CEA) in burn treatment: three decades later. Burns. 2007;33(4):405–13.
27. Cirodde A, Leclerc T, Jault P, Duhamel P, Lataillade JJ, Bargues L. Cultured epithelial autografts in massive burns: a single-center retrospective study with 63 patients. Burns. 2011;37(6):964–72.

28. Kym D, Yim H, Yoon J, et al. The application of cultured epithelial autografts improves survival in burns. Wound Repair Regen. 2015;23(3):340–4.
29. McHeik JN, Barrault C, Levard G, Morel F, Bernard FX, Lecron JC. Epidermal healing in burns: autologous keratinocyte transplantation as a standard procedure: update and perspective. Plast Reconstr Surg Glob Open. 2014;2(9), e218.
30. Heimbach D, Luterman A, Burke J, et al. Artificial dermis for major burns. A multi-center randomized clinical trial. Ann Surg. 1988;208(3):313–20.
31. Wainwright DJ. Use of an acellular allograft dermal matrix (AlloDerm) in the management of full-thickness burns. Burns. 1995;21(4):243–8.
32. Wainwright DJ, Bury SB. Acellular dermal matrix in the management of the burn patient. Aesthet Surg J. 2011;31(7 Suppl):13S–23.
33. Parcells AL, Karcich J, Granick MS, Marano MA. The use of fetal bovine dermal scaffold (PriMatrix) in the management of full-thickness hand burns. Eplasty. 2014;14, e36.
34. Strong AL, Bennett DK, Spreen EB, Adhvaryu DV, Littleton JC, Mencer EJ. Fetal bovine collagen matrix in the treatment of a full thickness burn wound: a case report with long-term follow-up. J Burn Care Res. 9 Dec 2014 [Epub ahead of print].
35. Boyce ST. Design principles for composition and performance of cultured skin substitutes. Burns. 2001;27(5):523–33.
36. Boyce ST, Goretsky MJ, Greenhalgh DG, Kagan RJ, Rieman MT, Warden GD. Comparative assessment of cultured skin substitutes and native skin autograft for treatment of full-thickness burns. Ann Surg. 1995; 222(6):743–52.
37. Boyce ST, Kagan RJ, Greenhalgh DG, et al. Cultured skin substitutes reduce requirements for harvesting of skin autograft for closure of excised, full-thickness burns. J Trauma. 2006;60(4):821–9.
38. Boyce ST, Kagan RJ, Yakuboff KP, et al. Cultured skin substitutes reduce donor skin harvesting for closure of excised, full-thickness burns. Ann Surg. 2002;235(2):269–79.
39. Boyce ST, Supp AP, Wickett RR, Hoath SB, Warden GD. Assessment with the dermal torque meter of skin pliability after treatment of burns with cultured skin substitutes. J Burn Care Rehabil. 2000;21(1 Pt 1):55–63.

Physical Rehabilitation

10

Ingrid Parry

Introduction

Rehabilitation after burn injury requires teamwork, communication and collaboration to maximize a patient's physical and psychological recovery. Advances in medical and surgical care have resulted in unprecedented rates of survival and patients withstanding more extensive burn injuries than ever before [1]. Patients with larger and more severe burn injuries have more scarring and therefore greater rehabilitation needs. Survival itself is no longer considered the end point of care, but rather the *quality* of a patient's survival is emphasized through rehabilitation efforts [2]. The overall goal of physical rehabilitation after a burn injury is to assist the patient in achieving the highest possible level of functional independence and maximal rehabilitation.

Physical rehabilitation begins on the day of admission and continues through scar maturation. For burn survivors with very severe injury, rehabilitation may continue for years due to ongoing reconstructive surgery and subsequent therapy-related needs, especially in growing children. Burn rehabilitation is typically provided by occupational and physical therapists (OT/PT) with special training in burn care. Although OTs and PTs have different professional training, the two disciplines work closely together in burn care and may overlap in their approaches to achieve distinct rehabilitation goals. For the purposes of this chapter, OTs and PTs will be referred to together as "burn therapists."

Rehabilitation Phases of Recovery

Although rehabilitation is a continuum of care provided throughout recovery from burn injury, the focus and emphasis of therapy shifts and can be described in three phases: acute rehabilitation, intermediate rehabilitation, and long-term rehabilitation [3]. The emergent care needs of the patient are extensive early in the recovery process and diminish over time, while the rehabilitative priorities and therapy needs gradually increase with time until maximal rehabilitation is achieved. It is helpful to understand the patient's rehabilitation needs in relationship to wound healing, surgery, and hospitalization.

Early Rehabilitation Phase

The early rehabilitation phase starts upon admission and continues until the patient's wounds are 50 % closed or skin grafting for wound closure has begun

I. Parry, M.S., P.T. (✉)
Department of Physical and Occupational Therapy, Shriners Hospital for Children, 2425 Stockton Blvd., Sacramento, CA 95608, USA
e-mail: iparry@parrypt.com

D.G. Greenhalgh (ed.), *Burn Care for General Surgeons and General Practitioners*,
DOI 10.1007/978-3-319-29161-1_10

[2]. Typically, burn therapists evaluate the patient within 24 h of admission and establish a rehabilitative plan of care. Early rehabilitation corresponds to the inflammatory phase of wound healing and the early proliferative phase when active wound contraction is occurring. Wound contraction, inflammation, and pain often restrict a patient's range of motion (ROM) and functional abilities during this phase. Therefore, the focus of therapy is to maintain ROM while promoting wound healing. "Appropriate therapy should not obstruct wound healing and would healing should not be allowed to prohibit rehabilitation" [4]. It is essential that the burn team coordinate their efforts to facilitate wound healing while preventing loss of function. Therapeutic interventions during this stage include wound care, edema management, anti-deformity positioning, splinting, ROM exercises, basic functional activities, and early ambulation.

Intermediate Rehabilitation Phase

The intermediate rehabilitation phase occurs until wound closure and/or acute skin grafting is complete [2]. This phase corresponds with the proliferative phase of wound healing when the tissue is re-vascularizing and re-epithelializing. Fibroblast are actively producing collagen, elastin, and glycosaminoglycans for the rebuilding and strengthening of scar tissue. The emphasis of rehabilitation in this phase is on maintaining ROM and restoring function as collagen is laid down in the wound while also avoiding mechanical trauma to newly healed tissue. Therapeutic interventions during this phase typically include the continuation of anti-deformity positioning, progression of splints to maintain ROM, ROM exercises, functional mobility, activities of daily living (ADLs), ambulation training, strengthening, early scar management, and initiation of basic cardiovascular/endurance training.

Long-Term Rehabilitation Phase

The long-term rehabilitation phase begins at wound closure until such time that the patient has received maximal benefit from rehabilitation services [2]. The patient may receive therapy within the acute hospital setting, a long-term rehabilitation facility, an outpatient therapy setting, or a continuum of all of these settings during this phase of care. Long-term rehabilitation corresponds with the maturation (or remodeling) phase of wound healing when the closed wound is developing strength, and collagen is being actively deposited and degraded. Therapeutic interventions during this phase emphasize minimizing scar contraction and hypertrophy and their impact on functional recovery. Common therapeutic interventions include anti-deformity positioning and splinting during times of inactivity or sleep, a progression of more complex and individually relevant functional tasks, physical agents/modalities, progression of functional mobility and ADLs, advanced ambulation activities, continued ROM and strengthening exercises, more demanding cardiovascular/endurance activities, sports and wellness activities, and scar management. During this phase, the interventions are transitioned to the patient and caregiver for eventual independence and compliance in their home setting.

Components of Rehabilitation

Positioning

Positioning is a fundamental part of any burn rehabilitation plan of care and the first line of defense against the formation of contractures. In the early rehabilitative phase of recovery, positioning is also important for the reduction of acute onset burn edema and protection of vulnerable tissues (i.e. exposed tendons, tissue over bony landmarks, skin grafts). An individualized positioning program is developed within 24 h of admission for each patient based on the distribution of the burn injury with consideration for associated injuries. The primary goal of a positioning program for the patient with burn injury is to maintain healing tissue in an elongated and anti-deformity position while protecting vulnerable structures. The involved body segment is placed in a position opposite the potential contracture based on wound distribution. For example, if the anterior hip crease or surrounding skin on the ventral surface

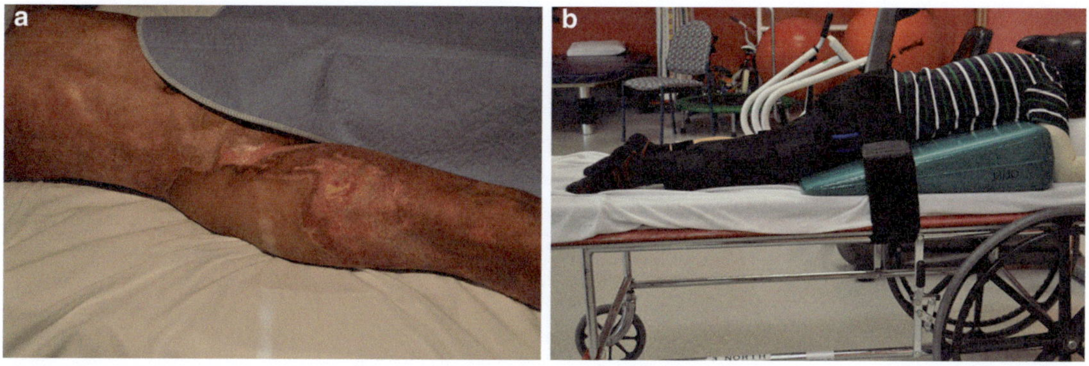

Fig. 10.1 (**a**) Distribution of burn injury. (**b**) Anti-contracture position

of the thigh and trunk is burned, then the anti-deformity position for that body segment would be full hip extension which can be achieved with a prone position (see Fig. 10.1a, b).

Patients tend to guard with pain after burn injury and assume a fetal like position with flexion of the extremities. It is well-known in burn care that the position of comfort is the position of deformity and standard anti-contracture burn positions have been defined [5]. Positions of function, however, are also important to consider and should be incorporated into any comprehensive positioning program. For example, the recommended position for a circumferential upper extremity burn that crosses the shoulder, elbow, and wrist joints is lying supine with the shoulder abducted and slightly horizontally flexed, elbow extended, and wrist supported in neutral. However, time in this position should be balanced with a position that encourages functional use of the upper extremities such as side-lying with the arms toward midline and the elbows flexed (functional position for feeding), (see Fig. 10.2a, b). There is currently no defined duration for a positioning schedule, so the best guide to determine how long any given position is beneficial is careful assessment of changes in the patient's ROM throughout the course of recovery.

Desired positions may be achieved and maintained with a variety of devices such as pillows, gel cushions, foam blocks, slings, bed modifications, and splinting devices. When possible, the patient should not be left supine in bed but should assume a combination of positions throughout the day including side lying, prone, sit, or stand in an effort to modify whole body positions and promote functional independence.

Splinting/Casting

Splinting is used in burn rehabilitation to protect vulnerable structures, minimize deformity, and maintain or increase tissue length of forming scar. Splints are used in situations where anti-deformity positioning alone does not sufficiently maintain ROM or when rapid loss of motion is anticipated. Although the use of splinting devices varies among burn centers [6–9], it is an accepted therapeutic treatment most often used in conjunction with active exercises and functional activities. Some burn centers prioritize mobility and only use splints when a loss in ROM is noted [10], while other centers use splinting more readily for immobilization and tissue elongation [11]. In 2011, Hollavanahalli et al. reported on the current trends regarding splinting in burn rehabilitation and found that therapists are using splinting more often to correct contractures than to prevent contracture [9]. That is, burn therapists tend to refrain from splinting joints that have full ROM, and instead, wait until there is a loss of motion observed before they splint, even with deep partial thickness and full thickness burns. Common splint-wearing schedules prescribed for the patient with burns are "2 hours on and 2 hours off" or "nights and naps in splints and active movement and function during daytime."

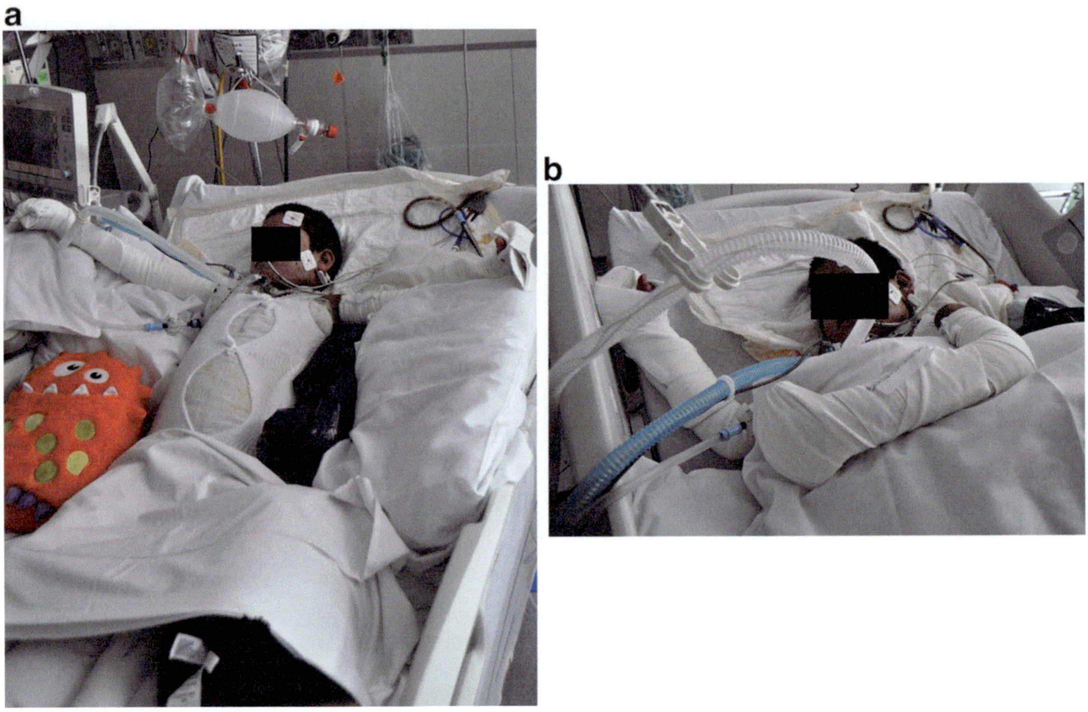

Fig. 10.2 (**a**) Standard anti-contracture position for upper extremity burns. (**b**) Functional positioning for upper extremity burns

The balance of time between wearing splints and removing splints for movement is typically dependent on the progress of the patient and is often determined by his/her ability to maintain ROM and functional independence during period when splints are not worn.

Despite a paucity of evidence on the effectiveness of splinting [12], the principles behind splinting are well-supported. Over 134 different splint designs have been described, likely a result of burn therapists' creativity to solve the many individualized problems that arise for patients with burn injury [13]. The actual splint type that is applied is less important than the limb position itself. Splints provide low load, prolonged duration forces intended to maintain elongation in scar and surrounding tissue [14]. Following the guidelines described for positioning, the forces of a splint should be applied in the opposite direction of the potential contracture.

Splints can be categorized according to the objective they are designed to achieve. Static splints aim to immobilize an area and therefore have no mobile parts. This type of splint may be used to protect tissue integrity, maintain joint alignment, provide opposing forces to forming scar contractures, or to maintain passive ROM [15]. Static splints are often used post-operatively over new skin grafts for immobility of the joint and protection of the graft. A static splint may also be made of immobile, but adjustable components, so that it can be remodeled to accommodate increases in ROM, in which case it is called a static progressive splint. In contrast, dynamic splints aim to mobilize a body part by utilizing the concept of tissue creep. That is, elastic parts are used to apply constant forces to forming scar tissue, thus progressively elongating the tissue over time [16]. Dynamic splints are used to provide prolonged stretch to tight tissue, apply controlled resistance for strengthening, or assist movement in weak muscles [15].

Serial casting, using plaster or fiberglass material, aids in tissue elongation and correction of burn scar contracture to areas non-responsive to other therapeutic interventions [17]. A cast is

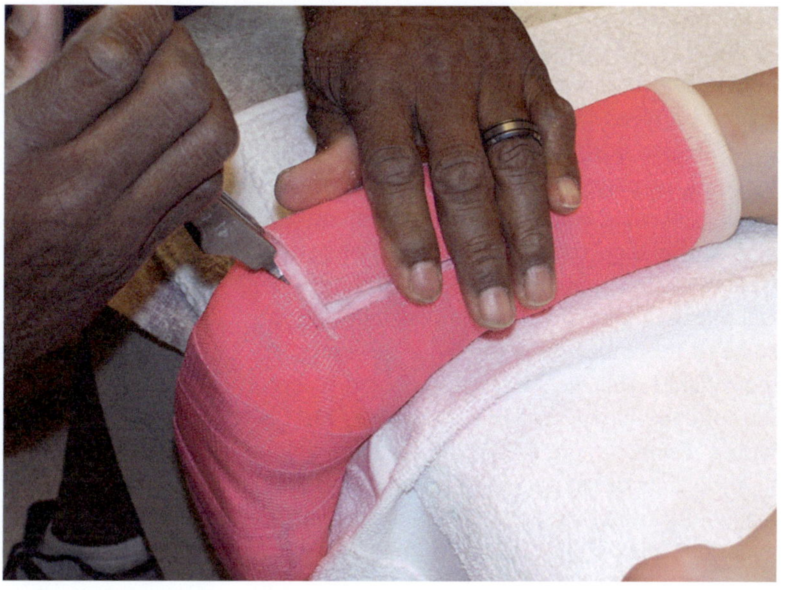

Fig. 10.3 A serial cast with a cut out for access to wound

applied circumferentially with evenly distributed pressure over the scars and positions the joint such that low load, prolonged corrective forces can be applied with minimal pain [18]. Casts are most often used with noncompliant patients or in children to prevent removal of the device. Casts may be safely used over non-infected skin grafts or open wounds [19]. They are typically applied and changed every 3–5 days when open wounds are present and every 7–10 days over healed scars. Windows may be cut in the cast to allow access to wounds if appropriate and necessary (see Fig. 10.3). Serial casting is a therapeutic option that has benefits to the patient with burn scar contracture when applied with skill and careful monitoring.

Range of Motion and Functional Exercises

Movement of burned areas after injury can be painful and result in muscle guarding and loss of motion. Exercise programs begin on the day of admission and continue throughout wound healing and scar maturation. ROM exercises can be active, active-assisted, or passive. Active exercise, where a patient independently moves a limb segment, is preferred in most situations because it provides sense of control, decreases perceived pain, and encourages active muscle contraction. Furthermore, active muscle pump reduces edema, promotes circulation [20], and mitigates muscle atrophy [21]. If a patient cannot achieve full ROM actively, then active-assisted exercises are used to manually assist the patient in moving through the segment of motion they cannot perform independently. With active-assisted ROM, patient may still receive the benefits of active exercises without compromising full available passive motion. Passive ROM is normally reserved for patients who are unable to participate in active motion either due to sedation, neuropathy, critical illness or other barriers. Passive ROM is applied in a slow, controlled manner, while caution is taken to monitor the local skin/tissue response and overall patient tolerance of the exercises.

Functional exercises are purposeful tasks that help to reinforce the ROM achieved while improving strength, endurance, and coordination. For example, feeding one's self with a utensil encourages grasp (hand ROM and strength) and elbow flexion and extension ROM, strength, and endurance while training coordination for an activity needed in daily life. The ultimate goal of OT/PT after a burn injury is to return the patient

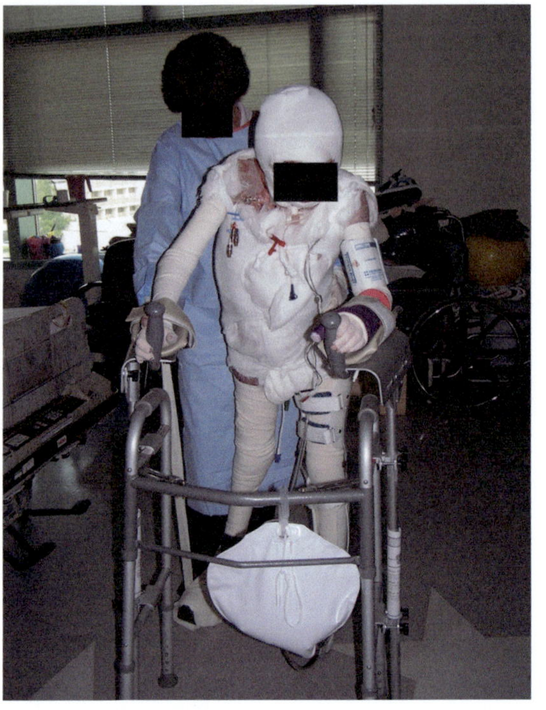

Fig. 10.4 Early ambulation in the ICU with a burn patient

to the pre-burn level of functional independence. In the very early phases of burn recovery, functional tasks are tasks related to self-care, feeding, and mobility, while in the later stages functional tasks involve skills related to work, school, family roles, or play/recreation in preparation for a patient returning home and to the community.

Bed mobility, transfers in and out of bed, as well as ambulation are all forms of functional tasks that require full body movement and are some of the initial skills trained after injury. As the patient is able, he/she begins to practice activities of daily living, such as self-hygiene and toileting. Focusing on ROM through functional tasks such as these, not only encourages maintenance of motion, strength, and muscular endurance, but allows the patient an opportunity for independence which often improves morale and confidence during the recovery process. In the long-term rehabilitation phase, higher level functional tasks such as advanced mobility skills (i.e. climbing stairs, floor transfers) or personal role tasks (i.e. cooking, work hardening) are emphasized.

Although the burn therapist is primarily responsible for implementing exercise programs and training patients toward independence with functional tasks, all team members are responsible for reinforcing independent movement whenever possible. For example, while in the intensive care unit (ICU), the nurse can encourage the patient to independently roll when placing a bed pan for toileting or during follow-up clinic visits, the surgeon can request the patient to demonstrate a functional task that he/she has mastered since the last visit.

Ambulation

Protocols for ambulation after burn injury and after skin graft surgery vary among burn centers. Research on early ambulation of critically ill patients demonstrates benefits such as fewer ventilator days [22], decreased pain [23], and decreased length of stay [24]. Early mobilization of critically ill patients has been shown to be both feasible and safe [25]. Upright mobility protocols in the burn ICU may begin with supported sitting in bed or a chair and gradual progression to standing and assisted ambulation. Equipment such as a cardiac chair and tilt table [26] may be helpful in facilitating more time in an upright position, while walkers or other assistive gait devices may enable longer ambulation distance (see Fig. 10.4). Adequate personnel and appropriate equipment is essential for keeping the patient and staff members safe when mobilizing large patients or patients on ventilators.

Early ambulation may be limited by the burn patient's need for surgery, in particular skin grafts. The majority of burn centers mobilize patients out of bed between post-operative day (POD) 2 and 5 after skin graft surgery to the legs and between POD 1 and 4 for skin grafts above the waist [9]. A recent prospective randomized controlled trial compared early ambulation (POD 1) to standard time to ambulate (POD 5) and found that there was no difference in graft loss between the groups and that the early ambulation group ambulated significantly more minutes per therapy session than the standard group [27].

A patient's ability to ambulate may initially be limited by edema, pain, decreased ROM, diminished strength, or fear and anxiety. Using elastic bandages wrapped in a figure-eight pattern on the lower legs provides vascular supports to new skin grafts and helps with pain. Using preparatory exercises such as isometric and concentric exercises in a variety of positions helps allay fear or anxiety about movement. As the patient gains independence with ambulation, higher level whole body balance and coordination activities should be incorporated into the therapy regimen according to the patient's pre-burn level of function and prior home, work, or recreational demands. As ambulation progresses, the focus on independent upright mobility shifts to one of increasing cardiovascular and endurance activity demands.

Strength and Conditioning Exercises

Patients with significant burn injury experience loss of lean muscle mass [28], decreased bone density [29], and fatigue [30]. When compared to non-burned children and adults, burn survivors show decreased aerobic capacity [31], strength [32, 33], and are generally deconditioned. Two factors contribute to this deconditioning following significant burn injury: (1) prolonged bedrest due to medical instability and need for multiple surgeries [34], and (2) prolonged hypermetabolic response which leads to muscle catabolism and atrophy [35].

Strength and conditioning activities are aimed to improve the ability of a burn patient to participate in daily/work-related/recreational activities for prolonged periods of time without fatigue [4] and are normally a major component of therapy in the long-term rehabilitation phase of recovery. Exercise programs that include strength and conditioning activities have been shown to reverse the effects of protein catabolism and immobilization after burns in both adults and children [36, 37]. Recent practice guidelines on exercise after burn injury recommend that strength and cardiovascular endurance be evaluated in individuals 7 years of age or older and a supervised resistance and/or aerobic exercise program implemented for those individuals testing below normal [38]. Strengthening may begin with active ROM or functional activities described previously, then progress to exercises that require greater muscular resistance and more cardiovascular demand. A variety of protocols exist for strength and endurance [39] training and may be initiated as early as immediately post-discharge to as late as 14 years post-burn. Exercise programs have shown benefit when implemented for 6–12 weeks in adults and up to 12 weeks for children [38].

Scar Management

Comprehensive scar management includes efforts to minimize scar contracture as well as scar hypertrophy. The previously described therapeutic interventions (i.e. positioning, splinting, exercise, etc.) are all aimed to mitigate contracture by providing elongation forces to the scar tissue that forms during dermal healing. This section will describe some of the non-surgical interventions that focus on reducing or preventing scar hypertrophy as well. Scar hypertrophy is an excess deposition of collagen resulting in an overgrowth of scar tissue.

Nonsurgical therapies to minimize scar hypertrophy aim to alter the mechanical or physical properties of the scar [40]. The most common interventions used clinically include massage, compression therapy, and insert/silicone application. Initiation of these interventions is determined based on assessment of the strength and integrity of the scar and may occur between 2 and 6 weeks after epithelialization or skin graft surgery. There is evidence that early intervention may have a greater influence on scar outcome [41, 42]. Duration of the intervention is based on scar maturation, which typically takes 12–18 months but may vary based on the individual. Scars progress from an immature state which is characterized by a red and raised appearance and rigid feel to a state of maturity which is characterized by a relatively paler color, planar disposition, and pliable feel. Clinically, scars are observed to thicken and rise the most at approximately 3–4 months after burn wound closure.

Massage and Moisturizing

Due to the imbalance in skin hydration, moisturizers play a key role in the early management of scars to hydrate the newly healed tissue, support damaged sebaceous gland function, and to mitigate the pruritic effect of dry skin [43]. Once burn scars have matured enough to tolerate sheering forces, scar massage using a moisturizing cream should be incorporated into the scar management regimen. A variety of techniques have been described and utilize principles of mobilizing scar tissue to reduce adhesions and improve pliability or friction to realign collagen fibers [44]. Scar massage has shown to benefit ROM and reduce itch, pain, and anxiety in burn patients [45–47]. Despite the lack of evidence for changes in physical scar characteristics, scar massage is still routinely used clinically in burn rehabilitation [9, 48].

Compression Therapy

The use of compression to control burn scar hypertrophy has a long history [49]. Despite conflicting evidence of the effectiveness of compression therapy [50], pressure garments and other compression devices are widely used in burn rehabilitation (see Fig. 10.5). A recent randomized within-wound comparison concluded that pressure garment therapy is effective, but that the clinical benefit is restricted to patients with moderate or severe scarring [51]. Patients with burn wounds that heal within 7–14 days (superficial partial thickness burn wounds) do not need compression therapy [51]. Those patients whose wounds heal within 14–21 days or require skin grafting are closely monitored and pressure garments are typically prescribed preventively [52, 53].

The appropriate amount of pressure to be applied to hypertrophic scar has not yet been determined [50]. Clinically, custom therapeutic pressure devices used for mitigation or prevention of scar hypertrophy average 24–40 mmHg of pressure, which is approximately equal to or greater than the capillary pressure (25 mmHg) [54]. Pressure garments are used throughout scar maturation and have been shown to have a positive effect on scar thickness when used for a minimum of 6 months [55]. Pressure garments are typically prescribed to be worn 23 out of 24 hours per day and should only be removed for bathing or during exercises if they interfere with movement. The garments should be replaced when the fabric is worn out or they no longer fit the patient (more frequently with growing children).

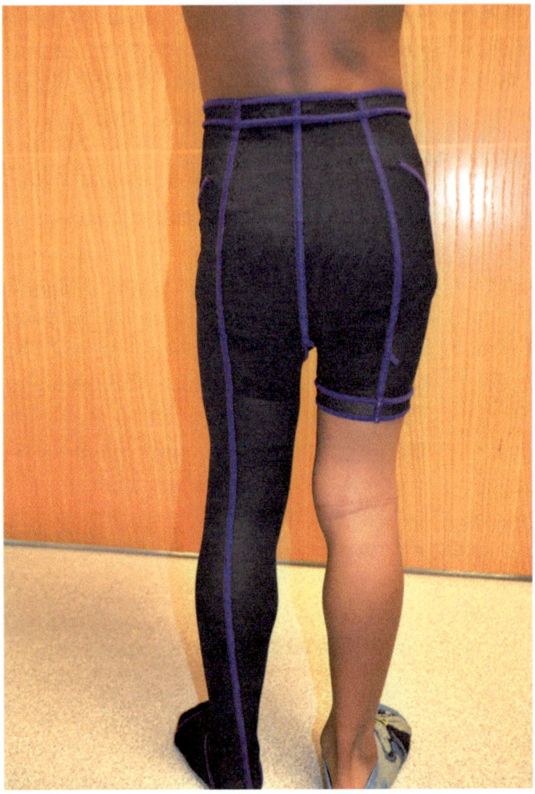

Fig. 10.5 Custom-fabricated pressure garment

Custom fit pressure garments can be costly and unavailable to all patients, in which case, other forms of pressure may be used if pressure is indicated. Alternative compression devices include elastic bandages, self-adherent stretch wrap, tubular compression bandages, or pre-fabricated compression garments.

Insert and Silicone Application

The human body has many areas of depression where continuous pressure with garments is difficult to achieve. Therefore, various insert materials are used to "fill the space" and create conformity

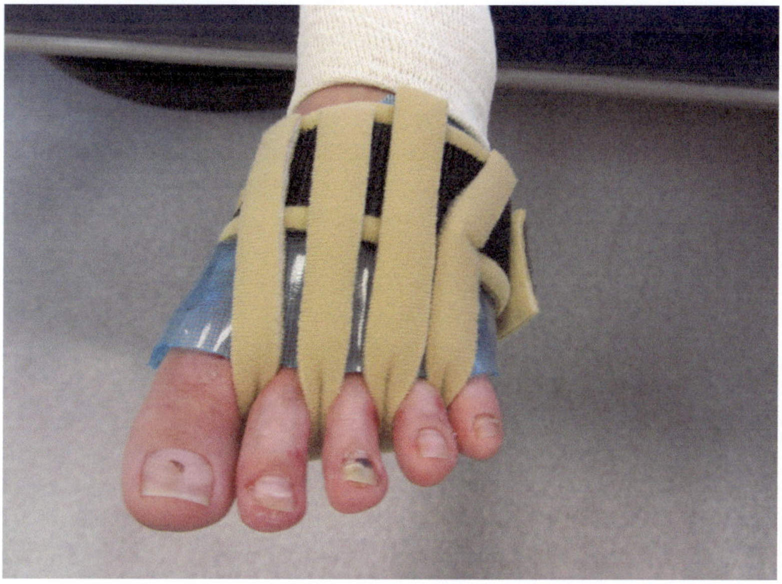

Fig. 10.6 Foam insert used in web spaces and silicone sheet applied to dorsum of foot

and compression in those areas of concavity such as the axilla, sternum, palm, web spaces of the finger/toes, and areas on the neck and face (see Fig. 10.6). Common insert materials used are foam, elastomer, putties, neoprene, or silicone sheets [18, 56]. The inserts may be placed directly on the scar or within a pocket in the garment.

Silicone gel sheets may function as an insert to improve continuous pressure, or according to some studies, the silicone material itself may benefit the scars [57–59]. Silicone gels or gel sheets have been recommended for use on scars that have a high probability of becoming hypertrophic [60, 61]. The exact mechanism of how silicone affects the burn scar is still not known, but some theories include hydration of the stratum corneum which facilitates regulation of fibroblast production, protection of scar tissue from bacteria-induced excessive collagen production, or modulation of growth factors [62]. Clinically, silicone has been observed to hydrate the burn scar, depress the height of hypertrophic scars, increase the pliability of scars, and improve pain and itch [63, 64]. Care should be taken when using inserts or silicone gel or gel sheets to clean the products regularly and monitor the skin for allergic reaction or maceration.

Scar Assessment

Evaluating scar characteristics is an important part of monitoring clinical progress throughout scar maturation and valuable in research for studying the effectiveness of interventions. A variety of subjective and objective tools exist to evaluate scars [65]. Subjective tools allow the clinician to systematically rate various aspects of the scar such as pliability, pigmentation, vascularity, and height and include additional patient self-rating of pain, itch, and satisfaction. Such scales are easy to administer and clinically feasible, but are subject to observer bias and have indeterminate or low-quality clinimetrics [66]. Commonly used subjective scar scales are the Vancouver Burn Scar Scale (VBSS), various modified versions of the VBSS, and the Patient Observer Scar Assessment Scale (POSAS) [67–69].

Objective scar tools provide a more objective and reliable evaluation with better reproducibility and inter-rater reliability than do subjective scales [70]. However, they measure only one aspect of the scar and are often not as feasible for clinical practice. Multiple objective scar tools are available including the cutometer (pliability), durometer (firmness), Chromameter or mexameter (color), ultrasound (thickness), and laser Doppler (perfusion) to name a few [65, 71].

Outcome Measures

Just as scar outcome is valuable to measure, so is functional outcome. A wide variety of outcome measures are used clinically in burn rehabilitation and for research. Using the World Health Organization International Classification of Functioning, Disability and Health, a few common outcome measures used after burn injury can be described [72]. Impairment (body functions and structures) outcome measurements commonly used for evaluation after burn injury include ROM (goniometry) and [73] strength (manual muscle testing or dynamometry) [74] and cardiovascular function (modified Bruce protocol) [39]. Activity limitations can be determined from functional ability such as hand function (Michigan Hand Outcomes Questionnaire) [75] and mobility (6 min walk test) [76]. Participation limitations are evaluated by a patient's ability to return to work or school [77, 78]. There are also many outcome measures used to evaluate the impact of burn injury on overall quality of life outcome [79, 80]. A recent consensus symposium on quality outcome indicators proposed that the following metrics be used to measure functional outcomes after burn injury: Burn Specific Health Scale-Brief (BSHS-B) (adults) and Health Outcomes Burn Questionnaires (children) [81].

Special Considerations for Rehabilitation

Specialized Areas of Treatment

Hands

Hands are one of the most common areas to sustain burn injury. Due to the complex anatomical and functional nature of the hands, a burn injury of any depth to this body part is considered significant and presents unique challenges to the burn therapist. Anticipated problems with the burned hand include edema formation, a multitude of possible hand deformities and functional problems, difficult scar management, and in children, impaired fine motor development. The burn therapist must diligently attend to early evaluation and treatment of hand burns. Special attention should be given to monitoring proper positioning and splinting to avoid disabling contracture formation. If contracture forms, it is essential to differentiate the involved structures and provide prompt and appropriate intervention. Additional considerations for therapy of the hands include early assessment of nerve injury, hand-specific functional training, maintenance of ROM and web spaces, and appropriate referrals for follow-up care.

Face

Due to the unique esthetic and functional nature of the face, it too presents unique challenges to the burn therapist when scarred. With facial burn injury, there is a high propensity to form contractures of the mouth (microstomia) and eyelids (ectropion), which can have a significant functional and cosmetic impact for the patient. The therapeutic interventions described previously (ROM exercises, splinting, massage, compression therapy, and silicone) are commonly used on the face, but consideration must be given to fragile facial features and complex anatomical curvatures. Compression therapy of the face is often provided with a clear, hard plastic material (transparent face mask) in order to provide continuous contact to facial curvatures and allow the patient to be seen through the material for more normal social interactions [82, 83].

Age-Related Rehabilitation Considerations

Children and the elderly require special consideration when rehabilitating from a burn injury. Children tend to have increased anxiety and a decreased attention span. They are a developing being physically and emotionally, which results in the need for the burn therapist to be adaptable, creative, and flexible. The child's decreased understanding of the benefits of therapy may lead to decreased compliance and the therapist must work closely with family members to ensure follow-up with the plan of care. In addition, frequent growth spurts may require ongoing modification of pressure garments or splints. Functional goals with the pediatric burn patient are directed at age appropriate play and school activities.

Elderly adults who sustain burn injury may have premorbid limitations in sensory (eye sight, hearing, skin sensation), motor (ambulation, balance, coordination), or cognitive (memory, judgement) abilities and will require special adaptations or assistance during rehabilitation to learn follow-up care. Skin function in the elderly may also be altered, resulting in delayed wound healing, susceptibility to infection, increased risk of pressure sores, and compromised thermoregulation [84]. Caution should be used with transfers to avoid shearing forces on the skin. Physiological response to therapy should be monitored closely in case of comorbidities affecting the heart, lungs, or circulation. Discharge planning may involve a return to a different living situation, in which case caregivers must be identified and trained.

Conclusions

Rehabilitation services are a critical part in recovery from burn injury and play a significant role in the restoration of a patient's physical function. Physical and occupational therapy should be prescribed on the day of admission and continue throughout acute hospitalization, long-term rehabilitation, outpatient, and follow-up care. Therapy must be implemented early and provided continuously throughout the stages of recovery for maximal benefit. The burn therapist is an integral part of the team and essential in facilitating the patient's physical rehabilitation.

References

1. Saffle JR, Davis B, Williams P. Recent outcomes in the treatment of burn injury in the United States: a report from the American Burn Association Patient Registry. J Burn Care Rehabil. 1995;16(3 Pt 1):219–32. discussion 88–9.
2. Richard RL, Hedman TL, Quick CD, Barillo DJ, Cancio LC, Renz EM, et al. A clarion to recommit and reaffirm burn rehabilitation. J Burn Care Res. 2008;29(3):425–32. Epub 2008/04/05.
3. Dewey WS, Richard RL, Parry IS. Positioning, splinting, and contracture management. Phys Med Rehabil Clin N Am. 2011;22(2):229–47. Epub 2011/06/01.
4. Ward RS. Physical rehabilitation. In: Carrougher GJ, editor. Burn care and therapy. St. Louis, MO: Mosby; 1998. p. 293–327.
5. Helm PKC, Lushbaugh M, Pullium G, Head MD, Cromes GF. Burn injury: rehabilitation management in 1982. Arch Phys Med Rehabil. 1982;63:6–16.
6. Richard R, Staley M, Miller S, Warden G. To splint or not to splint—past philosophy and present practice: part I. J Burn Care Rehabil. 1996;17(5):444–53. Epub 1996/09/01.
7. Richard R, Staley M, Miller S, Warden G. To splint or not to splint—past philosophy and present practice: part III. J Burn Care Rehabil. 1997;18(3):251–5. discussion 0. Epub 1997/05/01.
8. Richard R, Staley M, Miller S, Warden G. To splint or not to splint: past philosophy and current practice—part II. J Burn Care Rehabil. 1997;18(1 Pt 1):64–71. Epub 1997/01/01.
9. Holavanahalli RK, Helm PA, Parry IS, Dolezal CA, Greenhalgh DG. Select practices in management and rehabilitation of burns: a survey report. J Burn Care Res. 2011;32(2):210–23. Epub 2011/01/18.
10. Schnebly WA, Ward RS, Warden GD, Saffle JR. A nonsplinting approach to the care of the thermally injured patient. J Burn Care Rehabil. 1989;10(3):263–6. Epub 1989/05/01.
11. Kwan MW, Ha KW. Splinting programme for patients with burnt hand. Hand Surg. 2002;7(2):231–41. Epub 2003/02/22.
12. Kolmus AM, Holland AE, Byrne MJ, Cleland HJ. The effects of splinting on shoulder function in adult burns. Burns. 2012;38(5):638–44. Epub 2012/02/18.
13. Richard RJRMS. A compendium of customized burn splint designs. J Burn Care Rehabil. 2003;24:S142.
14. Richard R, Baryza MJ, Carr JA, Dewey WS, Dougherty ME, Forbes-Duchart L, et al. Burn rehabilitation and research: proceedings of a consensus summit. J Burn Care Res. 2009;30(4):543–73. Epub 2009/06/10.
15. Duncan RM. Basic principles of splinting the hand. Phys Ther. 1989;69(12):1104–16. Epub 1989/12/01.
16. Richard R, Shanesy 3rd CP, Miller SF. Dynamic versus static splints: a prospective case for sustained stress. J Burn Care Rehabil. 1995;16(3 Pt 1):284–7. Epub 1995/05/01.
17. Bennett GB, Helm P, Purdue GF, Hunt JL. Serial casting: a method for treating burn contractures. J Burn Care Rehabil. 1989;10(6):543–5. Epub 1989/11/01.
18. Serghiou M, Ott S, Farmer A, Morgan D, Gibson P, Suman OE. Comprehensive rehabilitation of the burn patient. In: Herndon D, editor. Total burn care. 3rd ed. Philadelphia: Saunders Elsevier; 2007. p. 620.
19. Ricks NR, Meagher Jr DP. The benefits of plaster casting for lower-extremity burns after grafting in children. J Burn Care Rehabil. 1992;13(4):465–8. Epub 1992/07/11.

20. Howell JW. Management of the acutely burned hand for the nonspecialized clinician. Phys Ther. 1989;69(12):1077–90. Epub 1989/12/01.
21. Alkner BA, Tesch PA. Knee extensor and plantar flexor muscle size and function following 90 days of bed rest with or without resistance exercise. Eur J Appl Physiol. 2004;93(3):294–305. Epub 2004/09/01.
22. Schweickert WD, Hall J. ICU-acquired weakness. Chest. 2007;131(5):1541–9. Epub 2007/05/15.
23. Partsch H, Blattler W. Compression and walking versus bed rest in the treatment of proximal deep venous thrombosis with low molecular weight heparin. J Vasc Surg. 2000;32(5):861–9. Epub 2000/10/29.
24. Mundy LM, Leet TL, Darst K, Schnitzler MA, Dunagan WC. Early mobilization of patients hospitalized with community-acquired pneumonia. Chest. 2003;124(3):883–9. Epub 2003/09/13.
25. Bailey P, Thomsen GE, Spuhler VJ, Blair R, Jewkes J, Bezdjian L, et al. Early activity is feasible and safe in respiratory failure patients. Crit Care Med. 2007; 35(1):139–45. Epub 2006/11/30.
26. Trees DW, Ketelsen CA, Hobbs JA. Use of a modified tilt table for preambulation strength training as an adjunct to burn rehabilitation: a case series. J Burn Care Rehabil. 2003;24(2):97–103. Epub 2003/03/11.
27. Lorello DJ, Peck M, Albrecht M, Richey KJ, Pressman MA. Results of a prospective randomized controlled trial of early ambulation for patients with lower extremity autografts. J Burn Care Res. 2014;35(5):431–6. Epub 2014/08/08.
28. Hart DW, Wolf SE, Chinkes DL, Gore DC, Mlcak RP, Beauford RB, et al. Determinants of skeletal muscle catabolism after severe burn. Ann Surg. 2000;232(4):455–65. Epub 2000/09/22.
29. Leblebici B, Sezgin N, Ulusan SN, Tarim AM, Akman MN, Haberal MA. Bone loss during the acute stage following burn injury. J Burn Care Res. 2008; 29(5):763–7. Epub 2008/08/13.
30. de Lateur BJ, Magyar-Russell G, Bresnick MG, Bernier FA, Ober MS, Krabak BJ, et al. Augmented exercise in the treatment of deconditioning from major burn injury. Arch Phys Med Rehabil. 2007;88(12 Suppl 2):S18–23. Epub 2007/12/06.
31. Willis CE, Grisbrook TL, Elliott CM, Wood FM, Wallman KE, Reid SL. Pulmonary function, exercise capacity and physical activity participation in adults following burn. Burns. 2011;37(8):1326–33. Epub 2011/05/03.
32. Ebid AA, Omar MT, Abd El Baky AM. Effect of 12-week isokinetic training on muscle strength in adult with healed thermal burn. Burns. 2012;38(1):61–8. Epub 2011/11/23.
33. Przkora R, Herndon DN, Suman OE. The effects of oxandrolone and exercise on muscle mass and function in children with severe burns. Pediatrics. 2007;119(1): e109–16. Epub 2006/11/30.
34. Ferrando AA, Lane HW, Stuart CA, Davis-Street J, Wolfe RR. Prolonged bed rest decreases skeletal muscle and whole body protein synthesis. Am J Physiol. 1996;270(4 Pt 1):E627–33. Epub 1996/04/01.
35. Pereira C, Murphy K, Jeschke M, Herndon DN. Post burn muscle wasting and the effects of treatments. Int J Biochem Cell Biol. 2005;37(10):1948–61. Epub 2005/08/20.
36. Al-Mousawi AM, Williams FN, Mlcak RP, Jeschke MG, Herndon DN, Suman OE. Effects of exercise training on resting energy expenditure and lean mass during pediatric burn rehabilitation. J Burn Care Res. 2010;31(3):400–8. Epub 2010/04/01.
37. Paratz JD, Stockton K, Plaza A, Muller M, Boots RJ. Intensive exercise after thermal injury improves physical, functional, and psychological outcomes. J Trauma Acute Care Surg. 2012;73(1):186–94. Epub 2012/06/20.
38. Nedelec B, Parry I et al. Practice guidelines for cardiovascular fitness and strengthening exercise prescription after burn injury. J Burn Care Res. Published ahead of Print, 2015
39. Suman OE, Spies RJ, Celis MM, Mlcak RP, Herndon DN. Effects of a 12-wk resistance exercise program on skeletal muscle strength in children with burn injuries. J Appl Physiol. 2001;91(3):1168–75.
40. Staley MJ, Richard RL. Scar management. In: Richard RSM, editor. Burn care and rehabilitation: principles and practice. Philadelphia: F.A. Davis Company; 1994. p. 380.
41. Parry I, Sen S, Palmieri T, Greenhalgh D. Nonsurgical scar management of the face: does early versus late intervention affect outcome? J Burn Care Res. 2013; 34(5):569–75. Epub 2013/07/03.
42. Leung P, Ng M. Pressure treatment for hypertrophic scars resulting from burns. Burns. 1980;6(4):241–4.
43. Bell PL, Gabriel V. Evidence based review for the treatment of post-burn pruritus. J Burn Care Res. 2009;30(1):55–61. Epub 2008/12/09.
44. Parry, I. Icaza I et al. Defining Massage Techniques used for Burn Scars. J Burn Care Res online http://journals.lww.com/burncareresearch/pages/videogallery.aspx?videoId=5&autoPlay=false, Accessed 19 Jan 2016.
45. Morien A, Garrison D, Smith NK. Range of motion improves after massage in children with burns: a pilot study. J Bodyw Mov Ther. 2008;12(1):67–71. Epub 2008/12/17.
46. Parlak Gurol A, Polat S, Akcay MN. Itching, pain, and anxiety levels are reduced with massage therapy in burned adolescents. J Burn Care Res. 2010;31(3):429–32. Epub 2010/05/11.
47. Field T, Peck M, Scd, Hernandez-Reif M, Krugman S, Burman I, et al. Postburn itching, pain, and psychological symptoms are reduced with massage therapy. J Burn Care Rehabil. 2000;21(3):189–93. Epub 2000/06/13.
48. Serghiou MA, Holmes CL, McCauley RL. A survey of current rehabilitation trends for burn injuries to the head and neck. J Burn Care Rehabil. 2004;25(6):514–8. Epub 2004/11/10.
49. Linares HA, Larson DL, Willis-Galstaun BA. Historical notes on the use of pressure in the treatment of hypertrophic scars or keloids. Burns. 1993;19(1):17–21. Epub 1993/02/01.

50. Anzarut A, Olson J, Singh P, Rowe BH, Tredget EE. The effectiveness of pressure garment therapy for the prevention of abnormal scarring after burn injury: a meta-analysis. J Plast Reconstr Aesthet Surg. 2009;62(1):77–84. Epub 2008/02/06.
51. Engrav LH, Heimbach DM, Rivara FP, Moore ML, Wang J, Carrougher GJ, et al. 12-Year within-wound study of the effectiveness of custom pressure garment therapy. Burns. 2010;36(7):975–83. Epub 2010/06/12.
52. Monstrey S, Middelkoop E, Vranckx JJ, Bassetto F, Ziegler UE, Meaume S, et al. Updated scar management practical guidelines: non-invasive and invasive measures. J Plast Reconstr Aesthet Surg. 2014;67(8): 1017–25. Epub 2014/06/04.
53. Deitch EA, Wheelahan TM, Rose MP, Clothier J, Cotter J. Hypertrophic burn scars: analysis of variables. J Trauma. 1983;23(10):895–8. Epub 1983/10/01.
54. Bloemen MC, van der Veer WM, Ulrich MM, van Zuijlen PP, Niessen FB, Middelkoop E. Prevention and curative management of hypertrophic scar formation. Burns. 2009;35(4):463–75. Epub 2008/10/28.
55. Li-Tsang CW, Feng BB, Li KC. Pressure therapy of hypertrophic scar after burns and related research. Zhonghua Shao Shang Za Zhi. 2010;26(6):411–5. Epub 2011/01/13.
56. Yelvington M, Brown S, Castro MM, Nick TG. The use of neoprene as a scar management modality. Burns. 2013;39(5):866–75. Epub 2013/01/15.
57. Karagoz H, Yuksel F, Ulkur E, Evinc R. Comparison of efficacy of silicone gel, silicone gel sheeting, and topical onion extract including heparin and allantoin for the treatment of postburn hypertrophic scars. Burns. 2009;35(8):1097–103. Epub 2009/09/22.
58. Momeni M, Hafezi F, Rahbar H, Karimi H. Effects of silicone gel on burn scars. Burns. 2009;35(1):70–4. Epub 2008/08/02.
59. Ahn ST, Monafo WW, Mustoe TA. Topical silicone gel for the prevention and treatment of hypertrophic scar. Arch Surg. 1991;126(4):499–504. Epub 1991/04/01.
60. Nedelec B, Carter A, Forbes L, Hsu SC, McMahon M, Parry I, et al. Practice guidelines for the application of nonsilicone or silicone gels and gel sheets after burn injury. J Burn Care Res. 2015;36(3):345–74. Epub 2014/08/06.
61. Mustoe TA. Evolution of silicone therapy and mechanism of action in scar management. Aesthetic Plast Surg. 2008;32(1):82–92. Epub 2007/10/31.
62. Puri N, Talwar A. The efficacy of silicone gel for the treatment of hypertrophic scars and keloids. J Cutan Aesthet Surg. 2009;2(2):104–6. Epub 2009/07/01.
63. Li-Tsang CW, Zheng YP, Lau JC. A randomized clinical trial to study the effect of silicone gel dressing and pressure therapy on posttraumatic hypertrophic scars. J Burn Care Res. 2010;31(3):448–57. Epub 2010/04/09.
64. van der Wal MB, van Zuijlen PP, van de Ven P, Middelkoop E. Topical silicone gel versus placebo in promoting the maturation of burn scars: a randomized controlled trial. Plast Reconstr Surg. 2010;126(2):524–31. Epub 2010/08/04.
65. Fearmonti R, Bond J, Erdmann D, Levinson H. A review of scar scales and scar measuring devices. Eplasty. 2010;10, e43. Epub 2010/07/03.
66. Tyack Z, Simons M, Spinks A, Wasiak J. A systematic review of the quality of burn scar rating scales for clinical and research use. Burns. 2012;38(1):6–18. Epub 2011/11/04.
67. Sullivan T, Smith J, Kermode J, McIver E, Courtemanche DJ. Rating the burn scar. J Burn Care Rehabil. 1990;11(3):256–60. Epub 1990/05/01.
68. Draaijers LJ, Tempelman FR, Botman YA, Tuinebreijer WE, Middelkoop E, Kreis RW, et al. The patient and observer scar assessment scale: a reliable and feasible tool for scar evaluation. Plast Reconstr Surg. 2004;113(7):1960–5. discussion 6-7. Epub 2004/07/16.
69. Nedelec B, Shankowsky HA, Tredget EE. Rating the resolving hypertrophic scar: comparison of the Vancouver Scar Scale and scar volume. J Burn Care Rehabil. 2000;21(3):205–12. Epub 2000/06/13.
70. Brusselaers N, Pirayesh A, Hoeksema H, Verbelen J, Blot S, Monstrey S. Burn scar assessment: a systematic review of objective scar assessment tools. Burns. 2010;36(8):1157–64. Epub 2010/05/22.
71. Verhaegen PD, van der Wal MB, Middelkoop E, van Zuijlen PP. Objective scar assessment tools: a clinimetric appraisal. Plast Reconstr Surg. 2011;127(4): 1561–70. Epub 2011/04/05.
72. Orgnization WH. International classification of functioning, disability and health. http://www.who.int/classification/icf/en/. Accessed 26 June 2015
73. Parry I, Walker K, Niszczak J, Palmieri T, Greenhalgh D. Methods and tools used for the measurement of burn scar contracture. J Burn Care Res. 2010;31(6): 888–903. Epub 2010/09/23.
74. Falder S, Browne A, Edgar D, Staples E, Fong J, Rea S, et al. Core outcomes for adult burn survivors: a clinical overview. Burns. 2009;35(5):618–41. Epub 2008/12/30.
75. Chung KC, Hamill JB, Walters MR, Hayward RA. The Michigan Hand Outcomes Questionnaire (MHQ): assessment of responsiveness to clinical change. Ann Plast Surg. 1999;42(6):619–22. Epub 1999/06/26.
76. Enright PL. The six-minute walk test. Respir Care. 2003;48(8):783–5. Epub 2003/08/02.
77. Staley M, Anderson L, Greenhalgh D, Warden G. Return to school as an outcome measure after a burn injury. J Burn Care Rehabil. 1999;20(1 Pt 1):91–4. discussion 0. Epub 1999/02/06.
78. Mason ST, Esselman P, Fraser R, Schomer K, Truitt A, Johnson K. Return to work after burn injury: a systematic review. J Burn Care Res. 2012;33(1):101–9. Epub 2011/12/06.
79. Cromes GF, Holavanahalli R, Kowalske K, Helm P. Predictors of quality of life as measured by the Burn Specific Health Scale in persons with major burn injury. J Burn Care Rehabil. 2002;23(3):229–34. Epub 2002/05/29.
80. Anzarut A, Chen M, Shankowsky H, Tredget EE. Quality-of-life and outcome predictors following

massive burn injury. Plast Reconstr Surg. 2005;116(3): 791–7. Epub 2005/09/06.
81. Gibran NS, Wiechman S, Meyer W, Edelman L, Fauerbach J, Gibbons L, et al. American Burn Association consensus statements. J Burn Care Res. 2013;34(4):361–85. Epub 2013/07/10.
82. Giele HP, Currie K, Wood FM, Hansen H. Early use of pressure masks to avoid facial contracture during the pregrafting phase. J Burn Care Rehabil. 1995;16(6):641–5. Epub 1995/11/01.
83. Shons AR, Rivers EA, Solem LD. A rigid transparent face mask for control of scar hypertrophy. Ann Plast Surg. 1981;6(3):245–8. Epub 1981/03/01.
84. Staley M, Richard R. The elderly patient with burns: treatment considerations. J Burn Care Rehabil. 1993;14(5):559–65. Epub 1993/09/01.

Burn Reconstruction Basics

11

Peter Kwan and Robert Cartotto

Introduction

Overview

Burn scar reconstruction is a rewarding endeavor for both patient and surgeon. The improvements to both aesthetics and function can be significant, and are a crucial aspect of returning quality of life to burn patients. Reconstructive procedures need not be complex to be effective; many problems can be tackled with skin grafts and simple Z-plasties. Other reconstructive problems or the anatomic areas affected are more complex and should be addressed by those with more extensive training and experience in plastic surgery.

We cover the major reconstructive options, with emphasis on those techniques within the scope of practice of most burn surgeons. We briefly mention more advanced reconstructive options and related considerations, as a guide to treatments that consultant plastic and reconstructive surgeons may offer.

P. Kwan, B.Sc.E., M.D., Ph.D., F.R.C.S.C. (✉)
Department of Burn Surgery, University of California Davis Medical Center and Shriners Hospitals for Children Northern California, Sacramento, CA, USA

Department of Plastic and Reconstructive Surgery, University of Alberta, Edmonton, AB, Canada
e-mail: Peter.Kwan@UAlberta.CA

R. Cartotto, M.D., F.R.C.S.C.
Department of Surgery, Ross Tilley Burn Centre, Sunnybrook Health Sciences Centre, University of Toronto, Toronto, ON, Canada

Caution

The discussion of reconstructive techniques in this chapter is not meant to imply they are either within or outside the scope of practice of any particular surgical specialty or subspecialty. As with all surgical procedures, they should be performed by practitioners who have the requisite experience, capability to handle potential complications, and good judgment to choose a safe course of action. The majority of reconstructive procedures rely on the principle of mobilizing and using donor tissue from one area to reconstruct another. The salient complication common to all reconstructive surgery is the simultaneous loss or failure of the donor tissue and the creation of a donor site defect. This very real possibility means the surgeon can easily violate a central tenet of medicine, "*primum non nocere*", or "first, do no harm" [1], and thus all reconstructive procedures are to be approached with the utmost caution and respect. Another issue that warrants caution is with respect to the timing of reconstructive surgery. The patient's desire for reconstruction usually occurs early after injury at a time that is not optimal from the standpoint of scar maturation, which takes place much later. Notwithstanding a severe debilitating contracture or deformity, the

D.G. Greenhalgh (ed.), *Burn Care for General Surgeons and General Practitioners*,
DOI 10.1007/978-3-319-29161-1_11

surgeon is well-advised to patiently rely on time and conservative measures such as splinting, pressure, intra-scar injection of steroids, and topical silicone gel [2], in order to avoid operating on active immature scars. This period of delay allows fresh scars to mature, and will help to increase the odds of a successful surgical outcome. Finally, careful preoperative consultation with the patient and an honest discussion of what is, and what is not possible is mandatory. Burn patients' expectations usually exceed the small and the sometimes subtle changes that occur following the majority of burn scar reconstruction.

Principles of Scars, Bands and Contractures, Scar Release, and Reconstructive Options

Principles

Fundamentally, contractures and shortage of tissue are the basis of many burn scar problems. Consequently, release of the scar involves surgical division of scar bands perpendicular to the line of pull of the contracture. This may be quite simple as in the case of a unidirectional contracture band divided by transverse division with darts (Fig. 11.1), or more complex as in the division of a contracture causing an ectropion where there are multidirectional lines of tension (Fig. 11.2). A key point is that scar contractures should be *incised* and rarely, if ever, *excised* as excision only augments the existing tissue deficiency. Once the release is created, the resulting defect will need to be closed. In general, scar contracture bands should be categorized as either broad and diffuse or as distinct and linear. Release of the broad diffuse contracture is usually not amenable to closure with local flaps or Z-plasties because these techniques rely on laxity of the surrounding soft tissues for mobilization. Conversely, linear distinct bands often have adjacent normal tissue that is loose and mobile (Fig. 11.3) allowing closure of the release using local flaps or Z-plasties. Finally, as a general principle all releases must be followed by a period of splinting combined with aggressive physiotherapy and stretching in order to maintain the release.

The reconstructive ladder (Fig. 11.4) is a time-honored method of approaching the reconstructive options available to the surgeon and patient [3]. Although the idea of proceeding from simple to complex reconstruction is sound, arguments can be made for skipping reconstructive rungs to choose a reconstructive technique with improved outcomes for the patient [3]. For example, although a skin graft can fill many contracture release defects, it may be preferable to jump immediately to the step of a local flap or a Z-plasty, if this is possible, in order to harness the shorter healing time, reduced pain, and improved texture that accompany the latter procedures.

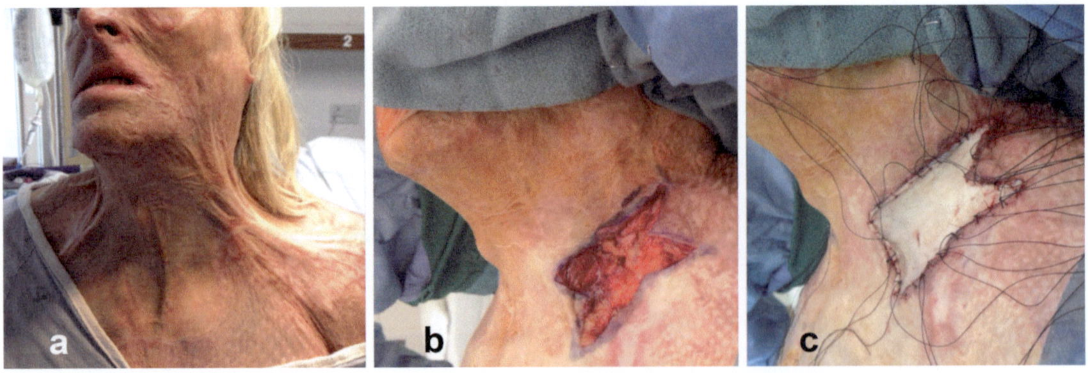

Fig. 11.1 Broad diffuse contracture across the neck showing transverse release pattern with darts placed perpendicular to the predominantly unidirectional line of pull (**a**), the typical "hourglass" shape of the release (**b**), and insertion of a full thickness graft to close the release (**c**). Photo courtesy of Robert Cartotto, MD, FRCSC

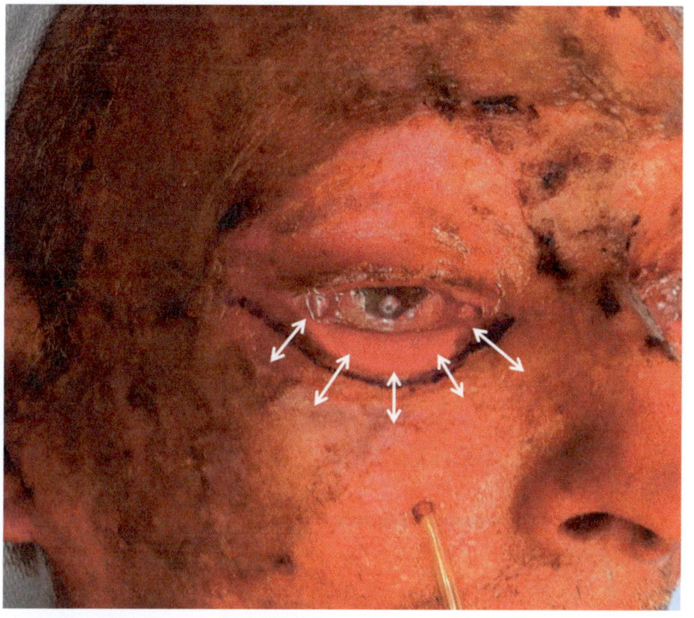

Fig. 11.2 Severe post-burn lower eyelid ectropion showing complex multidirectional lines of tension (*arrows*) with placement of the releasing incision markings. Photo courtesy of Robert Cartotto, MD, FRCSC

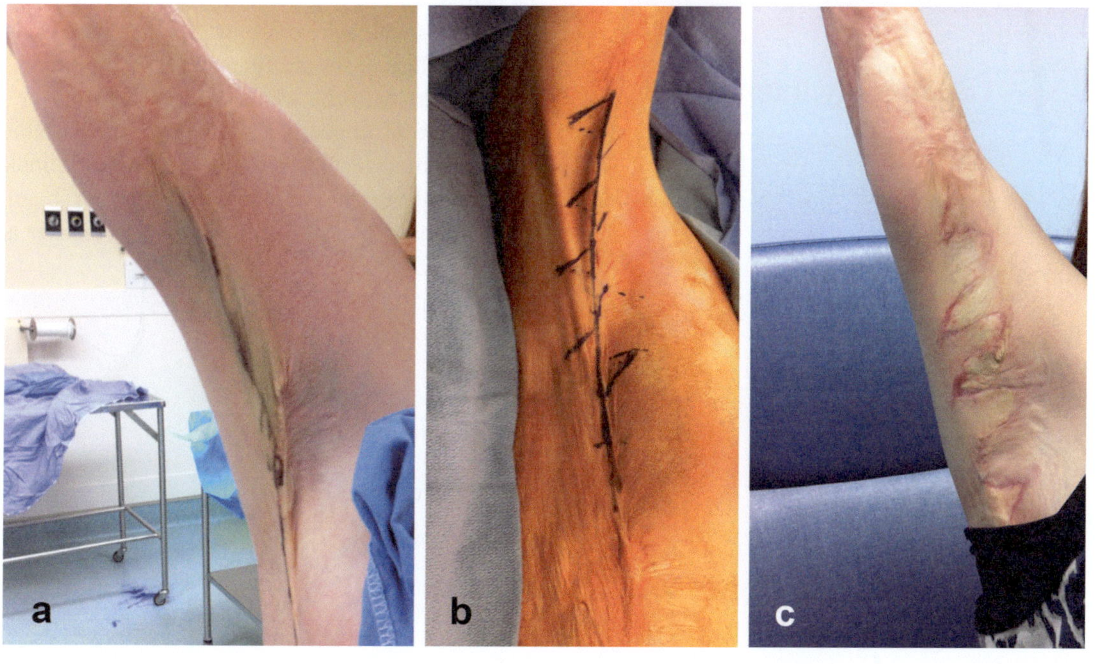

Fig. 11.3 Simple linear band post-burn contracture across the axilla with adjacent uninvolved lax skin (**a**), with placement of multiple Z-plasty markings (**b**), and postoperative result at 3 months (**c**). Photo courtesy of Robert Cartotto, MD, FRCSC

Choosing a Reconstructive Option

The choice of a reconstructive option should additionally be guided by patient factors such as personal preferences, clothing worn, and location of existing scars. One should also recognize that using a particular donor site may preclude its use for other applications in the future. For example, the frequently used full thickness skin graft groin donor site eliminates both the groin flap and

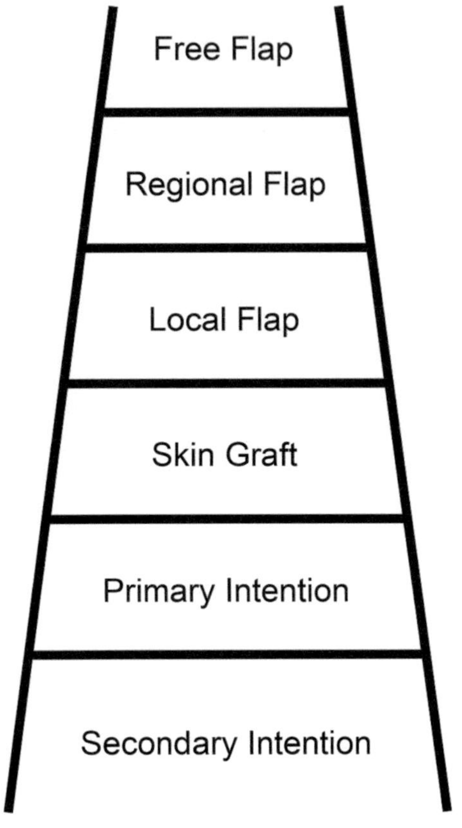

Fig. 11.4 Reconstructive ladder going from simplest to most complex option

superficial circumflex iliac artery perforator flap—very useful thin flaps which may be required later on.

Z-plasty

Z-plasties are based on the principles of trading width for length, and reorienting the lines of scar tension. The simple Z-plasty (Fig. 11.5) is the workhorse of burn reconstruction, and can be applied to a wide variety of reconstructive problems (Fig. 11.6) [4]. When designing the simple Z-plasty all limbs should be of equal length, and the angles should also be equal. The central ("contractural") limb is placed along the scar to be reoriented or contracture to be addressed (Fig. 11.5). A typical angle used is 60° which creates flap tips large enough to generally avoid ischemia, a good degree of lengthening, and produces flaps which are easily transposed with each other. Z-plasties should be marked in the preoperative area with the awake patient eliciting the contracture of concern. This allows one to take adjacent joints, which may be contributing, into account. Furthermore, the contracture or band may be less apparent once the patient is under a

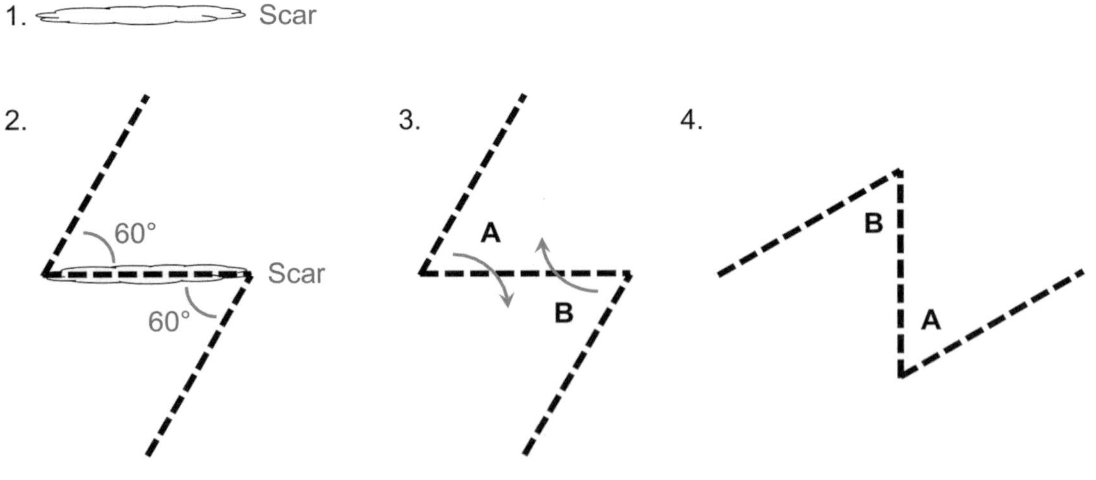

Fig. 11.5 Z-plasty designed for contracture release. All limbs are of equal length, and angles are 60°

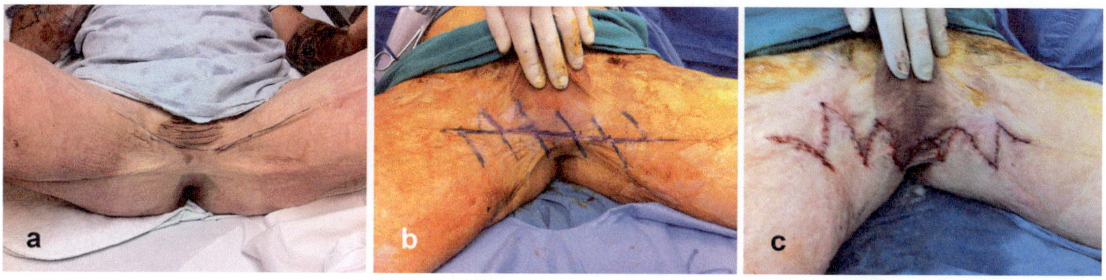

Fig. 11.6 Linear band contracture across the perineum (**a**), with planned release shown with multiple Z plasty markings which include planned flap elevation in areas previously burned and skin grafted (**b**), and final transposition and closure of the flaps (**c**). (Reprinted from Cartotto R, Cicuto BJ, Kiwanuka HN, Bueno EM, Pomahac B. Common postburn deformities and their management. Surg Clin North Am. 2014;94(4):817–37 [Reference [4]] with permission from Elsevier.)

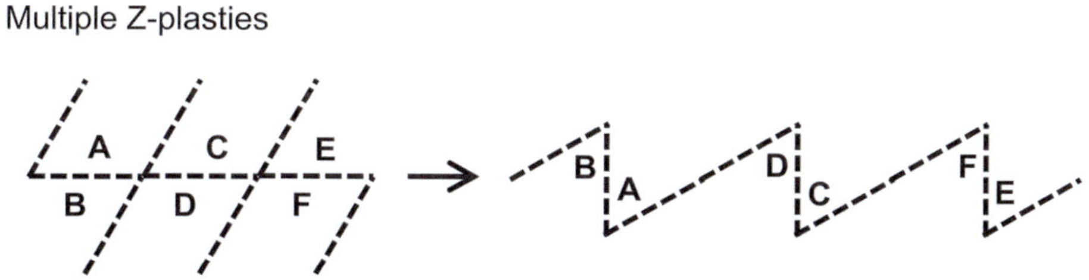

Fig. 11.7 Z-plasty variation for longer scars and contractures not suitable for a single Z-plasty release

general anesthetic. The flaps must be kept thick with an adequate amount of subcutaneous tissue in order to preserve the vascular supply. Z-plasties may be raised in areas of previous skin grafting as long as there is adequate subcutaneous tissue to support the flaps (Fig. 11.6) [4]. This requires the utmost caution and experience, as there is a higher risk of flap necrosis in this situation. When the contracture to be released is of such a length that a single Z-plasty would be too large, multiple Z-plasties may be designed in tandem to allow contracture release (Fig. 11.7).

Split Thickness Skin Graft

Split thickness skin grafts are a mainstay of many reconstructive procedures. They are readily harvested using the same techniques as during primary burn reconstruction, and can be used to cover large defects resulting from contracture release, or resurfacing. Donor sites can be chosen in areas such as the upper thighs or lower back, which may be easier to conceal with clothing. The main disadvantage of the split skin graft is that it is not very effective in inhibiting recurrent contracture formation. If it is utilized, it should be a medium to thick graft, typically in the range of 14–18/1000 inches thick.

Full Thickness Skin Graft

In contrast to the split graft, the full thickness graft is much more capable of inhibiting recurrent contracture formation. An important limitation with these grafts is the necessity of primary closure of the donor site, which limits the size that can be harvested. Also, take of the full thickness graft is less reliable than that of a split thickness graft, and demands an optimal recipient bed. Practically speaking, the two main sources of full thickness skin grafts are the abdomen, and the inguinal fold. The abdominal donor

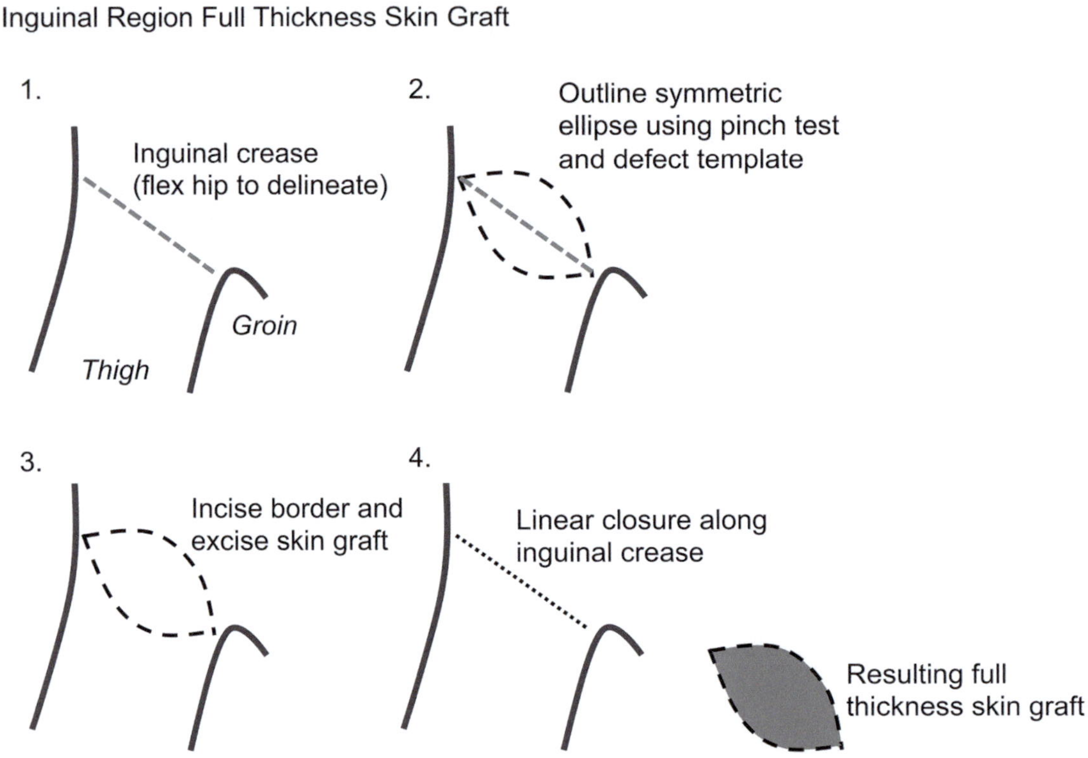

Fig. 11.8 Technique of full thickness skin graft harvest from inguinal crease

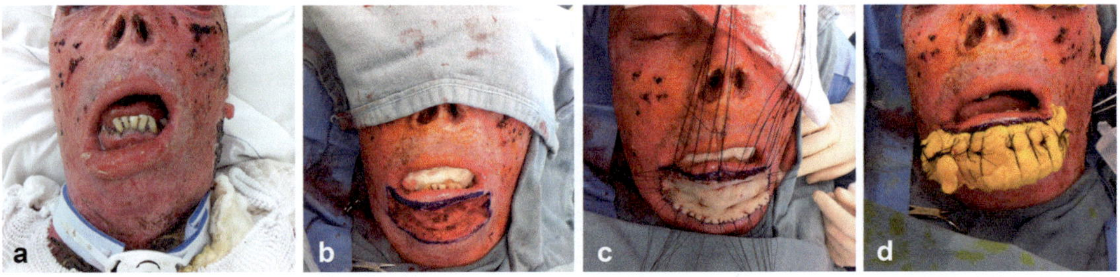

Fig. 11.9 Severe post-burn ectropion of the lower lip associated with oral incontinence (**a**), with extensive release performed which allows restoration of the lip to its normal position (**b**), followed by placement of full thickness skin graft with multiple tie-over bolster sutures placed around the graft perimeter (**c**), and graft secured with a tie-over bolster dressing (**d**). Photo courtesy of Robert Cartotto, MD, FRCSC

site has the advantage of providing more skin, but design and closure require a good understanding of abdominoplasty principles to avoid leaving an obvious donor site and ensuring proper positioning of the umbilicus. The groin is a preferred donor site as it provides a reasonably large amount of skin and, when designed along the groin crease, can be closed primarily with a good aesthetic result. By pinching the skin in equidistant amounts on both sides of the inguinal crease one can determine the maximal width that can be harvested allowing primary closure of the donor site. These steps are outlined in Fig. 11.8. Full thickness skin grafts are typically secured using bolster dressings, which remain intact for 5–7 days (Fig. 11.9).

Dermal Regeneration Templates

As an alternative to skin grafts, dermal regeneration templates (e.g., Integra® Dermal Regeneration Template, Integra LifeSciences, Plainsboro NJ, USA, or PriMatrix®, TEI Medical, Waltham, MA, USA) can be employed for reconstructive purposes. Typically the dermal regenerative matrix is placed into the defect that results from a scar release or a scar excision, and is then engrafted secondarily a few weeks later with a thin split thickness skin graft. The advantage of this approach is that the donor site requirements are reduced because only a thin autograft is required. This may be necessary when prior extensive burns have led to the availability of only a limited number of previously multiply re-harvested donor sites. This benefit must be weighed against the disadvantages of this approach including: cost, the need for two operations, and the higher risk of non-take of the template compared to a skin graft.

Local, Regional, and Free Flaps

The use of flaps is beyond the scope of this chapter. For local flap options, one may refer to a number of plastic and reconstructive surgery textbooks. The armamentarium of local flaps includes variations of transposition, rotation, and advancement flaps (usually requiring an advanced set of reconstructive skills), which will generally warrant referral to a plastic and reconstructive surgeon.

Excision and Serial Excision of Scars

When scarring, and not contracture, is the primary problem, some scars (such as areas of scalp burn alopecia) may be amenable to direct excision and closure, or serial excision and closure. Serial excision may allow patients to avoid tissue expansion and the accompanying temporary deformity. During planning, one can ascertain the approximate amount of tissue that can be excised by using a pinch test. While performing the excision, it is recommended to mark the desired area to be removed, but to begin the procedure by making the incision only along one border so that the dissected tissue may be advanced and the opposite border marked, thus confirming the limits of primary closure, before committing to the final excision. Serial excisions should be spaced out by 3–6 months, and a pinch test can be used to determine when sufficient tissue laxity exists to repeat the procedure.

Head, Neck, and Facial Reconstruction

Introduction

Facial reconstruction should not be undertaken lightly as both aesthetic and functional factors play a significant role. Typical burn deformities can include burn alopecia, various ear defects, varying degrees of nasal loss including alar rim loss or retraction, ectropion of upper and lower eyelids, microstomia and oral incompetence, and neck contractures, all resulting from scars.

Scalp

Scalp reconstruction is generally to restore hair bearing regions and eliminate alopecia. In general, the scalp can be expanded by 50 % before thinning is clinically and socially evident. Therefore, patients with deficits of more than 50 % of the hair bearing regions should be counseled that scalp reconstruction to restore all areas of hair is not possible [5]. For these patients, reorientation of existing hair is an option if this will improve aesthetics or the fit of hair-pieces. Depending on the degree of surrounding tissue laxity, small scalp defects (<3 cm width) can be directly excised and the resulting defect closed primarily. Larger defects are frequently more suitable for excision and closure with local flaps, serial excision, or tissue expansion. Of these options, serial excision is the safest option and least likely to produce further deformity or suffer complications. This comes at the expense of potentially requiring more operative procedures, and a limit to the ability to correct the alopecia defect completely. Tissue expansion is considerably more effective but requires a minimum of two surgeries and a prolonged period of temporary deformity. Many surgeons may recommend tissue expansion, if serial excision will likely require more than three procedures.

Auricular

The purpose of auricular reconstruction is to restore the external ear to an aesthetic normal, and generally has minimal functional impact, aside from the ability to support eyeglasses. Small ear defects may be amenable to excision and closure, with care to rebalance the overall proportions of the ear. Larger defects may be treated with a variety of local or regional flaps, or grafts from the contralateral ear [6]. Subtotal or total defects may be candidates for either osseointegrated prosthetics [7] or autologous reconstruction using rib cartilage according to the technique described by Nagata [8]. All of these techniques generally require referral to a plastic surgeon. If attempts are made to salvage the existing ear during acute burn treatment, these should not compromise future reconstruction efforts and should specifically avoid use of local skin or temporal parietal fascial flaps.

Nasal

The purpose of nasal reconstruction is to restore aesthetics, as the specialized functions of the nose, such as humidification and filtering, cannot be restored by today's reconstructive techniques. Attention should be given to restoration of the nose's lining, structural framework, and external cover. As local tissue options are usually limited, reconstruction may require use of the paramedian forehead flap [9] or a scalp flap. Alternatives for large or total defects would also include an osseointegrated prosthesis [10], or free flap reconstruction [11]. Again, such an undertaking is frequently complex and the patient should be referred to an expert in this area.

Ocular

Ectropion is a significant complication following burn injury, and can occur in patients with facial skin grafting, or in those with more superficial facial burns which are allowed to heal without surgery. In either case, the immediate goal is protection of the cornea, and this can be achieved temporarily with frequent administration of artificial tears and ocular lubricants. Those patients with a Bell's phenomenon (upward rotation of the globe during eye closure) will have a greater degree of corneal protection from exposure, but the goals of ocular protection remain the same. Ophthalmologic consultation may be warranted in these circumstances for assessment of the cornea. Ultimately, release of the ectropion and skin grafting of the resulting defect will be required to release the eyelid and allow complete closure of the eye. Usually full thickness skin grafts are used for the lower eyelid, while thick split thickness grafts are recommended for the upper eyelid. Full thickness skin graft donor sites can include the unburned contralateral upper eyelid (if it is available and there is sufficient laxity) pre- or post-auricular skin, and the upper medial arm. If available, a thick split thickness graft from the scalp works well for the upper lid. In general, ectropion reconstruction should be performed by reconstructive surgeons with experience operating around the eyelid and globe. This may warrant a consultation with an oculoplastic specialist or plastic surgeon.

Oral

Microstomia is a significant problem following oral commissure and surrounding cheek burns. Microstomia can interfere with oral hygiene, eating, and intubation for surgical procedures. Microstomia can be treated with serial splinting, but patient tolerance and compliance can be significantly limited. Local mucosal and tongue flaps are used to relocate the modiolis and correct microstomia while maintaining a relatively normal lip contour and color (Fig. 11.10). Again, these reconstructions should be undertaken by experienced reconstructive surgeons.

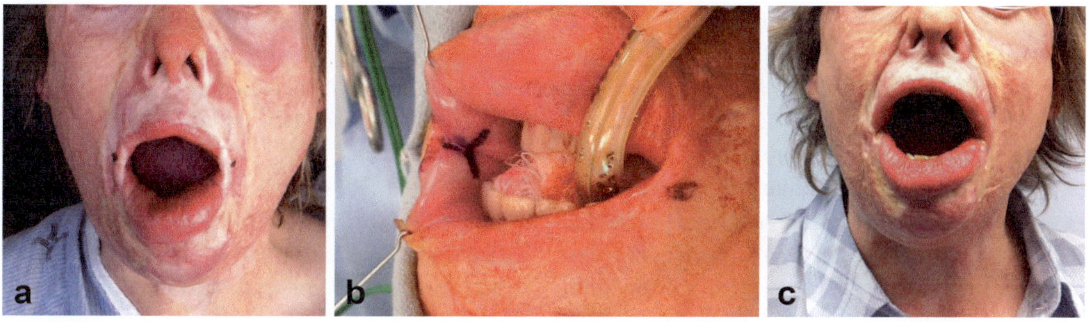

Fig. 11.10 Bilateral oral commissure contractures with *dots* identifying planned site of relocation of the modiolis (**a**), planned Y to V release utilizing oral mucosal flaps (**b**), with result at 3 months post-op (**c**). Photo courtesy of Robert Cartotto, MD, FRCSC

Neck

Flexion contractures of the neck can create significant functional and aesthetic defects. After neck contracture release the defect can be resurfaced using skin grafts, or local flaps of the neck or regional perforator flaps from the shoulder, if these areas are spared. If skin grafts are used, the patient can be placed on a bed that promotes neck extension for the first week postoperatively, or at the very least pillows should not be used. This will need to be followed by splinting of the neck in neutral or extension in order to maintain the release. One should be cautious and avoid combining simultaneous releases of both neck and axillary contractures, as the requirements of splinting for each procedure are antagonistic. In addition, an anesthesia consult prior to a planned neck release is prudent since patients with anterior neck contractures may be difficult to intubate.

Upper Extremity Reconstruction

Approach

The differential diagnosis of joint contracture in the setting of burn injury is complex, and not limited to skin and scar only. One must consider the possibility of heterotopic ossification, fracture, subluxation, arthritis, capsular contracture, tendon contracture, opposing tendon transection, and soft tissue attenuation either resulting from or contributing to overlying scar and burn contracture. Diagnosis of bony causes requires plain film X-ray. Diagnosis of tendon pathology can be made by examining other joints which are unaffected by scarring but which the tendon in question crosses. Alternatively, it may be possible to evaluate tendon gliding and excursion by placing adjacent joints in varying degrees of flexion and extension to change the relative distance the tendon must traverse. And finally, tendon ultrasound may be helpful in complex cases. Operative planning should include the possibility that multiple pathologies may need to be addressed simultaneously. Fortunately, if burn scar contractures are treated in a timely fashion, it is unlikely that enough time will have passed for soft tissue attenuation to occur, and contracture will generally be limited to skin scars, skin grafts, and subcutaneous tissues.

Axilla

Axillary contractures can significantly impair upper extremity function, yet are notoriously difficult to treat. If local or regional flaps options are available, these are preferable as they are least likely to undergo a recurrent contracture postoperatively. In contrast, skin grafting of the axilla frequently recontracts and thus postoperative splinting is essential to preventing recurrence.

Axillary contractures can occur along the anterior or posterior axillary folds, or in the dome of the axilla, and are common after skin grafting.

Axillary contractures can be classified as: adjacent scars, isolated anterior or posterior fold, anterior and posterior fold with spared apex, and total axillary involvement [12]. As the arm is abducted during axillary contracture release, the contents of the axilla: axillary vein, numerous peripheral nerves, and lymph nodes, are placed at risk of transection. Axillary releases can either occur through the zone of maximal contracture, or if one wishes to avoid the structures in the dome, then two releases (proximal and distal to the dome) can be performed. For smaller contractures with adequate surrounding soft tissue, Z-plasty or local transposition flaps work best to close the release (although one must avoid non-anatomic relocation of hair bearing areas), whereas larger contracture releases or those involving the apex will likely require skin grafting and a bolster dressing.

Elbow

Elbow flexion contractures are a frequent complication of burn injury to the region. The elbow is also the most frequent site of heterotopic ossification in burn patients [13], and so this potential cause of limitations in joint range of motion should be considered. During contracture release the contents of the cubital fossa: antecubital veins, radial and median nerves, and brachial artery, are all potentially at risk of injury. Therefore a combination of sharp and blunt dissection should be used during release. As with other joint releases, adequate surrounding soft tissue means the release can be treated with some variation of the Z-plasty, whereas larger releases or poor local tissue will lead to use of a skin graft for closure.

Hand

Principles

The main concern with operations of the volar digits is identification and preservation of the neurovascular bundles and flexor tendons. Careful release of contractures and blunt dissection are crucial to avoiding important structures, and if any concern exists that they are present in the surgical field, one should attempt to identify and protect the neurovascular bundles before proceeding with the remainder of the operative procedure.

If there is any concern that contractures are multifactorial or involve more than the skin and soft tissue, then referral to a plastic and reconstructive or hand surgeon is warranted.

Flexion Contractures

Flexion contractures can occur as a result of burn injury and contracture of the volar digit, or as a sequelae of either burn injury or iatrogenic injury of the extensor mechanism during excision and grafting. This distinction is important, as extensor mechanism injuries will not be corrected during volar contracture release, but must be addressed so that the contracture does not recur.

Flexion contracture releases are optimally treated with Z-plasties, but in many cases there is insufficient surrounding soft tissue and so full thickness skin grafts may be required instead (Fig. 11.11).

Webspace Contractures

Webspace contractures ("burn syndactyly") occur when adjacent digits are injured by burns and allowed to heal, or are skin grafted and subsequent scarring develops across the webspace. This can lead to significant aesthetic and functional deformity where the patient cannot abduct the digits. In the first webspace this can significantly impair the ability to oppose the thumb and grasp objects. Webspace contractures can be classified according to a schema proposed by Alexander et al. [14] based on the degree to which the contracture involves the proximal phalanx. Depending on the location and the extent of the scar, webspace contractures can be treated with release followed by full thickness skin grafts, simple Z-plasties, 4-flap Z-plasties, or a modified double opposing Z-plasty as described by Housinger et al. [15] (outlined in Fig. 11.12). In general, 50 % involvement or less can be treated with local flaps alone, whereas greater than 50 % involvement will likely require skin grafting.

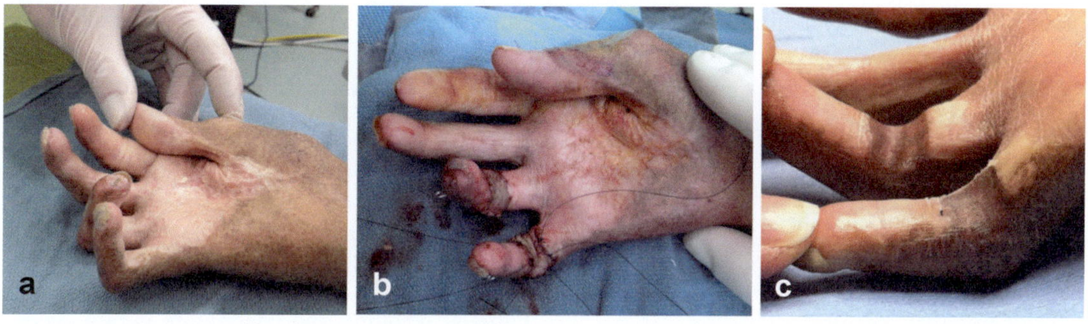

Fig. 11.11 Post-burn flexion contractures of the ring and small digits with planned transverse release marked (**a**), completion of release and insertion of full thickness skin grafts. Note the use of temporary K-wires across each proximal interphalangeal joint to maintain the release postoperatively (**b**), with result at 3 months (**c**). Photo courtesy of Robert Cartotto, MD, FRCSC

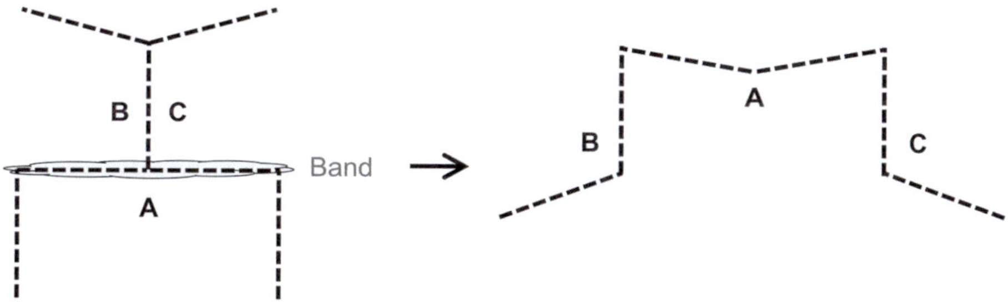

Fig. 11.12 Modified double opposing Z-plasty. This technique is particularly useful for webspace contractures ("burn syndactyly")

Miscellaneous

Missing digits and more proximal limb losses can be reconstructed through a variety of techniques. The classic examples for thumb loss including web space deepening, pollicization, and microvascular free tissue transfer such as toe-to-thumb, depending on the level of loss. Other, more exotic, reconstructions for burn amputation could include targeted muscle reinnervation with prosthesis, and hand transplantation. These types of reconstructions necessitate referral to a reconstructive plastic or hand surgeon.

Breast, Abdomen, and Perineum

Breast

Breast Mound

The breast can be of significant importance, particularly for female development from both an aesthetic and psychological perspective. Distortions of the breast requiring reconstruction are generally due to problems of development if acquired at a prepubertal age, or alterations of structure and form if injured by a burn after maturity. In the case of prepubertal injury, if the nipple areolar complex was damaged or removed, then the breast bud, which lies directly below it, may have been compromised. If the breast bud has been removed or is nonfunctional, then normal breast growth and development cannot occur. Alternatively, if significant scarring or skin grafting of the surrounding and overlying breast skin envelope has occurred with an intact underlying breast bud, then there can be significant retardation of normal breast development as the breast mound cannot expand. In these situations, release of the overlying skin can allow the breast to grow as puberty occurs. If breast deformity results from having portions removed or was skin grafted after maturity, then these contour irregularities may be due to either missing tissue or contracture. In all of these cases referral to a plastic surgeon is warranted. Reconstructive techniques can involve tissue expansion, placement of breast implants, resurfacing, or use of various flaps including those traditionally used for post-oncologic breast reconstruction such as the latissimus dorsi, and the wide range of pedicled and free abominally based flaps (for example the transverse rectus abdominis or deep inferior epigastric perforator flaps).

Nipple and Areola

Nipple reconstruction is performed for aesthetic purposes. There is currently no method of reconstructing a functional nipple, and reconstructions are limited to restoring some degree of projection and color. Projection can be restored using a variety of local flaps (for example the modified skate [16], and C-V [17] flaps) or free nipple grafts, and color can be restored with skin grafts or tattooing (which allows a greater degree of control over pigmentation). Again, such reconstructive efforts should be undertaken by an experienced breast reconstructive surgeon.

Abdomen

Abdominal scars may be amenable to revision or removal based on the availability of surrounding tissue and its laxity. Some scars can be removed using various modifications of abdominoplasty techniques, often when various life events or changes, such as pregnancy, have created a "natural" soft tissue expansion. Other scars will require the use of soft tissue expanders to allow for resurfacing, or serial excision. If these techniques are used, then one should attempt to place the resulting scars in inconspicuous areas such as below the underwear line. It is important to note that abdominoplasties are not similar to panniculectomies, in that the result should be aesthetically acceptable, the umbilicus is repositioned, and the goal is not simply removal of excess tissue. The abdomen can also be a source of significant full thickness skin graft as this can also be removed in an abdominoplasty style harvest, which allows for primary closure of the donor site.

Perineum

Perineal webbing and contracture is rare, as are perineal burns, but can have significant functional consequences. Perineal webs can prevent hip abduction, create difficulties with voiding and hygiene, and compromise sexual function. Generally these webs are large and may not always be amenable to correction with a Z-plasty although in appropriately selected cases Z-plasties or their variations may correct the deformity (Fig. 11.6) [4]. More significant contracture releases may require mobilization of abdominal and thigh skin flaps at the level of the fascia, or even myocutaneous flaps, but many also require skin grafts, and the operative plan should include this option. Care should be taken when mobilizing skin flaps not to compromise lymphatic drainage from the lower extremities. If skin grafts are used, bolster dressings may be the best option for improving adherence and preventing the shearing forces to which this region is prone.

Lower Extremity Reconstruction

In many ways lower extremity reconstruction is analogous to upper extremity reconstruction, and approaches to matching anatomic areas are similar. The same general principles and approaches apply to joints of the lower extremity, as they do to joints of the upper extremity.

Knees

Knee flexion contractures are similar in effect to elbow flexion contractures. The resulting primary disability is difficulty with ambulation, which can be improved with appropriate contracture release and skin grafting or Z-plasty as appropriate.

Ankles

Plantar flexion contractures may result from multiple causes including: foot drop, shortening of the Achilles tendon due to inadequate stretching and/or improper positioning during the acute burn phase, and posterior soft tissue contracture. Foot drop is common in critically ill patients, including burn patients [18, 19]. If this is the case, then serial splinting for foot drop, or referral to an orthopedic surgeon for fixed deformities may be warranted. Aggressive stretching and splinting should be undertaken when tendon shortening is identified. If the only cause appears to be posterior scar contracture, then Z-plasty or release and skin grafting should correct the deformity. Due to limited tissue availability in this region Z-plasty is less likely to be a viable option, and the need for skin grafting is higher.

Toes

Digital contractures and webspace contractures of the foot are dealt with using the same principles and techniques as in the digits of the hand. The anatomy is similar, and precautions to guard against tendon, digital nerve, and digital artery injury are the same. There may be less functional and aesthetic need to correct foot webspace contractures as compared to in the hand, but treatment should be guided by the patient, and it is not unreasonable to correct these deformities if they occur. The most common post-burn deformity is a dorsal foot contracture that pulls the toes into hyperextension at the MTP joints. These contractures may be broad and diffuse or may exist as linear bands to individual toes, and are dealt with using the aforementioned principles of scar release. Unlike in the hand, flexion contractures of the toes do not place them in a functional position, and these will need correction to allow proper ambulation and facilitate footwear fit.

Conclusion

While a wide variety of reconstructive techniques exist, in many cases straightforward techniques such as serial excision, skin grafting, and Z-plasty can have great benefit for patients. A thoughtful approach to reconstruction can help guide surgeons in determining when to attempt it themselves, what approach to use, and when referral to a plastic and reconstructive surgeon will be most appropriate.

References

1. Smith CM. Origin and uses of primum non nocere--above all, do no harm! J Clin Pharmacol. 2005;45(4):371–7.
2. Kwan P, Hori K, Ding J, Tredget EE. Scar and contracture: biological principles. Hand Clin. 2009;25(4):511–28.
3. Gottlieb LJ, Krieger LM. From the reconstructive ladder to the reconstructive elevator. Plast Reconstr Surg. 1994;93(7):1503–4.
4. Cartotto R, Cicuto BJ, Kiwanuka HN, Bueno EM, Pomahac B. Common postburn deformities and their management. Surg Clin North Am. 2014;94(4):817–37.
5. Buhrer DP, Huang TT, Yee HW, Blackwell SJ. Treatment of burn alopecia with tissue expanders in children. Plast Reconstr Surg. 1988;81(4):512–5.
6. Armin BB, Ruder RO, Azizadeh B. Partial auricular reconstruction. Semin Plast Surg. 2011;25(4):249–56.
7. Wilkes GH, Wolfaardt JF. Osseointegrated alloplastic versus autogenous ear reconstruction: criteria for treatment selection. Plast Reconstr Surg. 1994;93(5):967–79.
8. Ibrahim SM, Salem IL. Burned ear: the use of a staged Nagata technique for ear reconstruction. J Plast Reconstr Aesthet Surg. 2008;61 Suppl 1:S52–8.
9. Menick FJ. A 10-year experience in nasal reconstruction with the three-stage forehead flap. Plast Reconstr Surg. 2002;109(6):1839–55. discussion 56–61.
10. Wolfaardt JF, Wilkes GH. Craniofacial osseointegration. J Can Dent Assoc. 1994;60(9):805–9.
11. Menick FJ, Salibian A. Microvascular repair of heminasal, subtotal, and total nasal defects with a folded radial forearm flap and a full-thickness forehead flap. Plast Reconstr Surg. 2011;127(2):637–51.

12. Achauer BM. Burn reconstruction. New York: Thieme Medical Publishers; 1990.
13. Hunt JL, Arnoldo BD, Kowalske K, Helm P, Purdue GF. Heterotopic ossification revisited: a 21-year surgical experience. J Burn Care Res. 2006;27(4):535–40.
14. Alexander JW, MacMillan BG, Martel L. Correction of postburn syndactyly: an analysis of children with introduction of the VM-plasty and postoperative pressure inserts. Plast Reconstr Surg. 1982;70(3):345–54.
15. Housinger TA, Ivers B, Warden GD. Release of the first web space with the "goalpost" procedure in pediatric burns. J Burn Care Rehabil. 1993;14(3):353–5.
16. Hammond DC, Khuthaila D, Kim J. The skate flap purse-string technique for nipple-areola complex reconstruction. Plast Reconstr Surg. 2007;120(2):399–406.
17. Losken A, Mackay GJ, Bostwick III J. Nipple reconstruction using the C-V flap technique: a long-term evaluation. Plast Reconstr Surg. 2001;108(2):361–9.
18. Latronico N, Shehu I, Seghelini E. Neuromuscular sequelae of critical illness. Curr Opin Crit Care. 2005;11(4):381–90.
19. Richard R, Miller S, Staley M, Johnson RM. Multimodal versus progressive treatment techniques to correct burn scar contractures. J Burn Care Rehabil. 2000;21(6):506–12.

12 Outpatient Management of Burns

Daniel Goldberg and David T. Harrington

Introduction

In 2015, the American Burn Association reported a total of 486,000 burn injuries requiring medical treatment. Only 40,000 (8 %) of these burn patients required hospital admission for management of injuries—leaving approximately 92 % of the thermally injured patients to receive their care in an outpatient setting [1]. This low acuity population still requires careful evaluation and management. Though these patients do not require fluid resuscitation or need escharotomies, they still require monitoring of their healing wounds, adequate pain control, appropriate assessment of their emotional healing and societal reintegration.

Selection for Outpatient Burn Care

Successful treatment of burn injuries in the outpatient setting is dependent upon careful selection of appropriate patients. Key factors that must be taken into account include age, premorbid conditions, social circumstances, injuring agent, extent of burn, and depth of burn.

D. Goldberg, M.D. (✉) • D.T. Harrington, M.D.
Rhode Island Burn Center at Rhode Island Hospital, Alpert Medical School of Brown University, 593 Eddy Street, APC 443, Providence, RI 02903, USA
e-mail: dgoldberg@Lifespan.org; dharrington@usasurg.org

Extent of burn is the most important consideration when identifying patients that could potentially be managed as an outpatient. It is important to remember that the ABA criteria for referral to a burn center are exactly that, referral criteria, and are not admission criteria [2] (Table 12.1). At our institution, we see burns of greater than 10 % TBSA that are extremely superficial in depth in a patient with a high level of function that can be well managed as an outpatient.

Age is also an important consideration when deciding whether a patient can be safely managed as an outpatient. There is not an absolute age cut off for a child or senior that demands inpatient admission following burn injury, but patients at the extremes of age can pose undo challenges in the outpatient setting [3]. Careful selection is required. Young children often have wound care needs that outstrip the families and the visiting nurses resources. The older senior population can benefit from the daily wound care and rehabilitation that can be given in an inpatient burn center setting to maintain function.

A patient's premorbid medical problems can significantly affect the successful outcome of a burn injury. Chronic diseases such as heart failure, chronic obstructive pulmonary disease, cirrhosis, kidney disease, diabetes mellitus, and dementia are often found in burn patients and can affect the course of therapy and outcomes. The degree of control of underlying medical problems as well as support at home should be assessed. If the patient has

D.G. Greenhalgh (ed.), *Burn Care for General Surgeons and General Practitioners*,
DOI 10.1007/978-3-319-29161-1_12

Table 12.1 ABA referral criteria describe a range of conditions that require a referral to a burn center

ABA burn center referral criteria
1. Partial-thickness burns of greater than 10 % of the total body surface area
2. Burns that involve the face, hands, feet, genitalia, perineum, or major joints
3. Third-degree burns in any age group
4. Electrical burns, including lightning injury
5. Chemical injury
6. Inhalation injury
7. Burn Injury in patients with preexisting medical disorders that could complicate management, prolong recovery, or affect mortality
8. Any patients with burns and concomitant trauma (such as fractures) in which the burn injury poses the greatest risk of morbidity or mortality. In such cases, if the trauma poses the greater immediate risk, the patient's condition may be stabilized initially in a trauma center before transfer to a burn center. Physician judgement will be necessary in such situations and should be in concert with the regional medical control plan and triage protocols
9. Burned children in hospitals without qualified personnel or equipment for the care of children
10. Burn injury in patients who will require special social, emotional, or rehabilitative intervention

control of their premorbid conditions and a good support system at home, outpatient management can be attempted [4]. Unfortunately the patient's family and social support is often untenable in patients who suffer thermal injury. Without social support and a clean and safe home environment, patients and their wounds can rapidly deteriorate. A few days in the burn center to appropriately assess a patient's burn situation and suitability for transitioning to home care is often a wise investment. Secondary injuries such as smoke inhalation injury, skeletal fractures, or closed head injury often make inpatient care the only option. All patients should also be assessed for signs and symptoms of physical abuse or neglect. In our burn center we often admit these patients due to concern for their safety, which also allows us to do a careful social and home evaluation.

Outpatient Burn Wound Care

Minor burns should be treated immediately with cool running water and all inciting burn materials should be removed. The burn should then be cleansed. This includes using an antimicrobial soap. Our cleanser of choice is dilute chlorhexidine. Loose tissue and broken blisters should be debrided. Tense blisters, often occurring on the palms of hands and soles of feet should be deroofed. Non-tense intact blisters do not need to be de-roofed. Concurrently, adequate pain medication should be provided to allow tolerance of the initial burn debridement.

Following debridement, partial-thickness burns are covered with topical agents and dressings. The goal of these products is to minimize pain, decrease to risk of infection, promote wound healing, minimize cosmetic deformity, and preserve function. There are several topical agents and dressings on the market from which clinicians can choose. Silvadene cream is suitable for most all burns and is a time tested antimicrobial wound agent, however there are now many other products on the market that offer greater comfort to the patient and the convenience of less frequent dressing changes. A silver based dressing such as AquacellAG® (ConvaTech, Inc., Bridgewater, N.J.) or MepilexAG® (Molnlycke Healthcare, Norcross, GA) allows the dressing to remain in place for 7–10 days. These dressings have demonstrated faster healing, decreased pain, fewer dressing changes, and improved patient satisfaction. Silver impregnated dressing have also proven to be more cost-effective compared to traditional dressing methods such as daily dressing changes with silver sulfadiazine [5]. It is our practice to use these silver products preferentially in superficial dermal burns and use Silvadene for wounds at or deeper than the mid-dermis or in burns where the silver dressings are difficult to apply—axilla, neck, and diaper areas in infants.

Timing and frequency of follow-up for outpatient burns depends on the acuity of the burn. For acute superficial partial thickness burns, healing should occur at 2 weeks. This type of burn should be observed on a weekly basis. Assessment of wound healing, pain control, therapy compliance and teaching in the care of the healing wound occurs at these visits. Avoidance of harsh soaps, use of skin moisturizers and avoidance of unprotected sun exposure are important to teach and reemphasize often. These patients rarely need extended follow-up for the risk of scaring and other sequelae are rare. Longer periods of healing can be expected in patients with deeper injury (mid-dermal, deep dermal burns and full thickness burns) or patients who have concurrent medical problems that delay healing such as diabetes, immunocompromised states, chronic steroid use, or advanced age. These wounds should be assessed every week or every other week. Partial thickness burns that fail to heal at 2 weeks as well as deeper burns should be considered for surgery though the decision to operate is multifactorial and is dependent on not just depth of burn but location and size of wound, the age of the patient and the risk of donor site morbidity. It is important in these cases to review with the patient, your team, and yourself the benefits of excision and grafting of a wound: to reduce infection; to reduce time to healing (and return to work); to reduce the risk of functional scar; and to improve cosmesis. It is surprising how often running this list of benefits with the patient yields no clear indications for surgery.

In patients with healed burns, length between appointments can be extended typically to a monthly basis while scar maturation continues to occur. At these appointments, outcomes of scar maturation from compression garment and adherence to physical and occupational therapy can be assessed. Superficial burns and burns of small extent often mature by 3–4 months after burn. These patients have no detectable violaceous appearance to their healed wound and can be discharged from the clinic. Burns that have been grafted and spontaneously healed burns of mid and deep dermal depth should be followed for a longer periods. These appointments can be a 4–6 week intervals. At the completion of scar maturation, which usually occurs by 1 year, length between appointments can be further extended to one or two time a year basis [4].

Control of Pain and Pruritus

Pain control is essential for successful outpatient burn wound management. Appropriate pain control can usually be achieved through a combination of scheduled over the counter, nonnarcotic and short-acting, prescription narcotic medications. If adequate pain control cannot be achieved through these means, a long-acting prescription narcotic may be added to the patient's pain regimen to decrease spikes in pain. Low-dose anxiolytics can also be added to reduce anxiety associated with dressing changes. A nonsteroidal anti-inflammatory (NSAID) should also be part of the pain control regimen. A multitrack approach to pain control does not end with narcotics and NSAID, drugs in the class of antiepileptic and antidepressants can have a role in the control of pain. These medications act centrally and can provide a degree of pain control in burn patients who have difficult to manage pain. In the class of antidepressants selective serotonin reuptake inhibitors such as citalopram (Celexa) and sertraline (Zoloft) and Tricyclic antidepressants such as amitriptyline, desipramine (Norpramin), and doxepin (Silenor) and Serotonin and norepinephrine reuptake inhibitors such as venlafaxine (Effexor) and duloxetine (Cymbalta) should be considered. In terms of anticonvulsants, gabapentin (Neurontin), and pregabalin (Lyrica) can be considered [6]. Our center has seen good benefit with amitriptyline. Generally these antidepressants and anticonvulsant medications when used for pain control are not dosed at their full recommended levels. It is advisable to start at the lowest possible dose and titrate for effect. Additionally since many of these medications have a long half-life it sometimes takes days to weeks before the medication takes effect. Monitoring for side effects with these medications is necessary. For antidepressants symptoms such as blurry vision, constipation, difficulty urinating, dry mouth, and headache should prompt an evaluation and reduction or stopping of the medication. For anticonvulsants side effects such as drowsiness, dizziness, fatigue, and nausea should be monitored. Finally burn practitioners need to decide how alternative therapies might be utilized for control of pain in their patients. Acupuncture, guided imagery, yoga, hypnosis, biofeedback, aromatherapy, relaxation, and herbal remedies may benefit some patients.

Ensuring adequate pain and anxiety control in the outpatient setting requires careful planning. Patients and families need clear directions as to how to take their pain medications ½ to 1 h before their scheduled visit time and to have additional medications available for after the visit. Ideally an outpatient clinic should have the capacity and facilities to be able to administer IV or PO narcotics for patients with more extensive wounds and those who require cleaning of large wounds.

Part of outpatient pain and anxiety control is the discussion of the appropriate use of narcotics and the need to have a schedule for their tapering and eventual termination. This discussion needs to be highly individualized, for all patients will have their unique combination of burn size, size of wound, degree of functionally limiting scar, narcotic tolerance, and anxiety levels. No matter the need for individualization, this conversation about tapering and ending medications needs to be initiated early and goals should be set. Practitioners should be ready for reassessing targets of tapering and termination of these medications as conditions change. Ten to 20 % of trauma and burn victims are narcotic and cocaine positive on admission to the hospital and majority of those patients will have substance abuse problems [7, 8]. Preexisting addiction and patients who become narcotic dependant during burn treatment can pose a difficult management problem for the burn team. For these patients a referral to an outpatient detoxication program or even an inpatient rapid detoxification program will be necessary [9].

Pruritus is a common complication of burn injuries, observed in up to 90 % of patients during the first month following a burn. Successful control of pruritus requires a multifocal approach, addressing the underlying causes of pruritus. Known causes of pruritus following burns include histamine release, dry skin, and neuropathic causes. The first step is to review the patient's skin care regimen to ensure that they are still using a mild soap and are applying skin moisturizers 3–5 times a day. The release of histamine from mast cells occurs during healing. Histamine H-1 specific blockers have been found to be superior to lowering pruritus compared to nonspecific histamine receptor blockers [10]. Finally, neuropathic pruritus can be treated using medications used to treat neuropathic pain such as gabapentin, pregabalin, and duloxetine.

Telemedicine

The advent of telemedicine is another resource that can be utilized for the delivery of outpatient burn care to those patients without readily available access to a specialty burn center [11]. Telemedicine has been shown to provide accurate initial and follow-up assessments for burn wounds and patient and family satisfaction has been positive. It also provides a cost-effective solution for providing specialty burn care to rural communities [12]. Models of telemedicine in the USA in the field of dermatology have shown initial enthusiasm but over time over half these programs have closed. Of note the programs that remain open have seen their volumes of visit increase. For a program to be successful it has to overcome the hurdles of startup costs, cross state licensing, and inconsistent models for reimbursement [13].

The Outpatient Burn Team

As more and more thermally injured patients are managed as outpatients the scope of care that is delivered in the clinic needs to change. A doctor, nurse, and rehabilitation therapist would be considered a well-represented clinic in the past, but this neglects many other important aspects of burn care. The clinic is a place where patient's nutritional status should be assessed and where patients make the transition back into the workplace. Making sure that these issues are part of the conversation during clinic visits and having the resources to address patient's dietary status and reintegration into society will be an increasingly important part of the outpatient experience in a modern burn center.

Many advances in burn materials and new thinking on part of burn practitioners have lead to more and more burn patients getting their burn care as outpatients. Pressures on hospitals to reduce inpatient hospital costs and length of stays have been mounting on general hospitals as well as burn centers. Burn patients on average spend longer in the hospital than all other patients admitted to US hospitals with an average length of stay of 8.9 days versus 5.1 days. Thermally injured patient cost the system more than other conditions with an average in-patient cost of $173,000 versus $9000 for all other admissions to US hospitals [14]. Burn practitioners should be part of the solution in finding ways to reduce hospital costs and avoid unnecessary hospital admissions, but we need to be vigilant that the quality of care we deliver does not suffer. As the clinic takes on an increased volume of patients and patients with increased acuity the resources of the clinic need to be augmented. Materials, appropriate settings for wound care and analgesia, personnel to include nursing, rehabilitation therapists, nutritionists, social work need to be appropriately assigned to the outpatient burn clinic. To shift inpatient care to the outpatient setting without an appropriate increase in resources is a formula for less than optimal care.

Transitions of Care

Transitioning care from an inpatient to outpatient setting requires careful coordination of resources to assure smooth and safe transition of care. Factors that must be considered in the transition of a patient from inpatient to outpatient care include burn healing status, pain control needs, functional capacity, need for occupational and physical therapy, access to transportation, psychological needs, and the patient's financial/insurance status. These factors can be successfully addressed through a multifactorial, team approach utilizing input from the medical burn team, physical and occupational therapists, nutritionists, social workers, and case managers. Transitioning a patient from outpatient to an inpatient treatment setting should be considered in patients who have failed outpatient management of a burn or have severe complications related to their burn. This includes poor compliance with outpatient therapy, poor pain control, infection of a burn, or burns that require delayed surgical intervention. It also includes delayed healing of burns needing excision and grafting as well as complications related to scar maturation. An additional transition is the preparation of an outpatient burn patient for same day or ambulatory surgery. Establishing a good administrative process for these surgeries is necessary to eliminate patient frustration and unmet pain needs.

Quality Improvement

Quality Improvement and Process Improvement (QI/PI) should not begin and end at the doors of the burn center. While the vast majority of the criteria for successful verification of a burn center pertain to the care of inpatients, more and more burn patients receive their care in the outpatient setting. Burn centers should begin to look at their QI/PI process across the care continuum. Recovery and maintenance of weight, adequacy of pain control in the clinic, assessment and intervention of acute stress disorder and post-traumatic stress syndrome, and compliance with outpatient rehabilitation is just a partial list of elements that could be considered for an outpatient QI/PI program.

Conclusion

Medical care in the USA is in a time of great change and the burn community needs to be ready to respond while maintaining excellent patient care. Burn centers, which have been successful in building great inpatient burn centers, will need spend time building and resourcing robust outpatient clinics and begin to monitoring outpatient patient outcomes.

References

1. American Burn Association. Burn incidence fact sheet. 2015. http://www.ameriburn.org/resources_factsheet.php. Accessed 12 Jun 2015.
2. Committee on Trauma, American College of Surgeons. Guidelines for trauma centers caring for burn patients. In: Resources for optimal care of the injured patient. Chicago: The Burn Association; 2014. p. 101.
3. Saffle JR, Davis B, Williams P. Recent outcomes in the treatment of burn injury in the United States: report from the American Burn Association Patient Registry. J Burn Care Rehabil. 1995;16:219–32.
4. Warner PM, Coffee TL, Yowler CJ. Outpatient burn management. Surg Clin North Am. 2014;94:879–92.

5. Malic C, Verchere C, Arneja JS. Inpatient silver sulphadiazine versus outpatient nanocrystalline silver models of care for pediatric scald burns: a value analysis. Plast Surg (Oakv). 2014;22(2):99–102.
6. http://www.mdconsult.com/das/pharm/view/403939018-13/full/562/top
7. Soderstrum CA, Discharger PC, Kerns TJ, Kufera JA, Mitchell KA, Scalea TM. The magnitude of acute and chronic alcohol abuse in trauma patients. Arch Surg. 1993;128(8):907–12. discussion 912–3.
8. Soderstrom CA, Dischinger PC, Kerns TJ, Kufera JA, Mitchell KA, Scalea TM. Epidemic increases in cocaine and opiate use by trauma center patients: documentation with a large clinical toxicology database. J Trauma. 2001;51(3):557–64.
9. Maani CV, DeSocio PA, Jansen RK, Merrell JD, McGhee LL, Young A, Williams JF, Tyrell K, Jackson BA, Serio-Melvin ML, Blackbourne LH, Renz EM. Use of ultra rapid opioid detoxification in the treatment of US military burn casualties. J Trauma. 2011;71(1 Suppl):S114–9.
10. Bell PL, Gabriel V. Evidence of based review for the treatment of post-burn pruritus. J Burn Care Res. 2009;30:55–61.
11. Holt B, Faraklas I, Theurer L, et al. Telemedicine use among burn centers in the United States: a survey. J Burn Care Res. 2012;33:157–62.
12. Saffle JR, Edelman L, Theurer L, Morris SE, Cochran A. Telemedicine evaluation of acute burns is accurate and cost-effective. J Trauma. 2009;67(2):358–65.
13. Armstrong AW, Wu J, Kovarik CL, Goldyne ME, Oh DH, McKoy KC, Shippy AM, Pak HS. State of teledermatology programs in the United States. J Am Acad Dermatol. 2012;67(5):939–44. Epub 2012 Mar 28.
14. Agency for Research and Quality. Healthcare Cost and Utilization Project. Statistical Brief #25. [Internet] http://www.hcup-us.ahrq.gov/reports/statbriefs/sb25.pdf

Burns in Children

13

Robert L. Sheridan

Introduction

Most principles of burn care useful in the management of adults are equally applicable in pediatric patients. However, there are a number of important differences. The objective of this chapter is to detail the physiologic and anatomic differences that impact burn care and the practical technical differences that follow.

Epidemiology and Mechanisms

The mechanism of burn injury varies significantly with age and socioeconomic state. Young children are particularly vulnerable, with most being injured by scald in bathing and cooking accidents. In lower-income countries, scald injuries still predominate in young children, but flame burns are more common as are electrical injuries in older children [1, 2]. Young children are particularly prone to injury where open fires are in use ([3] and Fig. 13.1).

R.L. Sheridan, M.D., F.A.A.P., F.A.C.S. (✉)
Division of Burns, Massachusetts General Hospital,
Department of Surgery, Harvard Medical School,
Boston Shriners Hospital for Children,
51 Blossom Street, Boston, MA 02114, USA
e-mail: rsheridan@mgh.harvard.edu

Organization of Burn Care

Like most complex surgical problems, burns are most cost-effectively managed in dedicated programs [4]. The American Burn Association burn center transfer criteria include recommendations that all children with full-thickness components over 10 % of the body surface are transferred to a burn center [5]. Recent data has clearly demonstrated that survival is improved for burned children if they are managed in higher volume pediatric burn programs [6]. For individual children, burn care is a highly organized process going from resuscitation through reintegration that can be described in four distinct clinical phases [7]. A publically available set of clinical practice guidelines for burn care has been disseminated by the American military and has specific recommendations for initial pediatric care [8].

Burn Physiology

Burns are associated with both local injury and systemic response. When injury size is small, less than about 10 % of the body surface, the systemic effects are minimal. As burns become larger, the systemic effects can become quite profound and become a major clinical consideration. These issues apply to both adults and children,

D.G. Greenhalgh (ed.), *Burn Care for General Surgeons and General Practitioners*,
DOI 10.1007/978-3-319-29161-1_13

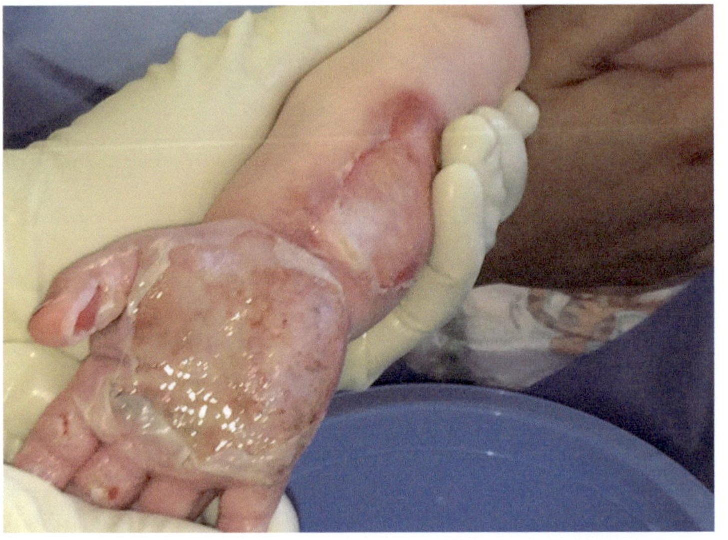

Fig. 13.1 Young children are susceptible to injury when open cooking methods are used. Coals in extinguished cooking fires can remain hot for days

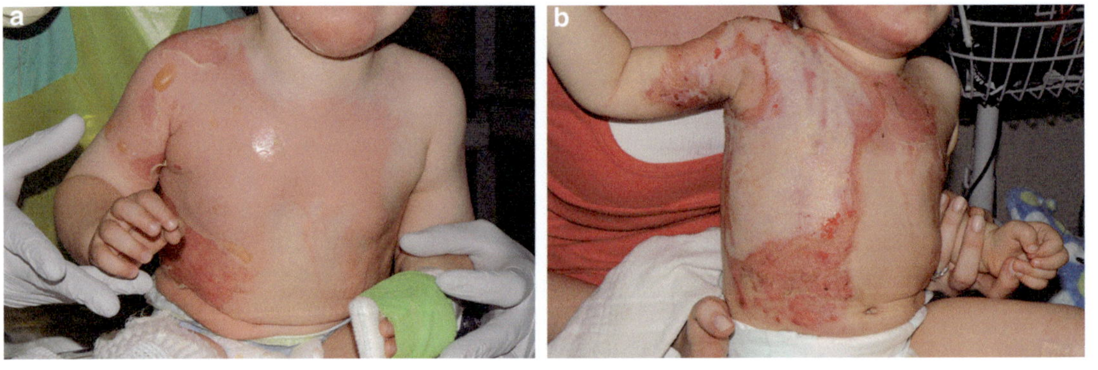

Fig. 13.2 Progression of microvascular injury can be clinically important, resulting in burns initially appearing more superficial than they ultimately will be. In this case, the difference in apparent burn depth between day 1 (**a**) and day 7 (**b**) was clinically important. This progression is not always easy to predict, even by experienced clinicians

but in infants and small children the clinical implications can be particularly important.

Local Response to Burning

The local response to burning involves both direct coagulation of tissue and surrounding microvascular vasoconstriction and thrombosis [9]. Progression of this microvascular injury commonly results in burns appearing initially more superficial than they ultimately will be (Fig. 13.2a, b). This progression is not always predictable with accuracy, even by experienced clinicians. This phenomenon is particularly common in young children with scald burns, the wounds appearing more superficial initially. Considering the possibility of burns appearing deeper after 3–5 days is important in children with scald burns. A number of devices have been introduced into clinical practice to help with early determination of burn depth [10], but none have proven entirely accurate nor have been universally adopted. Hypotension and hypothermia will compromise microvascular flow and may increase wound depth, so should be avoided during early care [11].

Systemic Response to Burning

The systemic response to burning is driven by a combination of neurohormonal changes, fluid losses across wounds, local colonization and systemic infection, hypoprotinemia, and wound colonization and infection [12]. The clinical consequences of these changes can be particularly exaggerated in young children, with some children suffering larger scald burns developing systemic inflammation and organ failures in the absence of sepsis. During the first 72 h, a relative hypodynamic state is common, with a decrease in cardiac output and metabolic rate [13]. In successfully resuscitated children, a sustained hypermetabolic response follows, This is characterized by a near doubling of cardiac output and resting energy expenditure. The magnitude of this response peaks in patients with injuries of 60 % or more of the body surface at as high as twice the normal basal metabolic rate [14]. The hypermetabolic response includes enhanced gluconeogenesis, insulin resistance, and increased protein catabolism. This catabolic state is particularly detrimental in children and requires nutritional monitoring and support [15]. Usual nutritional targets are 150 % of normal caloric and protein needs. There is a rich history of metabolic research in direct interventions to eliminate adverse components of hypermetabolic physiology, particularly protein catabolism. Beta-adrenergic agonists and antagonists, non-steroidal anti-inflammatory agents, recombinant growth hormone, insulin-like growth factor-1, and anabolic steroids have all been trialed in recent decades to modify this physiology in children [16]. The appropriate role of these substances is a controversial area in the field.

Unique Pediatric Anatomic and Physiologic Issues

Particularly important anatomic and physiologic differences between adults and children are highlighted in Table 13.1 [17]. The much smaller pediatric upper airway is rapidly occluded by progressive edema, which may prompt earlier intubation in small children. Children should be closely monitored for the development of stridor and retractions. The trachea of infant and young child is short, making mainstem intubation common. Bronchospasm is a frequent issue for young children after inhalation injury, but usually responds to inhaled beta-agonists. Infants have less mature renal concentrating ability and may require more fluid per unit body weight than predicted by common formulas for successful resuscitation [18]. It is relatively easy for fluid overload to occur in young children which should be prevented by cautious fluid support. Hypotonic fluids should be used with caution because young children are susceptible to cerebral edema if they become hyponatremic. Children have higher energy needs per unit body weight and rapidly go into negative nitrogen balance when starved, highlighting the importance of early nutritional

Table 13.1 Important anatomic and physiologic considerations in children

• The child's upper airway is smaller and more rapidly occluded by edema
• The child's trachea is short (7 cm in infants), making mainstem intubation more common
• Significant bronchospasm is more commonly following inhalation injury
• Infants have less mature renal concentrating ability
• Young children are more easily inadvertently fluid-loaded
• Younger children seem more prone to hyponatremia with secondary cerebral edema
• Children have higher energy needs per unit body weight
• Hypermetabolic children tolerate long periods of inadequate nutrition poorly
• The larger surface area to body weight ratio makes temperature control more difficult
• Children have thinner skin than adults complicating burn healing and donor harvesting
• Children have smaller vessels than adults complicating vascular access
• Children grow and will frequently outgrow good initial surgical results
• Children seem to form hypertrophic scar with greater intensity
• Pain and anxiety can be more difficult to access and manage
• School age children have schooling needs
• A child's recovery is strongly impacted by family dynamics

Fig. 13.3 There are a number of clinically important anatomic and physiologic differences between adults and children which have practical impact on therapeutic planning. Among these is that child's large surface area to mass ratio makes temperature control a constant issue

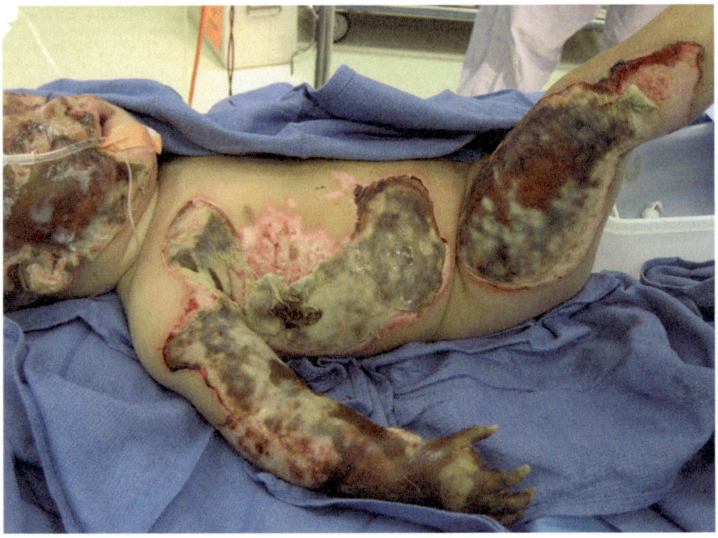

support. The child's large surface area to mass ratio makes temperature control a constant issue (Fig. 13.3). Children have thinner skin than adults, making mid-depth burns more likely to require surgical care and requiring greater skill with procurement of split-thickness grafts. Children have smaller vessels than adults complicating maintenance of vascular access. After initial care, children will grow and often very often need staged surgical revisions to optimize function and appearance. They have unique psychosocial and school reentry needs. Family dynamics play an important role in pediatric injury recovery [19, 20]. Family support is an important part of recovery planning.

Initial Evaluation and Management

The initial care of children with burns follows outlines presented elsewhere in this book. What follows are some of the unique considerations that apply to children who have been injured.

Primary Survey

Burned children should be initially approached as potential multiple trauma patients [21], following the guidelines of the Advanced Trauma Life Support Course [22]. Security of the airway is the highest priority issue during the initial evaluation. Fortunately, in most circumstances, airway access is not urgently needed, which allows for a thoughtful collaborative approach to airway evaluation, initial control, and maintenance (Fig. 13.4). A history of inhalation injury alone does not mandate intubation in otherwise stable children. Those who demonstrate progressive stridor, hoarseness, and/or retractions, or those obtunded from drugs, alcohol, trauma, or shock, should be intubated. Maintaining security of the endotracheal tube is critical and can be effected with a tie-harness or other device (Fig. 13.5). Cuffed endotracheal tubes should be used in all children [23]. Secure vascular access is required to safely transport and manage children with significant burns safe management. The intraosseous route is a good option if peripheral or central venous access cannot be reliably obtained, which is a particularly common problem in hypotensive young children. Placing intravenous or intraosseous lines through burns is acceptable initially, as wounds will be clean until colonized in the succeeding days (Fig. 13.6).

Burn-Specific Secondary Survey

A secondary survey is part of the evaluation of all injured patients. There are some issues unique

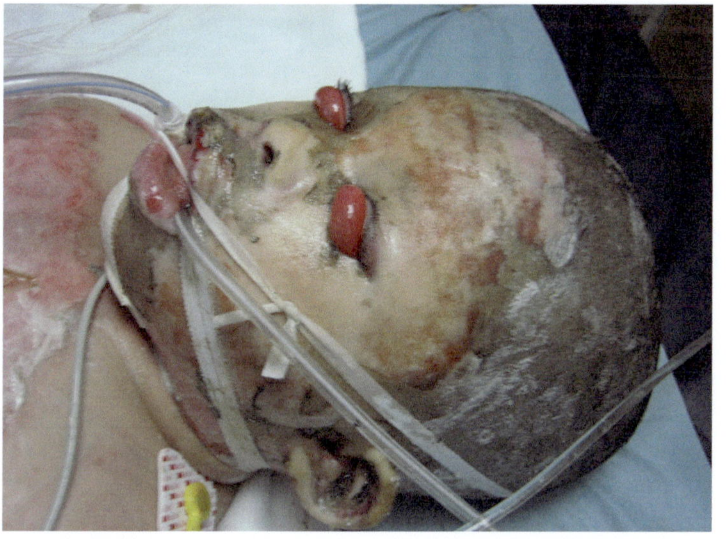

Fig. 13.4 Fortunately, in most circumstances, airway access is not urgently needed, which allows for a thoughtful collaborative approach to airway evaluation, initial control, and maintenance

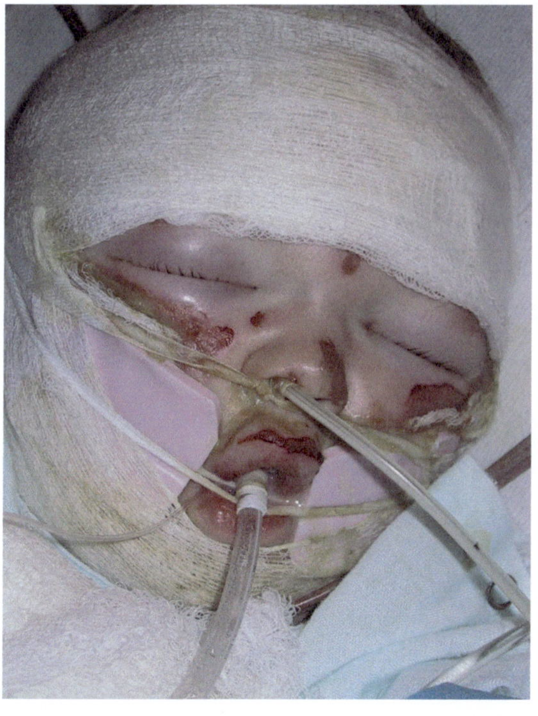

Fig. 13.5 Maintaining security of the endotracheal tube is critical. This can be effectively done with a tie-harness or other device

to burn-injured children that should be considered [24].

From a neurologic perspective, history and examination should be thorough as especially younger children cannot express themselves verbally. Those with larger injuries are frequently alert initially, but may become obtunded in the following hours because of pain medications required for management. If injury mechanism is consistent with possible head trauma, it is important to exclude intracranial injury by exam and/or imaging. Pain and anxiety control are important, but should be addressed cautiously with incremental small intravenous doses of analgesics and anxiolytics to prevent overmedication. Hypotonic fluids should be avoided during resuscitation to prevent hyponatremia with cerebral edema and seizures [25].

Initial otolaryngologic priorities are usually limited to documentation and management of corneal burns, treatment of external ear burns, and evaluation for intraocular hypertension secondary to retrobulbar edema. Deep corneal stromal burns are usually obvious by a clouded appearance. Corneal epithelial injury can be more subtle and only seen after fluorescein staining or slit-lamp examination. Alert older children will usually complain of significant pain and sensation of foreign body. This exam is best completed before eyelid edema makes a quality examination difficult. Initial management is application of viscous ophthalmic ointments. Untreated corneal burns can lead to desiccation, super-infection, and globe perforation (Fig. 13.7). Retrobulbar edema in the presence of non-elastic facial burns can result in

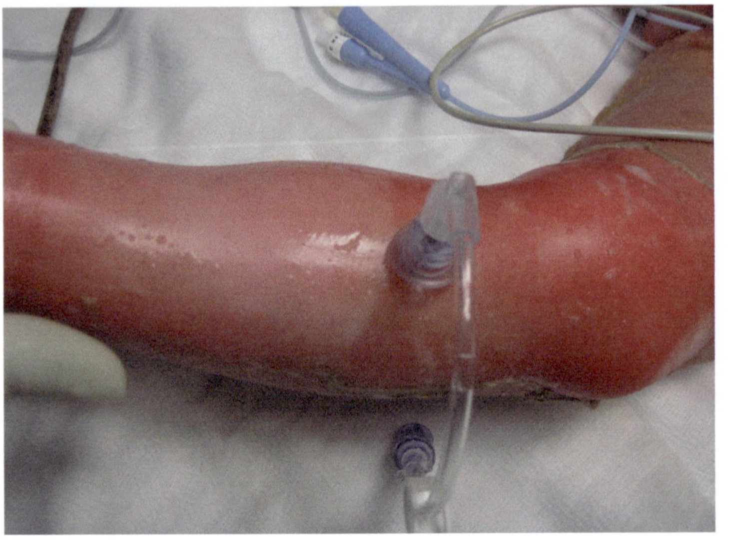

Fig. 13.6 Intraosseous lines are a good option when peripheral or central vascular access cannot be achieved for initial care. Initial placement through burns is acceptable

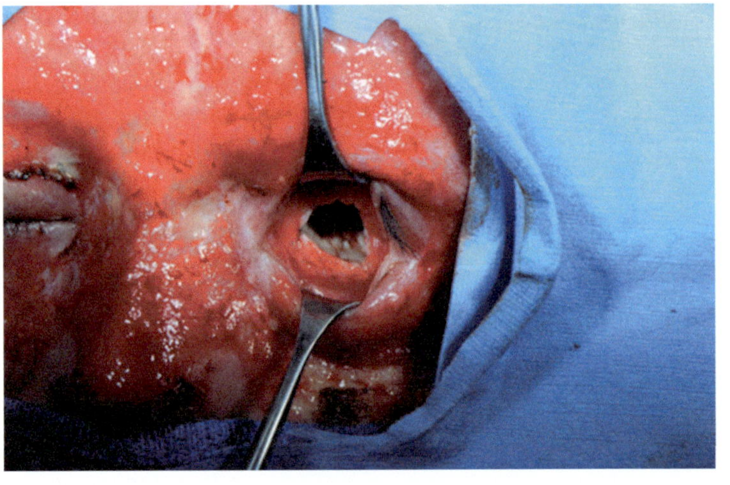

Fig. 13.7 Corneal ulceration can follow corneal burns or corneal exposure and can result in globe perforation and loss. Prevention of globe desiccation is essential and can generally be affected with frequent application of ophthalmic lubricants

secondary increased intraocular pressure and reduced retinal blood flow [26, 27]. This can be documented by tonometry and treated with bedside lateral canthotomy (Fig. 13.8). Deep burns of the external ear can be complicated by suppurative chondritis which will deform the ear. This complication is reduced with application of mafenide acetate [28]. Pressure on the burned ear should be avoided (Fig. 13.9).

In addition to the usual trauma issues, significantly decreased chest wall compliance can be caused by edema beneath near-circumferential eschar. This can sharply limit ventilation, particularly in non-intubated small children with their compliant chest walls. It can be markedly improved with chest and abdominal escharotomy. The diagnosis of inhalation injury in children is usually made by a history of closed-space exposure and physical examination demonstrating soot in the oropharynx. Bronchospasm is common in children with inhalation injury and generally responds well to inhaled beta-agonists.

In children, initial evaluation of the abdomen for non-burn trauma is done using standard ATLS protocols. Gastoduodenal ulcer prophylaxis is ensured with histamine-receptor blockers or proton pump inhibitors. Torso compliance is enhanced with liberal escharotomies when indicated. Children seem to be at particular risk for the complications of reduced torso compliance

Fig. 13.8 Retrobulbar edema with deep facial burns can cause vision-threatening intraocular hypertension. When documented, it can be treated with lateral canthotomy

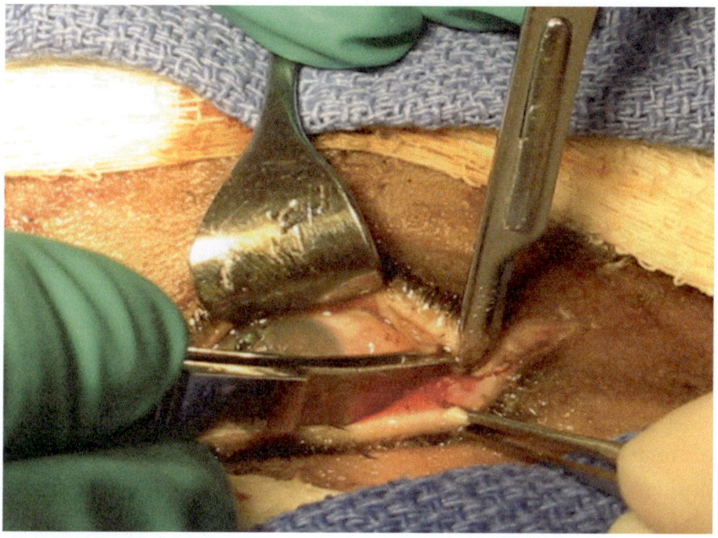

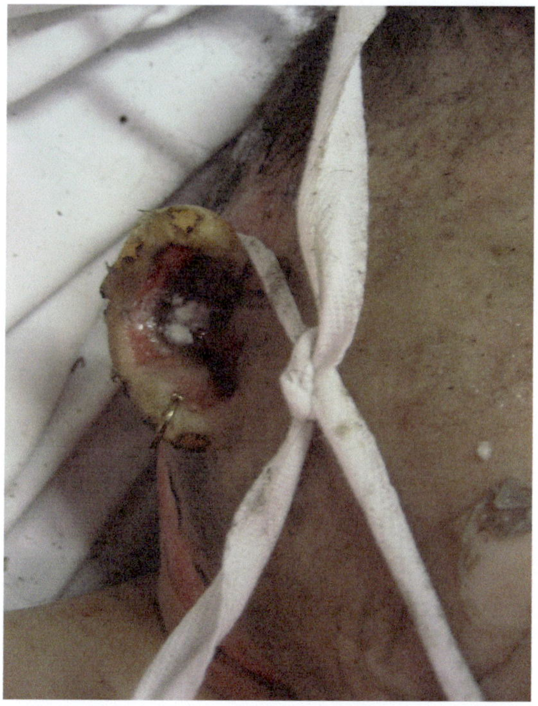

Fig. 13.9 Deep burns of the external ear such as pictured here initially require gentle debridement, removal of all jewelry, avoidance of pressure from bandages or tube securing tapes, and application of topical mafenide acetate cream

from near circumferential burns, which interferes with ventilation and occasionally causes abdominal compartment syndrome with hypotension, oliguria, and reduced ventilation [29]. Most patients respond to simple escharotomy. Rarely, abdominal decompression is required, typically in children with large burns who have received massive crystalloid resuscitation. Sometimes this is mostly peritoneal fluid which can be aspirated using ultrasound guidance. In other patients, the problem is visceral edema which responds to decompressive laparotomy. Ultrasound can be used to differentiate these two situations.

Immediate genitourinary priorities for children are usually limited to ensuring the foreskin is reduced over a bladder catheter to prevent difficult paraphimosis as soft tissue edema progresses and identification and management of pigmenturia in the presence of very deep thermal burns, high-voltage injury, crush injury, or compartment syndrome. Pigmented urine can generally be cleared with monitored volume administration. Intravenous bicarbonate can alkalinize the urine and facilitate pigment clearance. Rarely, mannitol or loop diuretics are needed.

Immediate musculoskeletal priorities include evaluating for non-burn trauma and ensuring distal perfusion. Non-burn trauma is excluded using usual physical examination and ATLS protocols. Extremity perfusion can be sharply reduced by edema beneath inelastic eschar or within muscle compartments with secondary ischemia, peripheral nerve injury, and tissue necrosis. This situation can be missed in children as they are less able to communicate the pain associated with tissue ischemia. Early identification of soft tissue ischemia is possible by identification and monitoring of extremities at risk through the resuscitation period. Extremities at risk of ischemia should be dressed to facilitate frequent examination and frequently assessed for temperature, pliability, voluntary motion, pain with passive motion, doppler signals, and oxygen saturation. Compartment pressure measurements are often impractical because of overlying wounds.

Laboratory and radiographic information are of limited utility in the early evaluation and monitoring of burned children. The mechanism of injury and need to access central line placement will drive radiographic needs. Laboratory studies immediately useful include arterial blood gas analysis for pH, base deficit, oxygenation, ventilation, and carboxyohemoglobin levels.

Initial Wound Evaluation: Burn Size and Depth

An accurate determination of wound size and depth (as a proxy for ability to heal) is the cornerstone of therapeutic decision making for pediatric burns. There is only a rough correlation between the physical depth of a burn and its propensity to heal. Burn depth is often underestimated on initial examination because microvascular thrombosis at the periphery of many wounds results in deepening over the days following injury. This assessment is particularly difficult in young children as their skin is inherently thin with fewer appendages and consequently a lesser ability to repopulate lost epithelium. Careful serial examination by an experienced examiner remains the most reliable method. Serial examination can be supplemented with a number of tools, such as the scanning laser doppler [10]. Determination of a burn's ability to heal is one of the most difficult and important decisions in caring for young children with mixed-depth injuries, such as scalds. Burn size is also more difficult to determine in children because body proportions change with age. For areas of irregular or non-confluent area burns, the palmar surface of the patient's hand represents approximately 1 % of their body surface [30]. The pediatric "rule-of-nines" or anthropometric charts can be useful in determining burned surface area (Fig. 13.10a, b). Circumferential, or near circumferential, components should be noted because they represent areas where special monitoring, and sometimes decompression, are needed.

Finally, the possibility of abuse and neglect must be considered during all pediatric burn evaluations. Delayed presentation for care, inconsistent stories, and prior engagement with state social services should prompt concern. Worrisome wounds include flexor sparing, immersion pat-

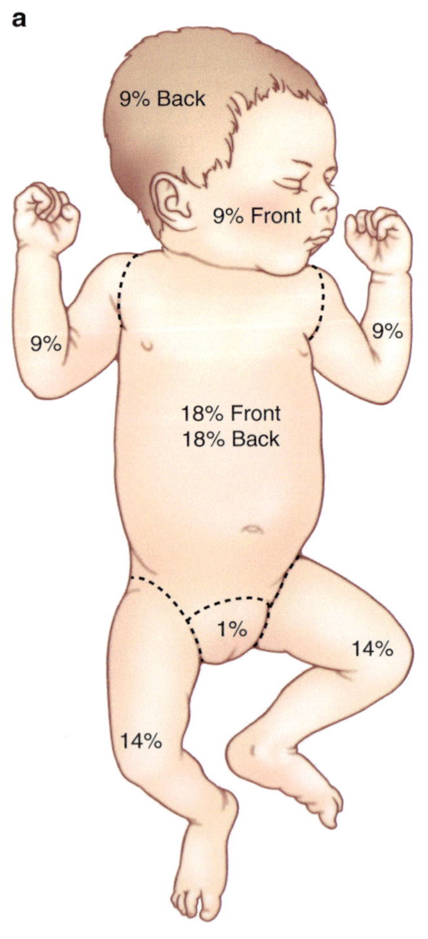

Fig. 13.10 (a) The "Rule-of-Nine" can be used to rapidly estimate the extent of burn in both adults and children. (b) The Lund-Browder diagram is useful to accurately record the extent of burn

b

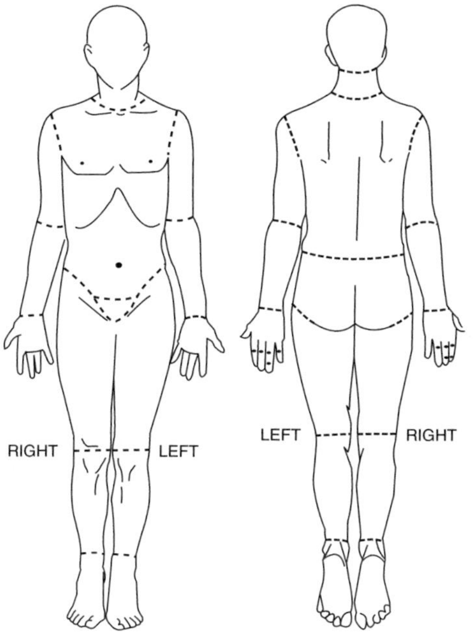

DATE

COMPLETED BY

X

SHALLOW		INDETERMINATE OR DEEP	
	+		= ___________

SHALLOW (PINK, PAINFUL, MOIST)

INDETERMINATE OR DEEP (DRY, LESS SENSATION, WHITE, MOTTLED, DARK RED, BROWN OR BLACK, LEATHERY .)

Percent Surface Area Burned
(Berkow Formula)

AREA	1 YEAR	1-4 YEARS	5-9 YEARS	10-14 YEARS	Y 15 YEARS	ADULT	SHALLOW	INDETER-MINATE OI DEEP
Head	19	17	13	11	9	7		
Neck	2	2	2	2	2	2		
Ant. Trunk	13	13	13	13	13	13		
Post. Trunk	13	13	13	13	13	13		
R. Buttock	2½	2½	2½	2½	2½	2½		
L. Buttock	2½	2½	2½	2½	2½	2½		
Genitalia	1	1	1	1	1	1		
R. U. Arm	4	4	4	4	4	4		
L. U. Arm	4	4	4	4	4	4		
R. L. Arm	3	3	3	3	3	3		
L. L. Arm	3	3	3	3	3	3		
R. Hand	2½	2½	2½	2½	2½	2½		
L. Hand	2½	2½	2½	2½	2½	2½		
R. Thigh	5½	6½	6½	8½	9	9½		
L. Thigh	5½	6½	6½	8½	9	9½		
R. Leg	5	5	5	6	6½	7		
L. Leg	5	5	5	6	6½	7		
R. Foot	3½	3½	3½	3½	3½	3½		
L. Foot	3½	3½	3½	3½	3½	3½		
TOTAL								

INITIAL BURN CHART

1994

Fig. 13.10 (continued)

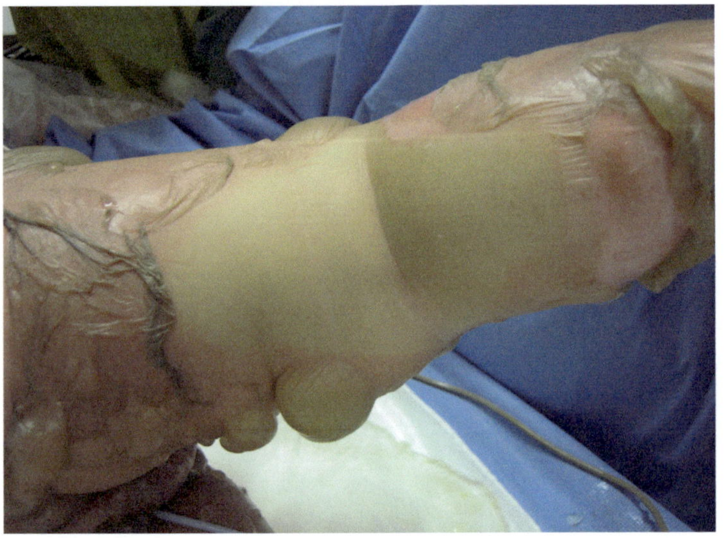

Fig. 13.11 In young children, the possibility of abuse must always be considered. This burn pattern demonstrates circumferential scalding with sharply demarcated margins which is potentially suspicious

terns, and contact burns (Fig. 13.11). Whenever these concerns arise, children should be admitted for safety and state social services alerted. A detailed non-judgmental history should be documented and wound photographs taken [31].

Initial Wound Care

Initial wound care in children does not differ greatly from that advised for adults as described elsewhere in this book. Initial wound cleansing and debridement may require some anxiolytic support as young children will not understand the need for these procedures. If wounds are large, judicious use of ketamine may be useful. Prolonged wound exposure should be avoided as hypothermia is more common in young children with their larger surface area to mass ratio. If in doubt about the child's immunization status, active and passive immunization should be administered. This is particularly true if burns are large, deep, or contaminated.

Decompression Procedures: Escharotomies and Fasciotomies

Peripheral nerve ischemia and even muscle necrosis can be caused by edema beneath inelastic near-circumferential eschar or within muscle compartments. Early signs and symptoms are easy to miss in pediatric patients, particularly pre-verbal young children. Early identification of extremities at risk, a high index of suspicion, and frequent reassessment will facilitate timely decompression and minimize occurrence of these complications. Escharotomies are described elsewhere in this book. In intubated children, they can be performed at the bedside using intravenous sedation and coagulating electrocautery. In children not requiring intensive care, escharotomies can be done under ketamine sedation or in the operating room. Fasciotomies, also described elsewere in this book, should ideally be done in the operating room as the anatomy is more complex, although in unstable patients they can be done in the intensive care unit.

Fluid Resuscitation

Burn physiology and fluid resuscitation have been covered elsewhere in this book. However, certain aspects are unique or exaggerated in children [32]. Perhaps the most important principle is that no two children are alike in their resuscitation needs. Small errors in volume cause greater morbidity in small patients. No formula can replace a conscientious bedside presence adjusting infusions to the individual needs of a burned child.

Most children with burns involving less than 15 % of the body surface do not develop a diffuse capillary leak and do not require resuscitation. Children with burns in this size range can be managed with fluid administered at 150 % of a calculated maintenance rate by the oral and/or intravenous route with close observation of the status of their hydration by weighing diapers and examining mucosal surfaces. Children with larger injuries will require resuscitation as described elsewhere in this book. Colloid is being more liberally used in recent years by many experienced burn care providers. Acknowledging the active controversy in this area, it is the routine practice of this author to begin colloid (5 % albumin) immediately at a maintenance rate in patients with burns over 30 % BSA, subtracting this amount from the crystalloid calculated for resuscitation. In patients with burns over 50 %, twice maintenance administration of 5 % albumin is administered. Although expert opinion remains divided regarding the timing and amount of colloid use in pediatric burn resuscitation, this author's personal belief is that early administration of colloid is associated with substantial decreased overall volume requirements and reduced morbidity from edema.

The particular resuscitation formula one chooses is nearly irrelevant to the quality of the resuscitation. The key element of resuscitation quality is vigilant bedside monitoring and adjustment of infusions based on resuscitation endpoints. Pediatric resuscitation endpoints are itemized in Table 13.2. The rate of infusion required will vary with the patient's weight, the size of the burn, the interval from injury to initiation of resuscitation, the depth of the injury, the vapor transmission characteristics of the particular wound, the presence of associated injuries, and the presence or absence of inhalation injury. Given all of these variables, it is not possible to accurately predict the fluid requirements of any individual with an acceptable degree of accuracy. This inherent inaccuracy of all fluid resuscitation formulas poses an increasing danger as body size decreases and burn size increases. In children, fluid resuscitation formulas are only useful to estimate the initial infusion rate. Infusions should be reassessed at least hourly and infusion rates increased or decreased in 10–20 % increments as indicated by endpoints.

Table 13.2 Pediatric burn resuscitation endpoints

• *Sensorium*: arouseable and comfortable
• *Peripheral Temperature*: warm peripherally
• *Systolic Blood Pressure*: for infants, 60 mmHg systolic, for older children, 70–90 plus two times age in years in mmHg, for adults mean arterial pressure over 60 mmHg
• *Pulse*: 80–180 per minute (age-dependent)
• *Urine Output*: 0.5–1 cc per kg per hour (glucose negative)
• *Base Deficit*: less than 2

Electrolyte monitoring and control is important in children with large burns. Serum electrolytes tend to mimic Lactated Ringers solution during the first 24 h because infusion rates are so high. Most patients will require approximately 150 % of a maintenance rate at 24 h, and at this point, electrolyte flux across the wound will have an increasingly important impact on serum electrolytes. Wounds treated with non-aqueous topical agents (such as silver sulfadiazine) generate a free water requirement, causing hypernatremia. This can be addressed with intravenous 5 % dextrose or enteral free water. In addition to the discomfort of extreme thirst, hypernatremia can cause adverse central nervous system effects, including intracranial bleeding, and should be avoided. Less commonly, wounds are treated with dilute aqueous topical agents (such as 5 % silver nitrate solution), which can be associated with electrolyte leeching and secondary hyponatremia that can be addressed with isotonic crystalloid and additional salt in enteral feedings. Cerebral edema and seizures can occur with severe hyponatremia [32]. Overly rapid correction of this hyponatremia may result in central pontine demyelinating lesions [33]. Serum potassium, ionized calcium, and magnesium should also be monitored in patients with larger injuries, as supplementation is commonly required to maintain normal levels.

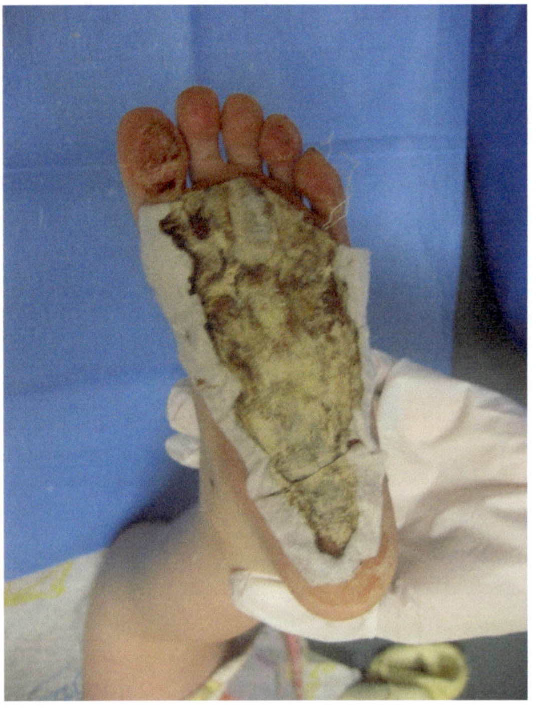

Fig. 13.12 An increasing variety of silver-releasing off-the-shelf dressings are available for burn care. All have been used to very good effect in the outpatient management of smaller partial-thickness burns. They will play an increasing role in the initial care of third-degree burns and in the definitive care of second-degree burns

Table 13.3 Elements of a successful pediatric burn outpatient program

Patient selection
• Airway is not threatened
• Monitored fluid resuscitation is not required
• The patient can eat and drink
• Community and/or family support is adequate for monitoring, wound care, and transportation
• The patient and/or family can verbalize understanding of the care plan
• There is no suspicion of abuse
• The wound does not unequivocally require surgery
Techniques of wound care
• Initial debridement of loose tissue
• Blisters should generally be debrided unless thick and intact
• Initial topical care or application of silver-releasing membrane
• Specific re-inspection of the wound at 24–72 h is planned
• Family and/or patient is taught cleansing and topical care plan
• A pain control plan is developed minimizing narcotic use
• Specific early return for hospitalization conditions are elaborated and understood
• Follow-up clinic visits are scheduled and tracked
• Long-term follow-up is arranged
• Liberal consultation to inpatient component of burn program

Resuscitation volume needs are increased by inhalation injury, delay in resuscitation, and unusually deep burns. Very small children may have reduced renal concentrating abilities and may require slightly more fluid per unit body weight than older children and adults. However, these same patients are frequently fluid-overloaded by artificially setting urine output targets of 2 cc/kg/h. Even in infants, 1 cc/kg/h generally suffices as a resuscitation endpoint. Over-resuscitation is more commonly seen as a complication of burn resuscitation than under-resuscitation. Both are associated with significant morbidity. Even in well-controlled resuscitations, total extra vascular water increases with the potential for limb-threatening ischemia in areas of circumferential eschar, hampered ventilation if there is circumferential torso burn, and elevations of compartment pressure in those with high voltage injuries or very deep extremity thermal burns. Monitoring for development of these problems is a priority during any burn resuscitation. In successful resuscitations, capillary integrity normalizes in 18–24 h. With hourly adjustment of volume infusions in response to urine output and other endpoints, infusion rates are generally in the range of 150 % of a maintenance rate at 24 h.

In remote, austere, or disaster settings, enteral burn resuscitation is a viable option to intravenous resuscitation of children. Although exact electrolyte content is debated, most authorities agree that the World Health Organization Oral Resuscitation Formula (WHO ORS) provides for the needs of most patients and is supported by significant clinical data [34]. Enteral burn resuscitation volume and rate can be calculated similar to intravenous resuscitation. The fluid can be delivered by gastric tube infusion or by frequent coached ingestion orally. Resuscitation endpoints are similar to intravenous resuscitation, most important in the austere setting being serial physical examination, vital signs, and monitoring of urine output.

Outpatient Care of Small Burns

The large majority of children with burns are managed as outpatients. Even children who require surgery will have significant parts of their course delivered in the outpatient setting. An increasing variety of silver-releasing dressings are available to facilitate outpatient burn care by decreasing the frequency of dressing changes (Fig. 13.12). All have been used to very good effect in the outpatient management of smaller partial-thickness burns. Most successful burn programs have developed programs with a seamless interface between the inpatient and outpatient setting and nearly continuous access to an outpatient team [35, 36].

Patient Selection

The most critical component of successful outpatient care is prudent patient selection (Table 13.3). The mechanism should be clear with no concern for coincident trauma or abuse. The airway should be unequivocally stable. The burn should be small enough that a formal fluid resuscitation is not needed. The child should be able to take fluid by mouth. Deep partial thickness burns of critical areas may not be optimally managed as outpatients initially until their true depth is clear. The child's family should be able to provide for wound care, monitoring, transport, pain control, and general care needs. Children with circumferential wounds with risks of sub-eschar ischemia should be admitted for monitoring until edema resolves. If pain cannot be adequately managed with judicious doses of narcotics, an initial inpatient stay is usually advisable. Deep wounds that obviously need surgery are best addressed early on, without a prolonged outpatient prelude. In many cases, availability of daily clinic visits will obviate the need for an inpatient care plan.

Techniques of Outpatient Care

General characteristics of a successful outpatient plan include (1) patient and family teaching, (2) wound cleansing and topical care, (3) pain control, (4) support services, (5) specific hospitalization conditions, (6) follow-up clinic visits, and (7) long-term follow-up. Initially, wounds should be gently cleansed using clean (not sterile) technique. Blister material is generally best removed unless blisters are intact and thick and ongoing frequent follow-up will be possible. There are innumerable specific methods of caring for small burn wounds, but certain principles are universal. Wounds should be kept generally clean with periodic inspection and removal of accumulated fibrinous debris and desiccated topical agent. Most small burns can be gently cleansed with clean lukewarm tap water and a bland soap. Parents and older children should be instructed in the signs of infection and told to return immediately should they occur (fever, erythema, swelling, drainage, malaise). Reasonable burn dressings prevent wound desiccation, decrease pain, reduce the incidence of wound colonization, and minimize physical trauma to the wound. Topical antimicrobials under gauze are commonly used to provide these functions, but the promulgation of silver releasing dressings of many types has changed the outpatient paradigm, allowing for less frequent dressing changes. Alternatively, there are many reasonable topical antibiotic containing agents in viscous carriers available that can be combined with clean gauze to provide quite similar benefits. In the vast majority of patients, adequate pain control is affected with judicious use of oral narcotics and over-the-counter non-narcotic analgesics. Elevation greatly facilitates pain control. Providing ready access to 24-h follow-up is an essential part of a successful outpatient program.

Definitive Care of Large Burns

Most children with large burns will be managed in verified pediatric burn centers as this is associated with improved survival [6]. Operative and critical care strategies are similar to those described elsewhere for adult patients, but certain aspects of pediatric management are worthy of emphasis.

Initial Excision and Biologic Coverage

Wound excision and biologic closure prior to the inevitable development of wound sepsis sharply truncates systemic infection and inflammation. Excision of deep burns is ideally completed in the first few days after injury and the resulting wounds closed with a combination of temporary biologic membranes, such as human allograft, and definitive split-thickness autografts [37]. In children, intraoperative hypothermia can develop quickly given the child's higher body surface area to mass ratio and often lesser subcutaneous fat layer. This must be prevented to avoid adverse impact on hemodynamics and coagulation. Although warming blankets, warmed intravenous and irrigating fluids, and hot-air pads should be used, heating of the operating room itself is the most effective way to maintain intraoperative euthermia.

Children are particularly vulnerable to hypovolemia given their lesser blood volume (approximately 80 cc/kg of body weight). It is critically important that hemostatic techniques of wound excision are used when operating on children [38]. As described elsewhere in this textbook, dilute epinephrine clysis should be used during torso excisions and extremity exsanguination with proximal tourniquet inflation used for extremity excisions. Fascial excisions should rarely be required and can be done with minimal blood loss using traction and coagulating electrocautery. Constant communication between the anesthesia and surgical teams will minimize the occurrence of intraoperative hypothermia and hypovolemia.

Pediatric Burn Critical Care Issues

A pediatric critical care capability should be a part of all pediatric burn programs. Organizationally, this can be done in two ways. Most commonly and perhaps most cost-effectively, the surgical team managing the wound is also managing the critical care in dedicated burn-trauma intensive care units. This facilitates communication and coordination between surgeons, nurses, rehabilitation therapists, psychologists, anesthesiologists, child life therapists, pediatricians, and other members of the burn team. The alternative is to provide critical care in a dedicated area of a general pediatric intensive care unit, taking great pains to ensure absolutely seamless flow of information between the surgical and critical care teams. Ensuring engaged collaborative management is difficult, but can be done. Common burn critical care issues are described elsewhere in this textbook. However, seriously burned children present the critical care team with a few unique but predicable issues that are highlighted here.

Endotracheal tube security is more difficult to maintain in small children with their short trachea and should be frequently reevaluated in all intubated children in the burn ICU, because facial and hypopharyngeal edema can make reintubation after unplanned extubation incredibly difficult. While multiple methods exist to secure tubes in children, a tie-harness system as illustrated in Fig. 13.5 has proven effective. Some authors advocate early tracheostomy for children requiring intubation [39], but protracted airway control via transoral intubation is also associated with good outcomes and avoids the short and long-term complications of tracheostomy [40]. This is one of many aspects of care that is program-dependent.

Adequate control of pain and anxiety is very difficult in children with serious burns. Opiate and benzodiazepine tachyphylaxis is common and dose escalation often required. Successful management is greatly aided by the use of program-specific guidelines [41]. Guidelines seem most effective when they use a limited formulary and emphasize dose ranging based on regular objective assessment of efficacy. Attention to the issue has physiologic as well as the psychological benefits. Reduced secretion of catecholamines may decrease systemic hypermetabolism, and treatment-related acute stress is reduced. If dose of benzodiazepines and opiates are excessive, a number of alternative drugs have proven useful, particularly dexmetatomidine, which is not a respiratory depressant and has proven particularly valuable during weaning and extubation [42]. Sleep regulation is also an important component of care of critically ill children with several practical environmental and useful pharmacologic adjuncts, including cyclic quiet and melatonin [43].

Young children do not communicate nor localize pain easily. Peripheral nerve injury due to compression or pressure may occur unless extremities at risk for compression are closely monitored and promptly decompressed and bandages and splints regularly examined for pressure points as edema waxes and wanes.

Nutritional support of children is complicated by their high metabolic rate [44]. Periods of fasting result in negative nitrogen balance quickly. Both underfeeding and overfeeding have adverse sequelae. Ideally, tube feedings are begun during resuscitation. Most children do well with continuous intragastric tube feedings. In children requiring resuscitation or vasopressor support, enteral nutritional support can be started through a nasogastric sump tube so that gastric residuals can be used to help determine feeding. Parenteral support is useful during periods when ileus is likely, such as during septic episodes or periods when high-dose vasopressor support is needed, or during the perioperative period. Transient parenteral support can be particularly important in hypermetabolic young children who are very catabolic and do not tolerate prolonged periods of fasting [45]. Consensus recommendations for support include approximately 2–2.5 g/kg/day of protein and a caloric load between 1.5 and 1.7 times a calculated basal metabolic rate or 1.3–1.5 times a measured (by indirect calorimetry) resting energy expenditure [15]. The role of anabolic agents in burned children has been an area of controversy for two decades. Currently, many programs advise use of anabolic steroids in particularly nutritionally depleted children, watching carefully for hepatic complications [46]. Serial physical examination, body weight, quality of wound healing, nitrogen balance, and indirect calorimetry can be integrated to assess the adequacy of support and help fine-tune the predictions of nutritional equations.

Finally, as described elsewhere in this textbook, infectious disease issues are similar in burned children and adults. However, young children have a propensity to develop high fever, even in the absence of systemic infection. At times, it can be difficult to know if a child with a high fever is infected or not [47]. At such times, physical examination of the child and wounds will guide initial therapy [48]. If children are hypotensive or lethargic or show obvious signs of infection on physical examination, cultures should be taken and broad spectrum antibiotics started. Culture results will guide subsequent therapy. In the absence of these findings, very close monitoring is appropriate.

Reconstruction and Reintegration

Children recovering from even massive burns can achieve a very high quality of life, but this requires long-term participation in a burn aftercare program to facilitate optimal function, appearance, and emotional health [49]. Children are offered a variety of functional and aesthetic reconstructive operations and associated rehabilitation and scar management programs. Integrated family support may be of value [19]. Efforts are made to address emotional needs with the objective of returning even seriously injured patients to a satisfying and productive life. A cohesive multidisciplinary burn team, so critical to successful acute care of seriously injured children, is equally essential to optimizing their long-term physical and emotional outcomes [50].

References

1. Cancio L, Lundy J, Sheridan RL. Burns and environmental injuries. In: Cannon J, editor. Injury care in deployed settings. Surg Clin North Am. 2012;92(4):959–86.
2. Gupta M, Gupta OK, Yaduvanshi RK, Upadhyaya J. Burn epidemiology: the Pink City scene. Burns. 1993;19:47–51.

3. Sheridan RL, Hoey ME, Daley WM, Lybarger PM. Childhood burns in camping and outdoor cooking accidents: a focus for prevention. J Burn Care Rehabil. 1997;18:369–71.
4. Sheridan R, Weber J, Prelack K, Petras L, Lydon M, Tompkins R. Early burn center transfer shortens the length of hospitalization and reduces complications in children with serious burn injuries. J Burn Care Rehabil. 1999;20:347–50.
5. Sheridan RL. Burn care: results of technical and organizational progress. JAMA Contempo Update. 2003;290(6):719–22.
6. Palmieri TL, Taylor S, Lawless M, Curri T, Sen S, Greenhalgh DG. Burn center volume makes a difference for burned children. Pediatr Crit Care Med. 2015;16(4):319–24.
7. Sheridan RL. The acutely burned child: resuscitation through reintegration. Part I Curr Probl Pediatr 1998;28(4):104–27; Part II Curr Probl Pediatr 1998;28(5):133–76.
8. United States Army Institute of Surgical Research Burn Clinical Practice Guideline: http://www.usaisr.amedd.army.mil/assets/cpgs/Burn_Care_13_Nov_13.pdf.
9. Shupp JW, Nasabzadeh TJ, Rosenthal DS, Jordan MH, Fidler P, Jeng JC. A review of the local pathophysiologic bases of burn wound progression. J Burn Care Res. 2010;31(6):849–73.
10. Resch TR, Drake RM, Helmer SD, Jost GD, Osland JS. Estimation of burn depth at burn centers in the United States: a survey. J Burn Care Res. 2014;35(6):491–7.
11. Bittner EA, Shank E, Woodson L, Martyn JA. Acute and perioperative care of the burn-injured patient. Anesthesiology. 2015;122(2):448–64.
12. Finnerty CC, Mabvuure NT, Ali A, Kozar RA, Herndon DN. The surgically induced stress response. J Parenter Enteral Nutr. 2013;37(5 Suppl):21S–9.
13. Atiyeh BS, Gunn SW, Dibo SA. Metabolic implications of severe burn injuries and their management: a systematic review of the literature. World J Surg. 2008;32(8):1857–69.
14. Tredget EE, Yu YM. The metabolic effects of thermal injury. World J Surg. 1992;16(1):68–79.
15. Rousseau AF, Losser MR, Ichai C, Berger MM. ESPEN endorsed recommendations: nutritional therapy in major burns. Clin Nutr. 2013;32(4):497–502.
16. Abdullahi A, Jeschke MG. Nutrition and anabolic pharmacotherapies in the care of burn patients. Nutr Clin Pract. 2014;29(5):621–30.
17. Sheridan RL. Burns at the extremes of age. J Burn Care Res. 2007;28(2):580–6.
18. Warden GD. Burn shock resuscitation. World J Surg. 1992;16:16–23. Review.
19. Sheridan R, Lee A, Kazis L, Shriners Pediatric Burn Outcome Group. Family characteristics impact long-term pediatric injury recovery. J Trauma. 2012;73(3):S205–12.
20. De Young AC, Hendrikz J, Kenardy JA, Cobham VE, Kimble RM. Prospective evaluation of parent distress following pediatric burns and identification of risk factors for young child and parent posttraumatic stress disorder. J Child Adolesc Psychopharmacol. 2014;24(1):9–17.
21. Gonzalez R, Shanti CM. Overview of current pediatric burn care. Semin Pediatr Surg. 2015;24(1):47–9.
22. American College of Surgeons – Committee on Trauma. Resources of optimal care of the injured patient. Chicago, IL: American College of Surgeons; 2014.
23. Sheridan RL. Uncuffed endotracheal tubes should not be used in seriously burned children. Pediatr Crit Care Med. 2006;7(3):258–9.
24. Sheridan RL. Comprehensive management of burns. Curr Probl Surg. 2001;38(9):641–756.
25. McManus WF, Hunt JL, Pruitt Jr BA. Postburn convulsive disorders in children. J Trauma. 1974;14(5):396–401.
26. Sullivan SR, Ahmadi AJ, Singh CN, Sires BS, Engrav LH, Gibran NS, Heimbach DM, Klein MB. Elevated orbital pressure: another untoward effect of massive resuscitation after burn injury. J Trauma. 2006;60(1):72–6.
27. Hurst J, Johnson D, Campbell R, Baxter S, Kratky V. Orbital compartment syndrome in a burn patient without aggressive fluid resuscitation. Orbit. 2014;33(5):375–7.
28. Mills DC, Roberts LW, Mason Jr AD, McManus WF, Pruitt Jr BA. Suppurative chondritis: its incidence, prevention, and treatment in burn patients. Plast Reconstr Surg. 1988;82:267–76.
29. Greenhalgh DG, Warden GD. The importance of intra-abdominal pressure measurements in burned children. J Trauma. 1994;36:685–90.
30. Sheridan RL, Petras L, Basha G, Salvo P, Cifrino C, Hinson M, McCabe M, Fallon J, Tompkins RG. Planimetry study of the percent of body surface represented by the hand and palm: sizing irregular burns is more accurately done with the palm. J Burn Care Rehabil. 1995;16(6):605–6.
31. Peck MD, Priolo-Kapel D. Child abuse by burning: a review of the literature and an algorithm for medical investigations. J Trauma. 2002;53(5):1013–22.
32. Sheridan RL, Remensnyder JP, Prelack K, Petras L, Lydon M. Treatment of the seriously burned infant. J Burn Care Rehabil. 1998;19:115–8.
33. Cohen BJ, Jordan MH, Chapin SD, Cape B, Laureno R. Pontine myelinolysis after correction of hyponatremia during burn resuscitation. J Burn Care Rehabil. 1991;12:153–6.
34. Kramer G, Michell MW, Oliveira H, Brown TLH, Herndon DN, Baker D, Muller M. Oral and enteral resuscitation of burn shock: the historical record and implications for mass casualty care. Eplasty. 2010;10:e56.
35. Sheridan R. Outpatient burn care in the emergency department. Pediatr Emerg Care. 2005;21(7):449–56.

36. Warner PM, Coffee TL, Yowler CJ. Outpatient burn management. Surg Clin North Am. 2014;94(4):879–92.
37. Sheridan R. Closure of the excised burn wound: autografts, semipermanent skin substitutes, and permanent skin substitutes. Clin Plast Surg. 2009;36(4):643–51.
38. Sheridan RL, Chang P. Acute burn procedures. Surg Clin North Am. 2014;94(4):755–64.
39. Sen S, Heather J, Palmieri T, Greenhalgh D. Tracheostomy in pediatric burn patients. Burns. 2015;41(2):248–51.
40. Kadilak PR, Vanasse S, Sheridan RL. Favorable short- and long-term outcomes of prolonged translaryngeal intubation in critically ill children. J Burn Care Rehabil. 2004;25(3):262–5.
41. Poh YN, Poh PF, Buang SN, Lee JH. Sedation guidelines, protocols, and algorithms in PICUs: a systematic review. Pediatr Crit Care Med. 2014;15(9):885–92.
42. Plambech MZ, Afshari A. Dexmedetomidine in the pediatric population: a review. Minerva Anestesiol. 2015;81(3):320–32.
43. Kudchadkar SR, Yaster M, Punjabi NM. Sedation, sleep promotion, and delirium screening practices in the care of mechanically ventilated children: a wake-up call for the pediatric critical care community. Crit Care Med. 2014;42(7):1592–600.
44. Prelack K, Dylewski M, Sheridan RL. Practical guidelines for nutritional management of burn injury and recovery. Burns. 2007;33(1):14–24.
45. Dylewksi ML, Baker M, Prelack K, Weber JM, Hursey D, Lydon M, Fagan SP, Sheridan RL. The safety and efficacy of parenteral nutrition among pediatric patients with burn injuries. Pediatr Crit Care Med. 2013;14(3):e120–5.
46. Diaz EC, Herndon DN, Porter C, Sidossis LS, Suman OE, Børsheim E. Effects of pharmacological interventions on muscle protein synthesis and breakdown in recovery from burns. Burns. 2015;41(4):649–57.
47. Vyles D, Sinha M, Rosenberg DI, Foster KN, Tran M, Drachman D. Predictors of serious bacterial infections in pediatric burn patients with fever. J Burn Care Res. 2014;35(4):291–5.
48. Parish RA, Novack AH, Heimbach DM, Engrav LR. Fever as a predictor of infection in burned children. J Trauma. 1987;27(1):69–71.
49. Sheridan RL, Hinson MM, Liang MM, Mulligan JL, Ryan CM, Tompkins RG. Longterm outcome of children surviving massive burns. JAMA. 2000;283(1):69–73.
50. Al-Mousawi AM, Mecott-Rivera GA, Jeschke MG, Herndon DN. Burn teams and burn centers: the importance of a comprehensive team approach to burn care. Clin Plast Surg. 2009;36(4):547–54.

Burns in the Geriatric Population

14

David G. Greenhalgh

Introduction

People are living longer, and with the persistence of the Baby Boomers, the population is shifting so that the elderly will soon be the dominant group. It has been estimated that, in 2050, one third of the population will be greater than 55 year [1]. Therefore, caregivers must know how to manage the medical issues that are specific for the elderly. In the past, an elderly patient with a sizeable burn was considered to have an unsurvivable injury so that we were provided comfort care and were allowed to die without resuscitation. While there is increased mortality with advancing age, more geriatric patients are surviving and living meaningful lives after injury. There are two main issues with the elderly that are important for the burn caregiver: anatomic changes that occur with aging and the gradual loss of reserve. This chapter will describe the changes in the skin, the changes in organ function that affect metabolic reserve, and finally burns that are typical for the aging population.

D.G. Greenhalgh, M.D. (✉)
Shriners Hospitals for Children Northern California, University of California, Davis Medical Center, 2425 Stockton Boulevard, Sacramento, CA 95817, USA
e-mail: dggreenhalgh@ucdavis.edu

Skin Changes with Aging

There are obvious changes that occur in the skin with aging [2–8]. These changes can be categorized into "*intrinsic*" and "*extrinsic*" factors. *Intrinsic factors* are the changes that occur in everyone with aging, no matter how hard they try to resist them. The aging processes can be accelerated by *extrinsic* behaviors and environmental factors. The most renowned extrinsic factor is exposure to ultraviolet light, but other destructive behaviors may contribute to accelerate aging in the skin. The metaphor is that it is *not just the years but also the miles* that contribute to aging changes. People who are chronically exposed to the sun or severe cold or have chronic alcohol/drug (especially methamphetamine) abuse tend to accelerate the aging of skin.

The *intrinsic* changes of skin are well-known to the general public (and are major money makers for those companies selling anti-aging products). Normally, the epithelium thins with aging, but with excessive sun exposure the opposite can happen. The epithelial–dermal junction flattens out as rete pegs become less prominent, which predisposes the skin to blistering. The number of skin adnexa decreases so that as oil and sebaceous glands decrease the skin tends to be dryer and more prone to cracking. A significant issue for burns is that the density of hair follicles decreases. Since the healing of partial-thickness burns

D.G. Greenhalgh (ed.), *Burn Care for General Surgeons and General Practitioners*,
DOI 10.1007/978-3-319-29161-1_14

depends on the density of hair follicles (and other skin adnexa), this decrease in adnexal density delays epithelial healing. Clearly, there is an increased risk for alopecia for the very elderly; but hair follicles throughout the body also decrease in number [7]. With fewer hair follicles, the rate of re-epithelialization is slowed and the risk for scarring is increased. The classic scenario occurs when an elderly person spills a hot liquid onto their thigh to produce a very superficial burn. If there are no hair follicles to resurface the thigh, the wound has no chance to re-epithelialize except from the edges. Since the basal epithelial cells can only migrate a short distance (around 2 cm), the rest of the healing must occur with contraction. Many caregivers will say that the superficial burn will get "converted" to a full-thickness injury; but in reality, with no skin adnexa to supply epithelial cells, it has no chance to re-epithelialize. The same issue is important to remember that when considering whether to graft a full-thickness burn in a very elderly patient, is the donor site going to heal? If the donor site is devoid in skin adnexa, grafting may need to be deferred. Fortunately, there are areas, such as the back, that have a better chance to re-epithelialize.

There also are age-related changes in the dermis. The dermis is more sensitive to damage from ultraviolet light than the epidermis, so extrinsic changes are more profound [2]. The dermis tends to thin out with age and there is a decrease in cellularity. The associated decrease in immune cells may predispose wounds to infection. The structure of collagen in the dermis undergoes changes, including fragmentation and disorganization. Skin tends to lose tensile strength and is more prone to tearing [9]. Everyone knows that skin becomes looser, more wrinkled and sags with aging. The increased looseness of skin may be somewhat advantageous since sizeable wounds can contract with decreased risks for contracture.

A significant problem in the elderly is the loss of sensation that tends to occur from "distal to proximal" in the extremities. The most prominent change is for cold/warm sensations, so the elderly may be less aware of pain when contacting hot surfaces [10]. The sensation changes are more pronounced in patients who have diabetes mellitus. Simply walking outside barefoot on a hot day may lead to burns. In addition, they tend to feel that their feet are cold, so there is a tendency to warm their feet in hot water or near heaters. We have treated dozens of diabetic patients with burns to their feet [11]. There are increases in complications and graft loss in these patients. Angiogenesis is also impaired, so healing is delayed and the new blood vessels tend to be more leaky, which leads to increased edema [12].

There are other anatomic changes that influence healing in the elderly. There is a tendency to lose muscle and fat so that there are increased bony prominences that increase the risk for pressure ulcers. Incontinence leads to maceration and increased risk for skin breakdown. People have slower reflexes and just move slower so that they are less capable of responding to a dangerous situation. There are many elderly patients admitted to the burn center who had practiced the same risky behavior for years, but finally could not respond quickly enough to escape. For instance, an elderly man may have used gasoline to ignite wet leaves for years, but this time the flames engulfed him. The slower response also increases the extent of the injury.

Any decline in neurologic status increases the risks for burn injuries. Clearly, with dementia there is a tendency to be less cautious than when fully alert. Forgetfulness also increases risks of burns. One may forget to turn off the stove or other heat-producing devices and thus increase the risk of fire. People who smoke and fall asleep are at increased risk for starting house fires. Fortunately, there are laws that require "fire-safe" cigarettes that self-extinguish when not used. These laws have greatly reduced fires and burns. Any neurologic disease may increase the risk for burns. People who have tremors may drop hot items. Anyone with epilepsy may have a seizure when in the shower or while cooking. These burns are often very deep as exemplified by a hand that is placed into a hot frying pan when seizing. Finally, when the elderly lose the ability to care for themselves, they are at a higher risk for being abused. As described in chapter 22, the elderly may suffer from similar "dip" burns as toddlers [13].

Typical Burns of the Elderly

For each age group, there are typical burn patterns that are seen. For instance, toddlers tend to explore their environment with their hands, so they are at risk for palm burns as they touch a hot item. For the elderly, there are common burns that are rarely seen in the younger population. One classic burn is the "home oxygen" burn. People who smoke while receiving nasal oxygen will often ignite the oxygen and sustain burns to the mid face. Fortunately, these burns tend to be limited to the face and will often heal on their own [14]. There is often a concern for smoke inhalation injury, but usually the injury is limited to the face and nasal passages. Since the patients require oxygen at home, there is often concern when oxygen saturations are not up to par. It is best to avoid intubation in this population if possible as, because of their underlying pulmonary disease, extubation may be very difficult.

Another classic burn occurs when an elderly woman with loose clothing (especially a nightgown) cooks over an open flame. The clothing then catches fire when leaning over the flame and burning the axilla, chest, and inner arm. Advising the elderly to avoid loose clothing when cooking may prevent these burns. As stated previously, people with insensate feet, especially with diabetes mellitus, suffer demarcated burns to the feet from either "warming" the feet in hot water or near a heater. Unfortunately, the elderly may also suffer from the massive burn that results from the inability to escape a fire. These burns are routinely fatal. The most difficult decision when dealing with these burns is whether to initiate resuscitation or not. Occasionally, the most humane treatment is comfort care.

Changes in the Ability to Handle Metabolic Stress

It is well-known that the elderly are less able to handle a large burn than the young. Classically, burn surgeons describe the LA50, which is the size burn that gives a specific age group a 50 % survival. For a teenager, the size burn that leads to a 50 % survival is around 85 % total body surface area (TBSA). As people age, the LA50 drops significantly. When the patient is greater than 80 years of age, the LA50 may drop to less than 10 % TBSA [15]. The cause of this inability to handle major stress with aging is not really known, but there are some possible explanations. First of all, burns are the most profound form of injury that anyone can sustain and still survive. The calories that are required to handle the metabolic demand have been stated to double above normal for any burn greater than 60 % TBSA [16, 17]. This is why aggressive feeding in all major burns is so important. In simple terms, the elderly patients may not have the "energy stores" to handle the increased metabolic demands. Investigators are starting to understand how aging affects the ability of an individual to repair cellular damage. There are studies that prove that there is increased damage to the DNA over time [3, 16–19]. Parallel to this increased damage, the ability of the DNA to repair itself is impaired. Even the epigenetic controls of DNA repair are altered [3]. If one looks at the skin of older people, there are many "age spots" that reflect altered gene expression. Each cell has a limited number of replication cycles before it can no longer divide. After a major stress, especially a large burn, the ability of major tissue beds to repair is limited. A second problem is that the mitochondria, which supply the energy to the cells, also lose the ability to repair themselves so that their dysfunction means that there are limitations to the fuel that can run the body [20]. One theory of the etiology of cardiomyopathy is that the cardiac muscle cells that power the heart "run out of fuel" [21]. A third problem is that minor injuries do not always result in complete regeneration of the tissues. When healing is compromised, fibrosis often occurs. Therefore, scarring of the organs, such as pulmonary fibrosis, cirrhosis, and scarring after a myocardial infarction, leads to impaired organ function.

I often tell patients that surviving a burn is like running a marathon. We can push a young person through the tremendous metabolic demand. An elderly person, however, may be willing, but they soon tire and are unable to "keep up" with the demand. Once there is insufficient energy to meet the demand of major stress, the tissues start to fail. This is why the elderly initially do well, but then they gradually develop some form of organ failure that expands to multiple organ dysfunction. Eventually, the multiple organ dysfunction results in death.

Burn Prevention for the Elderly

Burn prevention is the most important way to protect the elderly. As people slow down, they must avoid risky behavior even if they had "done it for years". They should avoid using accelerants on fires. Elderly people should never wear loose and flammable clothing around stoves or flames. It is probably a good idea to lobby for flame-retardant clothing for the elderly just as we do for infants. Setting water heaters at 120 °F is important for all households, but even more so for the elderly. Many more geriatric patients fall in showers or bathtubs and sustain burns because they are unable to escape than young people. Anyone with diabetes mellitus or other causes of vascular disease and neuropathies should avoid hot surfaces or liquids. Anyone with significant tremors or dementia should be careful with hot items. Simply living a healthy lifestyle by avoiding smoking, eating well, and maintaining physical fitness will prevent many burns and allow for a better chance for survival.

Conclusion

There are two populations at increased risk for burns and burn-related deaths—at the extremes of ages. The elderly have many risk factors that increase the inability to avoid injury, and if burned, less capability to survive. Fortunately, our ability to deal with burns in the geriatric population has improved tremendously. Since the population is shifting to be an older one, burn caregivers will be faced with more of these types of burns.

References

1. U.S Census Bureau Statistical Abstract of United States. 2012. Accessed 28 June, 2012 from http://www.census.gov/compendia/statab/2012/tables/12s0009.pdf.
2. Gosain A, DiPietro LA. Aging and wound healing. World J Surg. 2004;28(3):321–6.
3. Makrantonaki E, Bekou V, Zouboulis CC. Genetics and skin aging. Dermatoendocrinol. 2012;4(3):280–4.
4. Zouboulis CC, Makrantonaki E. Clinical aspects and molecular diagnostics of skin aging. Clin Dermatol. 2011;29(1):3–14.
5. Ramos-e-Silva M, Boza JC, Cestari TF. Effects of age (neonates and elderly) on skin barrier function. Clin Dermatol. 2012;30(3):274–6.
6. Wulf HC, Sandby-Moller J, Kobayasi T, Gniadecki R. Skin aging and natural photoprotection. Micron. 2004;35(3):185–91.
7. Birch MP, Messenger JF, Messenger AG. Hair density, hair diameter and the prevalence of female pattern hair loss. Br J Dermatol. 2001;144(2):297–304.
8. Greenhalgh DG. Management of the skin and soft tissue in the geriatric surgical patient. Surg Clin North Am. 2015;95(1):103–14.
9. Sussman MD. Aging of connective tissue: physical properties of healing wounds in young and old rats. Am J Physiol. 1973;224(5):1167–71.
10. Guergova S, Dufour A. Thermal sensitivity in the elderly: a review. Ageing Res Rev. 2011;10(1):80–92.
11. Barsun A, Sen S, Palmieri TL, Greenhalgh DG. A ten-year review of lower extremity burns in diabetics: small burns that lead to major problems. J Burn Care Res. 2013;34(2):255–60.
12. Greenhalgh DG. Wound healing and diabetes mellitus. Clin Plast Surg. 2003;30(1):37–45.
13. Greenbaum AR, Horton JB, Williams CJ, Shah M, Dunn KW. Burn injuries inflicted on children or the elderly: a framework for clinical and forensic assessment. Plast Reconstr Surg. 2006;118(2):46–58.
14. Robb B, Hungness ES, Hershko DD, Warden GD, Kagan RJ. Home oxygen therapy: adjunct or risk factor? J Burn Care Res. 2003;24(6):403–6.
15. Taylor SL, Lawless M, Curri T, Sen S, Greenhalgh DG, Palmieri TL. Predicting mortality from burns: the need for age-group specific models. Burns. 2014; 40(6):1106–15.
16. Ma Y, Li J. Metabolic shifts during aging and pathology. Compr Physiol. 2015;5(2):667–86.
17. De Gaudio AR, Rinaldi S, Chelazzi C, Borracci T. Pathophysiology of sepsis in the elderly: clinical impact and therapeutic considerations. Curr Drug Targets. 2009;10(1):60–70.
18. Kammeyer A, Luiten RM. Oxidation events and skin aging. Ageing Res Rev. 2015;21:16–29.
19. Pluquet O, Pourtier A, Abbadie C. The unfolded protein response and cellular senescence. A review in the theme: cellular mechanisms of endoplasmic reticulum stress signaling in health and disease. Am J Physiol Cell Physiol. 2015;308(6):C415–25.
20. Zang QS, Wolf SE, Minei JP. Sepsis-induced cardiac mitochondrial damage and potential therapeutic interventions in the elderly. Aging Dis. 2014;5(2):137–49.
21. Neubauer S. The failing heart—an engine out of fuel. N Engl J Med. 2007;356(11):1140–51.

Electrical Injuries

15

Nicole Gibran

An electrical injury represents a unique potentially devastating burn injury that often requires additional considerations from other burn injuries due to both short- and long-term sequelae. In 2006, the American Burn Association published a set of practice guidelines for the management of electrical burns that serve as an excellent resource [1] and should be considered when devising a practical management strategy. In general, the clinical plan for a patient with an electrical burn demands understanding of the local and systemic effects of an injury caused by electrical current. It is important to understand that many of the fundamental issues are controversial with minimal Level 1 evidence to support treatment regimens. However, optimal management benefits from center-specific algorithms for management of cardiac, soft tissue, and psychological sequelae. Acutely, electrical burns can be associated with cardiac arrhythmias and require an algorithm for determining which patients require cardiac monitoring. Since the visible cutaneous injury often represents only the tip of the iceberg, a decision tree is also necessary to identify patients who have established a potentially preventable neuromuscular damage; this requires a consistent plan for who needs compartment pressure measurements or fasciotomies. Additional considerations must include attention to late complications of high-voltage injuries, including cataract development, progressive nerve degeneration, and cognitive or psychological ramifications. Subsequently, electrical injuries should be referred to a specialized burn center per American Burn Association recommendations.

N. Gibran, M.D., F.A.C.S. (✉)
David & Nancy Auth - Washington Research Foundation Chair in Restorative Burn Surgery, Box 359796, 325 Ninth Avenue, Seattle, WA 98104, USA
e-mail: nicoleg@uw.edu

Electrical Injury Etiologies

Three forms of electrical injury include low-voltage injuries (<440 V), high-voltage injuries (>1000 V), and ultra-high voltage (lightning: 300,000 A; 100,000,000 V.). Injuries between 440–800 V behave variably with characteristics of either high- and low-voltage injuries. An alternative "electrical"—but non-contact—injury is an intense flash burn resulting from short-circuiting an industrial circuit with a metal tool. When the tool contacts an electric source, the metal component of the tool vaporizes and causes a flash burn that can lead to deep burns to the hand holding the tool and variable second- and third-degree burns on other parts of the body; these burns can be treated like other thermal burn injuries.

D.G. Greenhalgh (ed.), *Burn Care for General Surgeons and General Practitioners*,
DOI 10.1007/978-3-319-29161-1_15

High-Voltage Injury

Current exceeding 1000 V can cause massive tissue destruction due to conversion of the electrical energy to heat with tissue resistance. The smaller the body part, the more intense the heat is with less dissipation; fingers, hands, toes, and feet are especially at risk. Larger body surface areas such as the torso can dissipate enough current to prevent extensive internal injuries. Arc burns, caused by current traversing apposed skin surfaces across joints, commonly accompany the contact wounds; these deep burns often involve the volar aspect of the wrist, the antecubital fossa when the elbow is flexed, the popliteal fossa, and the axilla. Initial assessment of a patient with an electrical burn follows the standard work-up of a severely injured patient beginning with airway, breathing, and circulation. In addition to the obvious cutaneous and soft tissue injuries, associated injuries must be excluded including dislocations or fractures due to tetanic spasms of major muscle groups or from a concomitant fall; common injuries involve the lumbar spine and hips.

Lightning strikes represent a unique ultra-high voltage injury for a brief duration. The generated current may reach 300,000 A and 100,000,000 V, resulting in enormous quantities of energy passing through the body [2]. With a direct strike at a high flash strength, the insult may be instantaneously fatal or cause permanent impairment. Death immediately after a lightening strike usually results from respiratory center paralysis and cardiac standstill. Cardiac activity usually resumes spontaneously, but apnea lasts longer, sufficient to cause anoxic brain injury without pulmonary resuscitation. Cardiac and neurologic complications resemble those caused by other high-voltage injuries [3]. Another potential indirect insult due to lightening occurs when the lighting current strikes the ground and the high impedance of the ground causes the current to sidestep along other conduits such as tree roots or a person's legs. Finally, the lightning discharge produces an electromagnetic pulse, which can interfere with pacemakers. Fortunately, lightning strikes often create a "flashover" in which the current flows around the surface, rather than through, a body [4, 5]. Evanescent superficial dendritic skin burns known as "Lichtenberg's flowers" or "fractals"[6], sometimes seen immediately after the injury, represent superficial burns that heal rapidly without need for specific treatment and without sequelae. Ruptured tympanic membranes and vertigo can also occur [7, 8].

Low-Voltage Injury (Refs)

Low-voltage injuries are unlikely to leave permanent sequelae. In the USA, alternating current has generally replaced direct current for all commercial power applications because it is cheaper to transmit and can be more easily transformed to any required voltage. *The human body is three to four times as sensitive to alternating current as it is to direct current.* The threshold for 60-cycle alternating current in the hand is about 1.1 mA (MA), which is perceived as mild tingling. Skin resistance varies according to the thickness of the epidermal keratin layer, cleanliness, and moisture. As such, dry normal skin provides 5,000 Ω/in^2 resistance, wet skin only 1000 Ω/in^2, and calloused hands over 100,000 Ω/in^2 [9]. Above 2–4 MA, muscle contractions occur proportional to the current. At approximately 15 MA, the spasm prevents release of the hand gripping of the conductor in what is known as the "Let Go" reflex [10]. Above 20 MA, sustained spasm of the respiratory muscles develops leading to respiratory arrest, which can resume spontaneously, but may require CPR if the spasm lasts longer than four minutes. Ventricular fibrillation (VF) may occur if the threshold exceeds 30–40 MA. With increasing current, cardiac susceptibility to fibrillation increases and then decreases. At 1–5 A, the heart goes into sustained contraction, but usually reverts to sinus rhythm after current contact ends.

For an unconscious patient, the first responder should initially remove the current source, without becoming a victim, and then provide CPR including defibrillation if available. If sinus rhythm is restored, the patient should be evaluated for anoxic injury and undergo cardiac monitoring. Injury due to household current electric shock warrants an electrocardiogram; if normal, the patient does not require telemetry and can be discharged from the Emergency Department. The patient should be advised that muscle soreness will improve in 24–48 h and may be treated with analgesics, such as nonsteroidal agents.

One unique low-voltage electrical injury involves a mouth burn caused by chewing on a live electrical extension cord (usually at the connection with an extension cord) with the saliva completing the circuit between the positive and neutral leads [11]. The resulting electrical short circuit can cause significant tissue destruction of the lips, and/or tongue. These burns should be evaluated and treated by a burn specialist. Typically located at the oral commissure, the eschar often separates in a few days, resulting in bleeding from the labial branch of the facial artery. This can be very disconcerting to parents who should be forewarned and taught to pinch the lip between thumb and forefinger to provide hemostasis until definitive suture ligation can be performed. Non-operative and operative acute management have similar long-term outcomes [12, 13]. Regardless, aggressive stretching and sometimes splinting is necessary to prevent microstomia. Immediate coverage with flaps hastens the healing, but leaves a permanent scar and may sacrifice some normal tissue.

Resuscitation

Because the cutaneous injury is often only the "tip of the iceberg" with potential for extensive deep tissue damage, electrical contact burns may require significantly higher resuscitation fluid volumes than predicted by any of the usual predictive formula used for thermal injuries. However, initiating lactated Ringer's solution according to the Baxter (Parkland) burn formula is reasonable [14]. As with any estimation, ongoing intravenous fluid administration should be titrated according to urine output, mean arterial pressure ≥60 mmHg, and presence of metabolic acidosis [15]. Myonecrosis, due to the electrical injury itself and ongoing rhabdomyolysis due to compartment syndrome, generates elevated levels of circulating myoglobin and hemoglobin, which occlude the renal tubules and cause acute tubular necrosis; this has been reported to be associated with poor outcomes [16, 17]. No publications correlate specific myoglobin levels in the urine or the blood with renal failure. Furthermore, since myoglobin levels in the urine can be frighteningly elevated even in with clear yellow urine, the clinical relevance of quantitative urine levels of myoglobin is unclear. However, gross myoglobin in the urine warrants aggressive fluid hydration. If the urine is red or reddish black, increased fluid resuscitation to maintain a urine output goal of 1 ml/kg/h is indicated until the pigment clears; an osmotic diuretic such as mannitol (25 g bolus, followed by 12.5 g every 2–4 h) may be necessary to maintain this rate. Acidic conditions accentuate myoglobin precipitation in the renal tubules [18]. Theoretically, sodium bicarbonate administration to a targeted urine pH equal to 7 minimizes protein precipitation in the urine [19]; blood gases should be monitored to assure that the blood pH does not exceed 7.5. Whereas this treatment regimen has never been demonstrated to be clinically essential, it is fairly homeopathic and without significant adverse events.

Emergent Surgical Considerations

Three conditions warrant emergent surgery for a patient with a high voltage electrical burn: (1) evidence of compartment syndrome (2) evidence of nerve or vessel compression due to edematous compartment (3) ongoing rhabdomyolysis with myoglobinuria that threatens kidney failure. Depending on the specifics of the injury, early escharotomy and/or fasciotomy should be performed. An escharotomy is indicated for a circumferential third degree thermal burn with evidence of tissue compression and neurovascular compromise. Fasciotomies should be reserved for patients with compartment syndrome and evidence of ongoing myonecrosis or neurovascular compromise. Compartment pressure monitoring is mandatory, and a low threshold for escharotomy or fasciotomy is necessary with any deterioration in status. Routine compartment pressure measurements may be helpful, but any signs of impending compartment syndrome (increased pain, pallor, absence of pulse, decreased sensation, and tense swelling) mandate prompt compartment release.

Edema formation with even small upper extremity contact burns can cause median nerve compression necessitating urgent carpal tunnel decompression. If the tissue destruction at the contact point directly involves the volar wrist with evidence of median nerve injury, carpal tunnel release is unlikely to change the outcome and probably unnecessary. Monitoring neurovascular status in an awake patient is appropriate, but assessment in a non-responsive patient poses challenges; measuring compartment pressures in the carpal tunnel is highly unreliable and clinical judgment is paramount. If the injury is sufficiently devastating to cause a mummified hand, carpal tunnel release probably offers no benefit.

Wound Management

Cutaneous Wounds

Since most electrical injuries in the USA result from alternating current, "entrance" and "exit" sites are better referred to as contact points. These thermal burns result from heat generation as the electrical energy is converted to heat due to resistance to current flow in the tissues. Unlike flame burns, high-voltage electric current ($\geq$1000 V) burn injuries can be associated with greater deep-tissue injury than initially appreciated. As a result, these infrequent injuries [20] are associated with high amputation rates and greater use of resources than comparable %TBSA cutaneous burns. High-voltage current in contact with a dry hand may generate over 1000 °C, leading to tissue mummification. Delayed exploration and decompression in the compromised extremity may result in increased amputation rates along with increased organ failure and mortality [21, 22]. Conversely, unnecessary exploration increases morbidity, functional recovery, length of stay [23].

Sites of current arcing across joints should be treated like primary contact sites, because underlying damage can be just as severe. Contact points due to low-voltage injury rarely cause cutaneous burns that require treatment because the contact area dissipates the heat of the current with minimal underlying tissue destruction.

Large amounts of necrotic muscle due to high-voltage electrical contact injury and swollen muscle with resultant compartment syndrome and rhabdomyolysis necessitate surgical debridement to manage myoglobinemia and prevent acute kidney injury. If gross myoglobinuria does not clear after compartment release, aggressive hydration, and diuresis with mannitol, ongoing myonecrosis due to the electrical injury should be considered. Guillotine amputation may be a necessary and lifesaving intervention for obviously non-salvageable limbs. The goal of surgical procedures is to preserve viable tissue while removing neighboring dead tissue. As such, muscle of indeterminate viability should be spared and reexamined at a subsequent operation. Small, scattered areas of injured muscle will be replaced by fibrotic tissue. High fever and tachycardia, however, may indicate that remaining non-viable muscle has become infected and requires further debridement.

A peculiarity of electrical injuries, superficial extremity muscles may be viable and the deeper muscles along the radius, ulna, tibia, and fibula are necrotic. Since bone resists current flow, the heat generated causes a thermal injury to the muscle attachments.

Early aggressive debridement, followed immediately by reconstructive surgery with tissue transfer by rotation or free flaps to cover remaining viable tissue, nerves, vessels, and bone, may benefit early recovery. However, "early" has never been clearly defined. Many surgeons advocate immediate surgery on all patients with high-voltage electrical injuries to decompress soft tissues and debride necrotic muscle [21, 22]. The wounds are repeatedly debrided until suitable for closure with skin grafts or flaps.

However, delineation of dead from viable tissue is difficult during the first 24–72 h after injury and serial debridement can lead to removal of potentially viable tissue. Therefore, an alternative reported approach is to decompress those extremities that exhibit progressive peripheral nerve dysfunction, clinical manifestation of compartment syndrome, ongoing rhabdomyolysis, or resuscitation failure. Reports of this more conservative selective decompression approach suggest that delaying the initial operation for a few days minimizes the number of surgeries because the necrotic tissue can be recognized, excised, and the wound can be closed—often in a single procedure [23, 24]. No definitive data supports the concept that missing a deep injury leads to worse outcomes and more amputations or that immediate surgical decompression reduces the need for amputation.

The American Burn Association Practice Guidelines [1] management of electrical injuries recommend that (1) any patient with an electrical injury to the upper extremity be referred to specialized burn centers experienced with these injuries and (2) indications for surgical decompression include progressive neurologic dysfunction and vascular deterioration.

Extremity Injuries

Because extremities are the most common site to be injured and are at increased risk for compartment syndrome or muscle compression, they warrant special comment. There are several methods to evaluate the injured extremity. Extremity muscle compartment pressures may be measured as an adjunct to clinical examination. Tissue pressures higher than 30 mmHg or within 10–20 mmHg of diastolic blood pressure suggest compartment syndrome and potential deep-tissue injury, indicating the need for emergent surgical decompression. Measuring pressures in the carpal tunnel or Guyon's canal is not reproducible and unreliable. There is no evidence that nuclear scans, plethysmography or vascular Doppler scans, reliably indicate which extremities require decompression [1].

Cardiac Injuries

Immediate cardiac arrest is the most common cause of death due to electrical injury. High-voltage injuries are more likely to produce cardiac standstill, but low-voltage injuries can cause ventricular fibrillation, which is more likely to require defibrillation [25, 26]. However, the most common ECG abnormality involves nonspecific ST-T changes; atrial fibrillation is the most common dysrhythmia [27, 28].

The potential for cardiac dysrhythmia and myocardial injury has driven a tradition that all patients with an electrical injury undergo cardiac evaluation in the Emergency Department cardiac with a low threshold for admission and telemetry monitoring. Whereas an ECG is a well-established component of the early evaluation of patients after electrical injury, the indications for further cardiac work-up and duration of telemetry monitoring have been less clear. Consensus and review of the literature suggest that patients with low-voltage injuries who have normal ECGs and no history of loss of consciousness or evidence of dysrhythmia at the scene can be discharged from the Emergency department [26]. After high-voltage injuries, patients who have a history of loss of consciousness, ECG abnormalities, or other injuries that would otherwise require treatment are admitted to the hospital and monitored for 24 h. Several reviews report monitoring for 24 h after resolution of dysrhythmias or after admission, if there were no ECG abnormalities [29, 30]. At least one publication reported that all patients with dysrhythmias resolved within 48 h of admission either spontaneously or with pharmacologic intervention [31]. However, their data are insufficient to formulate management guidelines for electrical monitoring.

According to the 2006 American Burn Association Guidelines for the Management of Electrical Injuries [1]:

1. Individuals who sustain low-voltage electrical injuries, with no ECG abnormalities, no history of loss of consciousness, and no other injuries be discharged from the emergency department.

2. Individuals with history of loss of consciousness or documented dysrhythmia should be admitted for telemetry monitoring.
3. There was insufficient data on troponin levels after electrical injury to formulate a guideline.

Neurologic Complications

Neurologic complications represent common sequelae of high-voltage electrical injuries, affecting the central nervous system and peripheral nerves. Immediate but frequently transient symptoms include unconsciousness, respiratory paralysis, and motor paralysis. Loss of consciousness accounts for most CNS sequelae in patients with high-voltage injuries. Permanent changes include cortical encephalopathy due to the electrical injury itself or hypoxia due to cardiac or respiratory arrest. Spinal cord injuries are rare, but may occur at the time of the injury due to spinal fractures or present as later due to progressive muscular atrophy, amyotrophic lateral sclerosis, or transverse myelitis [32]. Late spinal cord paralysis progresses slowly and may occur months after the injury. [33, 34] Although recovery has been reported, the prognosis is usually poor [35, 36].

Peripheral neuropathies are relatively common in burned extremities, either from direct nerve injury or fibrosis surrounding the nerves. Reflex sympathetic dystrophy is not uncommon. Many patients suffer aches, headaches, chronic pain, and various non-anatomic neurologic complaints for some months after injury [37, 38].

A rare but reported complication is keraunoparalysis, in which one or more extremities appears blue, mottled, cold, and pulseless due to vascoconstriction and sympathetic nervous system instability. It is usually short lived, rarely lasting more than 24 h and more often resolves within an hour [39].

Cataracts

Premature cataract development occurs in 5–10 % patients after high-voltage electrical injury [40–42], but is not associated with contact points on the face or head. They can occur within a few weeks or may present years after the injury with an average time till presentation of 6 months [40] Complete ophthalmologic examination is warranted at the initial hospitalization and with subsequent decreased visual acuity. For injuries on the job, an eye exam shortly after the injury is indicated to verify normal lens transparency at the time of the injury.

Psychological Sequelae

Posttraumatic stress syndrome is common following electrical burns than after thermal burns [43]. Furthermore, patients with electrical injuries often face barriers to returning to work with significant emotional distress and subsequently poor quality of life [44]. While at least one study has reported that patient reported quality of life is similar between thermal and electrical burns [45], more research is needed in this area to validate these observations. Patients with electrical burns warrant screening for depression and posttraumatic stress.

Laboratory and Radiologic Evaluation

Thorough evaluation of the patient sustaining an electrical injury depends on the extent of injury, but may require additional laboratory tests. All patients with evidence of conductive injury or significant surface burns should have the following tests: Complete blood count, electrolyte levels, blood urea nitrogen level, creatinine level, and urinalysis with special attention to the presence of myoglobin. If intubated or with evidence of significant tissue injury, arterial blood gas determinations are indicated. If early debridement or decompression is indicated, a blood cross and screen is also appropriate. While creatine kinase levels are often obtained after electrical injury with the MB subunit reported to be more specific for myocardial injuries, several studies suggest that creatine kinase-MB levels poorly predict cardiac injury due to high background levels with the skeletal muscle injury [28, 46].

Radiographs of the cervical spine should be performed if spinal injury is suspected and a head CT is indicated if the patient is unresponsive. If there is evidence of other trauma, radiographic work-up for bony injury and CT scans for other spine, intraabdominal, or thoracic injuries are indicated.

Hospital Admission After an Electrical Injury

Most patients with low-voltage injuries and normal ECG can be discharged from the emergency department; the possible exceptions include patients with other injuries that require hospitalization or children with an oral commissure burn that would require monitoring for labial artery bleeding. Admission for cardiac monitoring of patients with history of loss of consciousness, ECG abnormalities, soft tissue destruction, or other injuries is a standard practice in published reviews of electrical injuries. Given that several retrospective publications have documented that monitoring patients with a normal ECG identified no serious dysrhythmia, a negative initial cardiac evaluation could obviate the need for hospital admission solely for cardiac monitoring.

Summary

Patients with electrical injury should be referred to Burn Centers for definitive care. No level 1 evidence exists for any clinical recommendations regarding cardiac or soft tissue management. However, some generalizations about safe management of patients with electrical injuries are feasible.

1. Most patients with low voltage can be discharged from the Emergency Department after evaluation for dysrhythmia or other injuries.
2. Patients with high-voltage electrical injuries should be admitted for monitoring if they have loss of consciousness or cardiac arrest in the field, documented cardiac arrhythmia, abnormal ECG, or other soft tissue injuries requiring wound care or surgery.
3. Unless there is evidence of compartment syndrome, conservative debridement of injured tissue after the extent of injury has declared itself avoids unnecessary surgery without compromising functional recovery.
4. Patients with high-voltage injuries should be screened for neurologic deficits and cataracts.
5. Patients with high-voltage injury should be followed long-term for delayed neurologic and psychologic sequelae.

References

1. Arnoldo B, Klein M, Gibran NS. Practice guidelines for the management of electrical injuries. J Burn Care Res. 2006;27:439–47.
2. Ritenour AE, Morton MJ, McManus JG, Barillo DJ, Cancio LC. Lightning injury: a review. Burns. 2008;34:585–94.
3. Muehlberger T, Vogt PM, Munster AM. The long-term consequences of lightning injuries. Burns. 2001;27:829–33.
4. Milzman DP, Moskowitz L, Hardel M. Lightning strikes at a mass gathering. South Med J. 1999;92:708–10.
5. Graber JU-WH-H. Lightning accident with eight victims: case report and brief review of the literature. J Trauma. 1996;40:288–90.
6. ten DHJ, Klasen HJ, Nijsten MW, Pietronero L. Superficial lightning injuries—their "fractal" shape and origin. Burns Incl Therm Inj. 1987;13:141–6.
7. Ogren FPE-AL. Neuro-otologic findings in the lightning-injured patient. Semin-Neurol. 1995;15: 256–62.
8. Jones D, Ogren F, Roh L, Moore G. Lightning and its effects on the auditory system. Laryngoscope. 1991;101:830–4.
9. Fish RM, Geddes LA. Conduction of electrical current to and through the human body: a review. Eplasty. 2009;9, e44.
10. Fish RM, Geddes LA. Medical and bioengineering aspects of electrical injuries, 2nd edn. Tucson AZ: Lawyers and Judges; 2009.
11. Canady JW, Thompson SA, Bardach J. Oral commissure burns in children. Plast Reconstr Surg. 1996;97:738–44. discussion 45; 46–55.

12. Milano M. Oral electrical and thermal burns in children: review and report of case. ASDC J Dent Child. 1999;66:116–9. 85.
13. Thomas SS. Electrical burns of the mouth: still searching for an answer. Burns. 1996;22:137–40.
14. Colic M, Ristic L, Jovanovic M. Emergency treatment and early fluid resuscitation following electrical injuries. Acta Chir Plast. 1996;38:137–41.
15. Luce E, Gottlieb S. True high-tension electrical injuries. Ann Plast Surg. 1984;12:321–6.
16. Gupta KL, Kumar R, Sekhar MS, Sakhuja V, Chugh KS. Myoglobinuric acute renal failure following electrical injury. Ren Fail. 1991;13:23–5.
17. Rosen CL, Adler JN, Rabban JT, et al. Early predictors of myoglobinuria and acute renal failure following electrical injury. J Emerg Med. 1999;17:783–9.
18. Slater MS, Mullins RJ. Rhabdomyolysis and myoglobinuric renal failure in trauma and surgical patients: a review. J Am Coll Surg. 1998;186:693–716.
19. Zager RA. Studies of mechanisms and protective maneuvers in myoglobinuric acute renal injury. Lab Invest. 1989;60:619–29.
20. Vazquez D, Solano I, Pages E, Garcia L, Serra J. Thoracic disc herniation, cord compression, and paraplegia caused by electrical injury: case report and review of the literature. J Trauma. 1994;37: 328–32.
21. d' Amato TA, Kaplan IB, Britt LD. High-voltage electrical injury: a role for mandatory exploration of deep muscle compartments. J Natl Med Assoc. 1994; 86: 535–7.
22. Parshley P, Kilgore J, Pulito J, Smiley P, Miller S. Aggressive approach to the extremity damaged by electric current. Am J Surg. 1985;150:78–82.
23. Mann R, Gibran N, Engrav L, Heimbach D. Is immediate decompression of high voltage electrical injuries to the upper extremity always necessary? J Trauma. 1996;40:584–7. discussion 7–9.
24. Engrav LH, Gottlieb JR, Walkinshaw MD, Heimbach DM, Trumble TE, Grube BJ. Outcome and treatment of electrical injury with immediate median and ulnar nerve palsy at the wrist: a retrospective review and a survey of members of the American Burn Association. Ann Plast Surg. 1990;25:166–8.
25. Purdue GF, Hunt JL. Electrocardiographic monitoring after electrical injury: necessity or luxury. J Trauma. 1986;26:166–7.
26. Searle J, Slagman A, Maass W, Mockel M. Cardiac monitoring in patients with electrical injuries. An analysis of 268 patients at the Charite Hospital. Dtsch Arztebl Int. 2013;110:847–53.
27. Das KM. Electrocardiographic changes following electric shock. Indian J Pediatr. 1974;41:192–4.
28. Housinger T, Green L, Shahangian S, Saffle J, Warden G. A prospective study of myocardial damage in electrical injuries. J Trauma. 1985;25:122–4. Published erratum appears in J Trauma 1986 Jul;26(7):659.
29. Bailey B, Gaudreault P, Thivierge RL. Experience with guidelines for cardiac monitoring after electrical injury in children. Am J Emerg Med. 2000;18:671–5.
30. Lewin RF, Arditti A, Sclarovsky S. Non-invasive evaluation of electrical cardiac injury. Br Heart J. 1983;49:190–2.
31. Arrowsmith J, Usgaocar RP, Dickson WA. Electrical injury and the frequency of cardiac complications. Burns. 1997;23:576–8.
32. Levine NS, Atkins A, McKeel Jr DW, Peck SD, Pruitt Jr BA. Spinal cord injury following electrical accidents: case reports. J Trauma. 1975;15:459–63.
33. Ratnayake B, Emmanuel ER, Walker CC. Neurological sequelae following a high voltage electrical burn. Burns. 1996;22:578–9.
34. Kanitkar S, Roberts AH. Paraplegia in an electrical burn: a case report. Burns Incl Therm Inj. 1988;14:49–50.
35. Koller J, Orsagh J. Delayed neurological sequelae of high-tension electrical burns. Burns. 1989;15: 175–8.
36. Varghese G, Mani MM, Redford JB. Spinal cord injuries following electrical accidents. Paraplegia. 1986;24:159–66.
37. Isao T, Masaki F, Riko N, Seiichi H. Delayed brain atrophy after electrical injury. J Burn Care Rehabil. 2005;26:456–8.
38. Selvaggi G, Monstrey S, Van Landuyt K, Hamdi M, Blondeel P. Rehabilitation of burn injured patients following lightning and electrical trauma. NeuroRehabilitation. 2005;20:35–42.
39. Ten DHJ, Klasen H, Reenalda P. Keraunoparalysis, a 'specific' lightning injury. Burns. 1985;12:54–7.
40. Saffle JR, Crandall A, Warden GD. Cataracts: a long-term complication of electrical injury. J Trauma. 1985;25:17–21.
41. Biro Z, Pamer Z. Electrical cataract and optic neuropathy. Int Ophthalmol. 1994;18:43–7.
42. Reddy SC. Electric cataract: a case report and review of the literature. Eur J Ophthalmol. 1999;9:134–8.
43. Mancusi UHRJ, Tarbox AR, Wainwright DJ. Posttraumatic stress disorder in electric burn patients. J Burn Care Rehabil. 1986;7:521–5.
44. Noble J, Gomez M, Fish JS. Quality of life and return to work following electrical burns. Burns. 2006;32: 159–64.
45. Cochran A, Edelman LS, Saffle JR, Morris SE. Self-reported quality of life after electrical and thermal injury. J Burn Care Rehabil. 2004;25:61–6.
46. Ahrenholz DH, Schubert W, Solem LD. Creatine kinase as a prognostic indicator in electrical injury. Surgery. 1988;104:741–7.

Chemical Burns

16

Robert Cartotto

Introduction

Chemical burns are challenging to manage for a variety of reasons. They account for only 3–8 % of all burn injuries [1] and this infrequency limits the surgeon's accumulation of experience with any given chemical. Equally problematic is that there are over 25,000 possible chemicals that may be used in the household and in industry, many of which can cause burns [2]. The injuries range from minor burns sustained at home to major life-threatening injuries following industrial accidents. While most chemical burns are small and involve only a few percent of the TBSA, the face and hands are most frequently affected. Determination of depth of injury can be particularly difficult, and despite their small size, almost 20 % of chemical burns eventually require surgical debridement and skin grafting [1, 3]. Unfortunately, a rising number of chemical burns now develop as a result of domestic assault in which various acids or alkalis are deliberately sprayed into the face of the victim frequently resulting in facial disfigurement and permanent ocular damage [4]. Finally, chemical agents may increasingly be used in war, terrorism, and production of weapons of mass destruction.

Because of the complex and heterogeneous nature of chemical burns, the surgeon should have a set of basic principles of management that can be applied to *any* chemical burn. This chapter will primarily focus on those principles, but it will also describe the management of some specific chemical burns that may be encountered including hydrofluoric acid, sulfuric acid, hydrochloric acid, lyes, and cement.

Mechanism of Injury

Unlike thermal burns where the extent of injury is related to only two factors (temperature and duration of exposure), the extent of cutaneous injury from a chemical contact is related to multiple factors. Chief among these is the duration of contact [3, 5, 6]. Chemicals continue to produce injury for as long as they are in contact with the skin and may continue to act hours after the initial contact. This is in contrast to thermal injuries where exposure to heat is usually transient and rapidly terminated. Chemical injury to the skin is also dependent upon the specific nature of the chemical and its action upon biological systems. Chemicals may act as oxidants (that denature protein by inserting oxygen), reducing agents (which denature proteins by binding free electrons), corrosives (which

R. Cartotto, M.D., F.R.C.S.C. (✉)
Department of Surgery, Ross Tilley Burn Centre, Sunnybrook Health Sciences Centre, University of Toronto., 2075 Bayview Avenue, Room D 712, Toronto, ON, Canada, M4N 3M5
e-mail: robert.cartotto@sunnybrook.ca

D.G. Greenhalgh (ed.), *Burn Care for General Surgeons and General Practitioners*,
DOI 10.1007/978-3-319-29161-1_16

Table 16.1 Chemicals that burn

Mechanisms	Classes of chemicals	Determinants of severity
Oxidation (e.g., NaOH)	Acids (coagulation necrosis)	Duration of contact
Reduction (e.g., HCl)	Alkalis (liquification necrosis)	Mechanism of action
Corrosion (e.g., Phenol)	Organic solutions (dissolve lipid membranes)	Quantity
Protoplasmic poison (e.g., HF)	Inorganic solutions (bind to proteins and form salts)	Concentration
Vessicant (e.g., Mustard Gas)		Penetration ability
Desiccant (e.g., H_2SO_4)		Exothermic properties

directly denature protein), protoplasmic poisons (which form esters with proteins or which inactivate essential organic ions), vesicants (that cause ischemic necrosis), or desiccants (which dehydrate tissues) [2, 6]. Many chemicals can exert more than one of these actions simultaneously. Other factors that affect the severity and extent of a chemical burn include the chemical's concentration, quantity, lipid solubility, and penetration capabilities [2]. Finally, some chemicals have exothermic properties allowing them to inflict an accompanying thermal injury [6].

A simple and practical approach to classifying and understanding the mechanism of action of most chemicals is to consider if the chemical agent is (1) an acid or a base, and (2) if it is an organic or inorganic solution (Table 16.1). Usually, acids with a pH less than 2 create coagulation necrosis of the skin and soft tissue. This results in a less severe and more confined injury than alkalis with a pH greater than 11.5, which create more expansive and diffuse liquification necrosis. This liquification of tissues loosens tissue planes and allows on-going chemical penetration and, as a result, alkali burns are generally more serious than acid burns [2, 6]. Organic solutions are lipid-soluble and create more destruction and penetration because of their ability to dissolve cell membranes than inorganic solutions which bind to the skin and form various salts [2].

Basic Principles of Management

Protect Yourself!

When responding to a patient with a chemical contact, providers should always take precautions to prevent exposure of themselves to the chemical agent. This can occur by touching the contaminated skin or clothing of the patient or by splashing during the process of irrigation. At a minimum, personal protective equipment should include gloves and eye protection. Plastic aprons or gowns provide an additional level of protection when dealing with patients exposed to large quantities of chemical, more extensive chemical burns, or burns from more dangerous chemicals such as hydrofluoric acid.

Airway First!

Infrequently, chemical burns may include chemical injury to the airway. Typically, this occurs when chemicals explode and become aerosolized or when a patient has aspirated deliberately or accidentally ingested chemicals. Always carefully look for peri-nasal and peri-oral burns, dysphonia, wheezing, stridor, excessive mucus or saliva production, and signs of respiratory distress. Clinical suspicion of significant chemical inhalation should prompt endotracheal intubation for airway protection and/or support of respiration [7].

Remove the Chemical

The most important determinant of a chemical burn's severity is the duration of contact of the chemical with the skin. Tissue injury continues to occur for as long as the chemical agent is present [2, 3, 5, 6], and complete removal of the chemical has been shown to reduce the severity of chemical burns [5]. Chemical removal can be summarized by remembering the motto "Strip, Remove, and Flush" [7]. Contaminated clothing, including footwear, must be removed immediately. Residues or deposits of dry chemical materials, powders, or particulate debris should be removed next by brushing these off the skin before liberally flushing the area with water. Lavage with water should be copious and should be initiated at the scene and continue for at least 30 min. Irrigation should be repeated on arrival to the hospital. Sterile solutions are not needed and tap water at body temperature is always preferred. It is essential to carefully control splashing and runoff during irrigation to ensure that the chemical agent is not inadvertently dispersed to uninvolved body areas. Always ensure that the irrigation effluent doesn't collect in pools around the patient or within a soft tissue fold [2]. Immersion of affected parts in a tub is not recommended as this only serves to spread the agent.

It is not uncommon to need to continue water irrigation anywhere between 30 min and several hours, as in the case of alkali contacts [2, 8]. One may use pH testing strips to evaluate the effluent as an approximate guide to the adequacy and duration of irrigation, aiming to achieve a pH between 5 and 11 [2]. While some chemicals are not water-soluble (e.g., Phenol), or produce heat when combined with water (e.g., concentrated hydrochloric acid and sulfuric acid), as a general rule, copious irrigation with water will be beneficial and will rarely cause harm [7]. Table 16.2 lists the rare exceptions to immediate water lavage among relatively common encountered chemicals where an intervention strategy prior to water lavage is recommended.

Table 16.2 Occasional exceptions to immediate water lavage

Chemical	Problem	Strategy prior to water lavage
Calcium oxide (CaO, "Dry Lime")	Forms the strong alkali CaOH with water	Thoroughly brush off dry lime powder from the skin prior to water lavage
Phenol	Insoluble in water	Wipe phenol off the skin with 50 % polyethylene glycol prior to water lavage [11]
Concentrated hydrochloric or sulphuric acid	Exothermic on contact with water	Neutralize with a soapy solution prior to lavage if possible [6]

Know the Chemical

It is essential to obtain as much information on the chemical as possible. This can be obtained from a variety of sources, including the labels on containers or the chemical if these have been brought in, from the industry itself (in the case of workplace injuries), internet searches, and consultation with the local poison control centre. Critical information about a chemical includes its pH, concentration, and systemic toxic effects. The use of chemical testing strips to determine the pH of a chemical agent, when it is unknown, is generally to be avoided as these can be inaccurate [7].

Antidotes and Neutralization Are Usually not Indicated

Antidotes have the theoretical appeal of inactivating a chemical, thus limiting skin and soft tissue damage. However, a number of factors limit the practical usefulness of antidotes. First, the specific antidotes may not be readily available. Second, antidotes themselves may have their own adverse effects and toxicities. Third, occasionally the neutralization reaction is exothermic creating the potential for an associated thermal injury. Thus, as numerous authors have stated, dilution with copious amounts of running water, rather than neutralization, is the key to therapy [5, 9, 10]. The most important exception to this general rule is the hydrofluoric acid burn where rapid neutralization of the free fluoride ion is critically important (discussed below).

Systemic Toxicity Is Wide-Ranging

In the scenario of a chemical burn, it is important to remember that the agent can be absorbed systemically through the skin, by inhalation, or by ingestion. While systemic toxicity usually results from large surface area exposure to the chemical, significant and even life-threatening systemic toxicity may occur from smaller contacts (e.g., concentrated hydrofluoric acid). Systemic toxicity is as diverse and varied as the range of chemicals themselves and can affect the neurological, respiratory, cardiovascular, hematologic, renal, and hepatic systems alone or in combination. Consequently, it is imperative to have a clear identification of the chemical agent and information on its systemic effects. In the author's experience, the local poison control centre has provided the most rapid and accurate information on any given chemical agent's toxicity. Once the systemic toxicity is identified, appropriate diagnostic and therapeutic strategies can be undertaken.

Diagnosis of Burn Depth Is Difficult

In general, determination of the depth of the burn is more difficult than in thermal burns. Some chemicals may tan or discolor the skin (e.g., phenol, and potassium permanganate), compromising the usual visual clues to burn depth. Some chemicals may induce vesicle or blistering formation (e.g., mustard gas, and lewsite), or hardening of the skin (e.g., sulfuric acid). Other chemicals have local anesthetic properties (e.g., phenol) rendering pain and loss of sensation useless as diagnostic tools to assess burn depth [6, 11]. Consequently, repeated evaluation of the burn and surgical excision only when the extent of depth and demarcation is clear is warranted. In some instances, following surgical debridement of the chemical burn wound, temporary closure with allograft to "test" the wound bed for viability prior to definitive autografting is advisable.

Supportive Care: Treat the Chemical Burn Patient Like a Burn Patient

Notwithstanding the general principles described above, care of the patient with a chemical burn may proceed as it would for a patient with a thermal burn. Fluid resuscitation is administered if the burn is $\geq$15–20 % TBSA with appropriate monitoring of endpoints and titration as needed. Once the chemical is completely removed by irrigation, the wounds may be covered with an antimicrobial dressing. For most chemical burns, opioid analgesics should be provided to alleviate pain. However, in some selected instances such as the hydrofluoric acid burn, pain is indicative of ongoing tissue injury and should not be masked with analgesics but rather eliminated by specific inactivation of the chemical (see hydrofluoric acid burns below). Tetanus prophylaxis should be administered if the patient's immunization is not up-to-date. Early excision of clearly non-viable tissue is advised, recognizing (as described above) that assessment of injury depth can be difficult and may require a period of observation.

Check The Eyes!

Patients with a chemical burn may also have sustained a chemical contact to the eyes. It is imperative to identify an ocular chemical contact because any delay in removal of the chemical from the ocular surface may lead to significant and potentially permanent visual disturbances [12, 13]. Alkali ocular burns from agents such as lye, ammonia, potassium hydroxide, magnesium hydroxide, and lime are the most common and serious [12]. As with cutaneous burns, alkali eye burns are more destructive than acid burns because of their lipophilic nature and ability to penetrate and produce saponification necrosis readily leading to penetration of the agent through the cornea and sclera [12, 14]. Patients with an ocular chemical burn typically present with intense eye pain, marked conjunctival injection, epiphora, photophobia, and blepharospasm. The first principle is to remove the chemical. The ocular surface, including the conjunctival fornices, should be examined for any particulate debris and this debris should be removed first. Sweeping the fornices with a glass rod may facilitate removal of solid material [13]. Following this, copious lavage of the eye with isotonic saline or Ringer's lactate should be initiated before proceeding with the ophthalmologic evaluation [13]. Topical anesthetics may facilitate irrigation of the eye in patients when involuntary blepharospasm interferes with effective lavage. Similarly, a Morgan Lens may be used in patients who have trouble tolerating lavage [12, 13]. A minimum of 30 min of lavage is needed for each eye, provided simultaneously if there is a bilateral contact [12]. More prolonged irrigation using volumes of 20 l or more may be needed, especially for severe alkali chemical burns. Testing the effluent using chemical-testing pH strips may help to evaluate the adequacy and duration of irrigation. Neutralizing agents are not indicated [12]. All ocular chemical burns should be considered a true ophthalmologic emergency and an ophthalmology consult should be urgently obtained to direct further treatment. This may include provision of adequate analgesia, intra-ocular pressure control, optimization of corneal epithelial healing, and use of anti-inflammatory and anti-microbial therapies [12].

Specific Chemical Burns

Hydrofluoric Acid

Hydrofluoric acid (HF) is an inorganic acid which may be found in the home in heavy-duty cleaning agents for stone and metals, rust removal solutions, and glass-polishing material [15–17]. In industry, HF is used in the manufacturing of semi-conductors, plastics, fertilizers, and refrigerant fluids [15, 17]. HF is also utilized in various research laboratory settings. HF exists in aqueous concentrations ranging from less than 10 % up to 90 % solutions and rarely may exist as 99 % pure HF referred to anhydrous HF [17]. HF burns are not uncommon, and in general, the majority of these burns occur from household contact with less than 20 % HF resulting in small burns usually to the hands [17, 18]. In contrast, industrial HF burns typically result from more concentrated HF and involve larger surface areas and pose an immediate life-threatening danger [19, 20].

HF damages tissue through two mechanisms. At concentrations less than 50 %, it is a weak acid and it exerts a corrosive effect which becomes considerably strong at concentrations greater than 50 % where HF acts as a strong acid. The second, and far more important mechanism, is that HF acts as a protoplasmic poison [6]. HF is highly lipophilic and readily and continuously penetrates into soft tissues as well as bone, creating a liquification necrosis as it dissociates into free hydrogen ions and free fluoride ions [15]. The free fluoride ion is highly destructive to intra and extra-cellular structures and its presence elicits intense pain. Furthermore, free fluoride ions are absorbed into the systemic circulation and bind available calcium and magnesium, potentially leading to life-threatening hypocalcaemia and/or hypomagnesaemia. The primary toxicity of HF is from hypocalcaemia-induced ventricular dysrhythmias including ventricular fibrillation and Torsades de Pointes [20].

The clinical presentation of HF burns varies depending on the concentration and the extent of the area exposed. The hallmark of all HF burns is intense pain, which, in many cases, appears to be out of proportion to the cutaneous injury [15]. Contact with less than 20 % HF may not produce any immediate symptoms and patients often present as late as 24 h after contact with a burn consisting of localized erythema but with intense pain. This is highly typical of household contacts that result from cleaning or rust removal solutions where faulty gloves or failure to use protective equipment occurred [15, 17, 21]. Patients with a burn from greater than 20 % HF typically present within 1–8 h with more immediate evidence of tissue destruction and severe pain [15]. The burns may appear as simple erythema (from less concentrated HF), to the more classical wound with a hard grayish to silver eschar surrounded by erythema and blisters. The wound may ulcerate and local tenosynovitis or even osteolysis can result if the HF is concentrated [15]. In cases of large burns or burns from concentrated HF, the main systemic manifestation is from hypocalcaemia and hypomagnesaemia. Paradoxically, classic signs of hypocalcaemia such as tetany, Chvostk's, and Trousseau's signs may be absent [15, 22, 23] with the earliest manifestation being QT prolongation on the ECG. This is an ominous sign that precedes fatal ventricular arrhythmias. Other laboratory abnormalities may include acidosis, fluorosis, and hyperkalemia [17, 20].

The immediate treatment of any HF burn is copious water lavage at the scene for 15–30 min. Treatment personnel should protect themselves from self-contamination by wearing double gloves, eye protection, and plastic aprons or gowns, if possible. On arrival to the hospital, it is essential to identify patients at high risk of fatal systemic toxicity as identified in Fig. 16.1. Both high- and low-risk HF burns should receive further copious water lavage, but high-risk patients should immediately be placed on an ECG monitor and be given empiric intravenous calcium and magnesium prior to checking serum electrolyte levels [17, 20]. The purpose of systemic calcium delivery is to correct hypocalcaemia and not to achieve neutralization of the free fluoride ion. Further calcium and magnesium may be administered as guided by monitoring of plasma levels of these electrolytes. Potassium and blood gas analysis should also be obtained in high-risk contacts.

The next step in both high and low-risk HF burns is to neutralize free fluoride locally in the wound. The aim of this is to halt tissue destruction and relief of pain is the most reliable end-point that indicates successful neutralization of the free-fluoride ions. The simplest initial approach is to apply 2.5 % calcium gluconate gel to the burns for a 30 min period, initially massaging this into the skin then repeating application as needed if pain persists. A surgical glove containing the gel is a useful way to topically treat hand and digital HF burns. Some authorities recommend this therapy can be repeated every 4 h for 4 days [15, 24], repeating if needed if pain redevelops.

Although simple and noninvasive, calcium gluconate gel's effectiveness is limited by its ability to penetrate into the skin. This has led to the direct injection of 10 % calcium gluconate into and surrounding the eschar. Generally, this is only considered for more severe burns with concentrated HF or where irrigation and topical gel have not

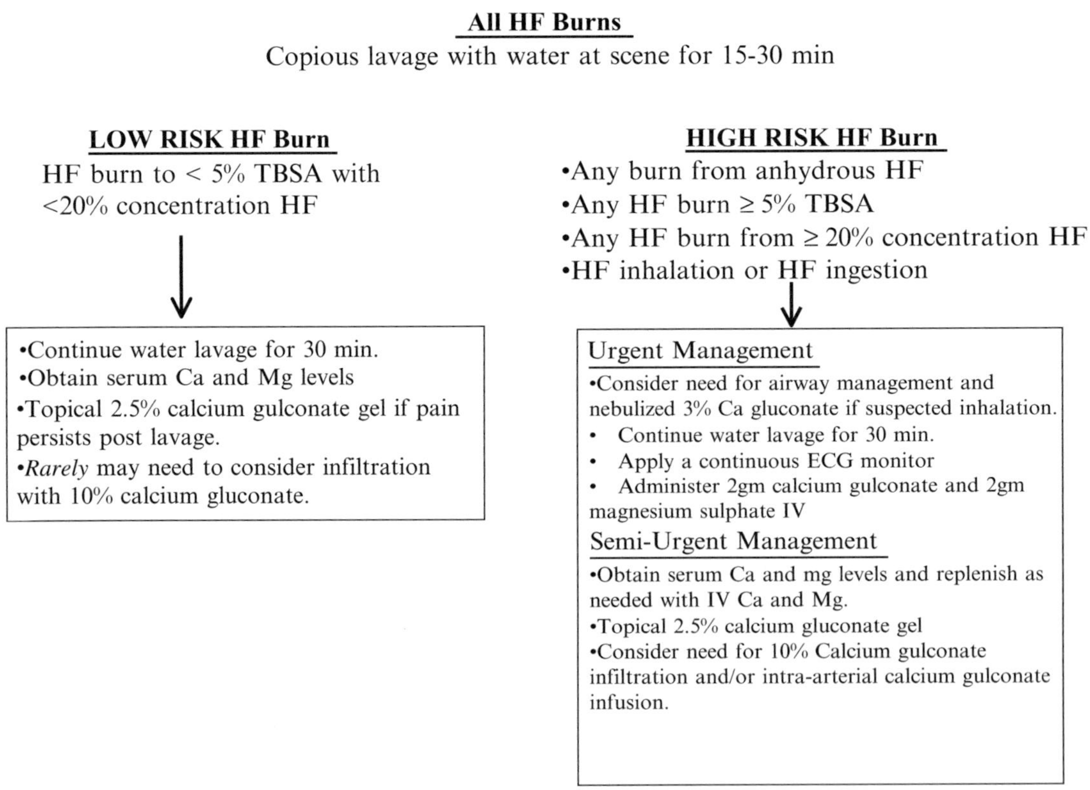

Fig. 16.1 Algorithm for the management of hydrofluoric acid burns

relieved pain. Most agree it is not necessary for contacts with less than 20 % HF [17]. A 27-G or 30-G needle is used to inject a maximum of 0.5 mL/cm^2 beneath and around the involved skin. This can be quite painful for the patient and great caution must be taken when injecting digits or near fascial compartments because of the well-recognized risk of causing pressure necrosis, ischemia, or compartmental syndromes [18]. Theoretically, local anesthetics may be used to alleviate the pain of infiltration, but this is problematic and highly controversial because the anesthetic confounds accurate assessment of pain alleviation. Also, injection for a digital block itself causes increased tissue pressure, which may then limit how much calcium gluconate can be injected. If local anesthesia is used, it should be short-acting and allowed to wear off before deciding if pain has been relieved. Special considerations for a digit include limiting injections to only 0.5 mL per phalanx and use of repeated small injections rather than one large single dose [15, 25]. Subungal HF penetration with HF burns to the fingertips or nail folds may necessitate nail removal under a digital block followed by topical or infiltration calcium therapy to the nail bed [15].

In the case of HF burns to the hands and digits, intra and para-lesional calcium gluconate infiltration poses several disadvantages including pain, additional trauma, risks of tissue or compartmental injury from pressure, limitations to the volume of calcium gluconate that can be injected, and the need to remove the nail(s) for subungal injuries [21]. Intra-arterial infusions of calcium gluconate are an effective way to deliver neutralizing calcium to the hand and digits while avoiding the risks from direct soft-tissue injection of calcium gluconate. Depending on the distribution of the burn in the hand, either a radial or brachial artery 20-G catheter is inserted percutaneously [15, 23, 26, 27]. Next, 1–2 g of calcium gluconate is infused over 4 h. In the original protocol [27], 50 mL of 4 % calcium gluconate was used, whereas others have used 10 mL of 10 % calcium gluconate in 40 mL saline [21, 27, 28]. This cycle is then repeated every 4–12 h if pain is not alleviated [21, 27, 28].

Intra-arterial calcium infusion is not without risk and should only be considered for severe hand and digital burns from concentrated HF. The technique has also been adapted for HF burns to other body areas including the arm (axillary artery), lower extremities (femoral artery), and face (carotid artery) [29].

Inhalation of HF fumes can occur easily because HF is highly volatile [20]. Therefore, it should be suspected whenever a patient presents with extensive HF burns, clothing soaked in HF, burns from highly concentrated HF (>50 %), or head and neck burns [20]. Suspected HF inhalation should be managed as a high-risk HF burn and specific pulmonary treatment includes prophylactic intubation, provision of 100 % oxygen, and inhalational delivery of nebulized 3 % calcium gluconate [20].

Very rarely, immediate surgical excision of severe burns from concentrated HF may need to be considered in situations where systemic toxicity is not brought under control through the above-described methods of local neutralization with systemic calcium replenishment [15].

Lye Burns

Lyes are strong corrosive alkalis and include sodium hydroxide, potassium hydroxide, ammonium hydroxide, and calcium hydroxide [6]. These strong alkalis are commonly found in household cleaning solutions and drain cleaners. Because of their wide availability, lyes are also frequently used in suicide attempts by ingestion and as a weapon in personal assault [4]. Lyes penetrate skin and soft tissue easily and demand more aggressive and prolonged irrigation as compared to other chemicals. Ocular lye burns are particularly serious and have the greatest potential to inflict severe damage to the eye. Therefore, heightened attention to the eyes is necessary when initially treating a patient with lye burns.

Cement Burns

Calcium oxide (CaO), also known as "quicklime," is a major component of cement and when combined with water it forms calcium hydroxide, one of the potent alkalis (Lyes) described above. Wet cement causes burns usually when there is prolonged contact of soaked clothing or boots with the worker's skin [2, 30]. Alternatively, dry lime dust may collect around a worker's wrist at the glove line or leg at the sock line and be activated to the injurious calcium hydroxide by perspiration. These burns develop insidiously with little pain being noticed and recognition of the burn may occur hours or even days after the injury [30]. Again, due to the potent penetrating capability of calcium hydroxide, these burns may end up being very deep and often require surgical care (Fig. 16.2).

Sulfuric Acid Burns

Sulfuric acid burns are probably the commonest type of acid burn. Also known as "oil of vitriol," sulfuric acid is found in commonly available acidic drain cleaners and in lead acid batteries. Again, because of its availability, it is frequently used by assailants attempting to injure and maim victims. This corrosive and strong desiccant produces painful burns which rapidly form a hard, dry eschar [6]. While copious water lavage is always helpful and rarely causes harm, there is some exothermy when concentrated sulfuric acid mixes with water. Therefore, it is sometimes

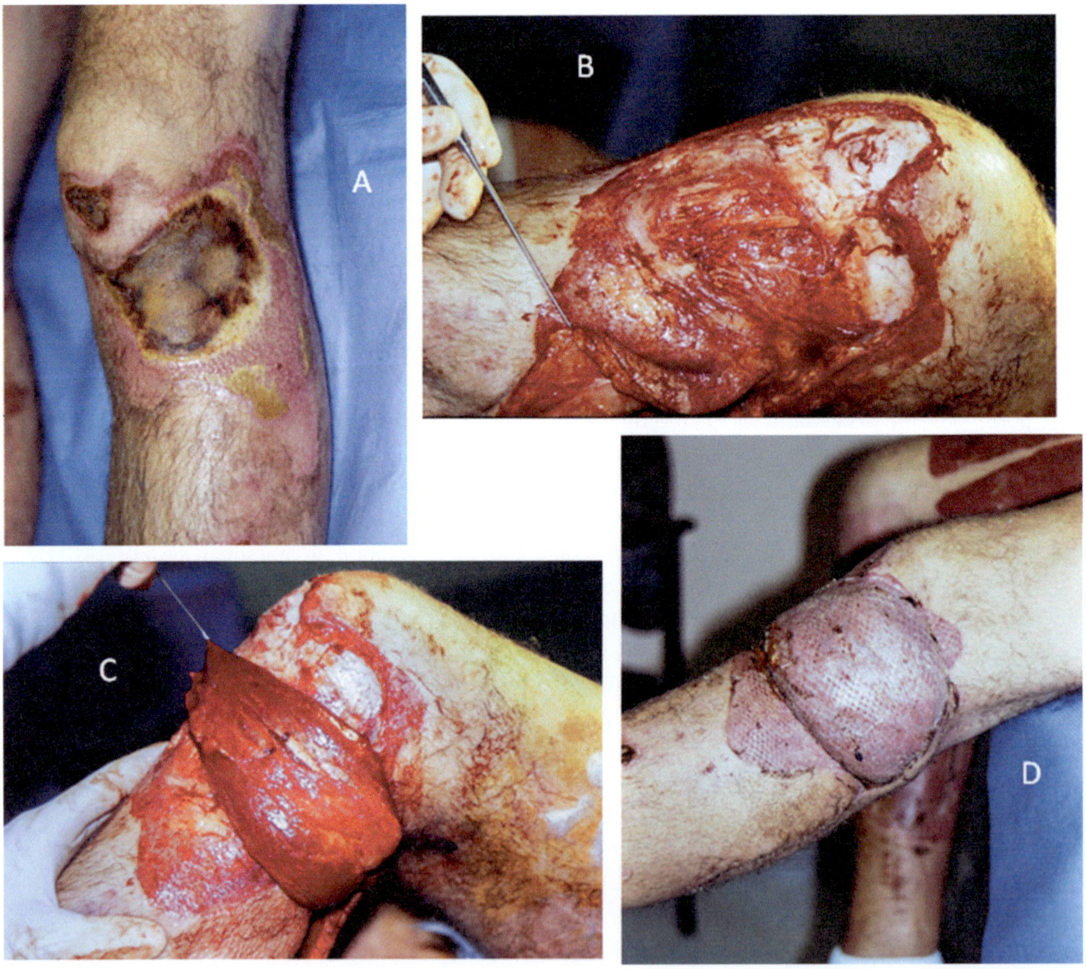

Fig. 16.2 (**a**) Cement burn to the left knee that went unrecognized initially with the worker presenting 48 h later. (**b**) Extremely deep injury at debridement with exposure of patella and knee joint. (**c**) Immediate coverage with lateral gastrocnemius muscle flap. **d**) result at 1 month with full knee extension actively

recommended to attempt neutralization by scrubbing first with a soapy solution before proceeding with copious water lavage [6].

Hydrochloric Acid Burns

Hydrochloric acid which, in its highly concentrated form, is called muriatic acid is used in a variety of settings including some household cleaners, industrial plastic manufacturing, pool water neutralization, and leather processing. It is a strong, corrosive, and desiccant and, like sulfuric acid, produces painful hard leathery eschars and ideally is neutralized with a soapy solution in conjunction with copious water lavage [6].

White Phosphorus Burns

White phosphorus is commonly encountered in military or terrorism settings as it is a key component in munitions. However, in the civilian sector, white phosphorus is also found in fertilizers and fireworks. White phosphorus injuries are considered both thermal and chemical burns and usually following an explosion white phosphorus particles end up embedded in the skin and soft tissues [31]. This induces not only a chemical injury as white phosphorus acts as a corrosive, but also as a thermal injury when it auto-ignites on exposure to air [31]. White phosphorus also causes life-threatening systemic toxicity from hypocalcaemia and/or hyperphosphatemia [31]. These burns should initially be managed by copious lavage with cool water and the wounds should be kept covered with continuously moist saline compresses or dressings. Visible white phosphorus particles should be removed and placed in cold water as they will auto-ignite on exposure to air and immediate surgical debridement is frequently indicated [31]. Topical copper sulfate is not used as a neutralizing agent, but rather it is applied to turn the embedded white phosphorus particles and debris black in order to help with identification and debridement.

References

1. Hardwicke J, Hunter T, Staruch R, Moiemen N. Chemical burns-an historical comparison and review of the literature. Burns. 2012;38:383–7.
2. Palao R, Monge I, Ruiz M, Barret JP. Chemical burns: pathophysiology and treatment. Burns. 2010;36: 295–304.
3. Sykes RA, Mani MM, Hiebert JM. Chemical burns: retrospective review. J Burn Care Rehabil. 1986;7:343–7.
4. Mannan A, Ghani S, Clarke A, Butler PEM. Cases of chemical assault worldwide: a literature review. Burns. 2007;33:149–54.
5. Leonard LG, Scheulen JJ, Munster AM. Chemical burns: effect of prompt first aid. J Trauma. 1982;22:420–3.
6. Jelenko C. Chemicals that "burn". J Trauma. 1974;14:65–72.
7. Kearns RD, Cairns CB, Holmes JH, Rich PB, Cairns BA. Chemical burn care: a review of best practices. EMS World. 2014;43(3):40–5.
8. Wolfort FG, DeMeester T, Knorr N, Edgerton MT. Surgical management of cutaneous lye burns. Surg Gynecol Obstet. 1970;131:873–6.
9. Cartotto RC, Peters WJ, Neligan PC, Douglas LG, Beeston J. Chemical burns. Can J Surg. 1996;39:205–11.
10. Saydjari R, Abston S, Desai MH, Herndon DN. Chemical Burns. J Burn Care Rehabil. 1986;7:404–8.
11. Horch R, Spilker G, Stark GB. Phenol burns and intoxications. Burns. 1994;20:45–50.
12. Bunker DJL, George RJ, Kleinschmidt A, Kumar RJ, Maitz P. Alkali-related ocular burns: a case series and review. J Burn Care Res. 2014;35:261–8.
13. Fish R, Davidson RS. Management of ocular thermal and chemical injuries including amniotic membrane therapy. Curr Opin Ophthalmol. 2010;21:317–21.
14. Brodovsky SC, McCarty CA, Snibson G, et al. Management of alkali burns. Ophthalmology. 2000;107:1829–35.
15. Kirkpatrick JJR, Enion DS, Burd DA. Hydrofluoric acid burns: a review. Burns. 1995;21:483–93.
16. Seyb ST, Noordhoek L, Botens S, Mani M. A study to determine the efficacy of treatments for hydrofluoric acid burns. J Burn Care Rehabil. 1995;16:253–7.
17. McKee D, Thoma A, Bailey K, Fish J. A review of hydrofluoric acid burn management. Plast Surg (Oakv). 2014;22:95–8.
18. Burd A. Hydrofluoric acid-revisited. Burns. 2004;30:720–2.
19. Welder V, Guggenheim M, Moron M, Kunzj W, Meyer VE. Extensive hydrofluoric acid injuries: a serious problem. J Trauma. 2005;58:852–7.
20. Dunser MW, Ohlbauer M, Rieder J, Zimmermann I, et al. Critical care management of major hydrofluoric acid burns: a case report, review of the literature, and recommendatoons for therapy. Burns. 2004;30: 391–8.

21. Vance MV, Curry SC, Kunkel DB, Ryan PJ, Ruggeri SB. Digital hydrofluoric acid burns: treatment with intraarterial calcium infusion. Ann Emerg Med. 1986;15:890–6.
22. Mayer TG, Gross PL. Fatal systemic fluorosis due to hydrofluoric acid burns. Ann Emerg Med. 1985;14:149–53.
23. Mullett T, Zoeller T, Bingham H, et al. Fatal hydrofluoric acid cutaneous exposure with refractory ventricular fibrillation. J Burn Care Rehabil. 1987;8:216–9.
24. Trevino MA, Herrmann GH, Sprout WL. Treatment of severe hydrofluoric acid exposures. J Occup Med. 1983;25:861–3.
25. Edelman P. Hydroflouric acid burns. Occup Med. 1986;1:89–103.
26. Lin TM, Tsai CC, Lin SD, Lai CS. Continuous intra-arterial infusion therapy in hydrofluoric acid burns. J Occup Environ Med. 2000;42:892–7.
27. Köhnlein HE, Achinger R. A new method of treatment of hydrofluoric acid burns of the extremities. Chir Plast. 1982;6:297–305.
28. Siegel DC, Heard JM. Intraarterial calcium infusion for hydrofluoric acid burns. Aviat Space Environ Med. 1992;63:206–11.
29. Nguyen L, Mohr W, Ahrenholz D, et al. Treatment of hydrofluoric acid burns to the face by carotid artery infusion of calcium gluconate. J Burn Care Rehabil. 2004;25:421–4.
30. Poupon M, Caye N, Duteille F, Pannier M. Cement burns: retrospective study of 18 cases and review of the literature. Burns. 2005;31:910–4.
31. Barillo DJ, Cancio LC, Goodwin CW. Treatment of white phosphorous and other chemical burn injuries at one burn center over a 51 year period. Burns. 2004;30(5):448–52.

Cold Injuries

17

Amalia Cochran

Nonfreezing Cold Injury

Pernio, or chilblain, is a mild form of nonfreezing cold injury resulting from cold-induced vasculitis and associated with repeated non-immersive exposure to temperatures just above freezing. Patchy areas of erythema and cyanosis with purple-hued plaques and nodules characterize it; no freezing of the tissue occurs. Pernio is most commonly seen on the face, anterior tibia, and hands and feet. Treatment in the period surrounding a pernio injury is to get the patient to warm shelter where they can gradually rewarm. It is often self-limited with resolution within 2 weeks of injury, but areas of epidermal injury may blister, ulcerate, scar, or atrophy [1]. Patients may experience pain, pruritis, and recurrence of dermopathy with future cold exposures.

Nonfreezing injury of the feet and hands is commonly referred to as trenchfoot or immersion foot. Chronic or repeated exposure to wet conditions at temperatures between 1 and 10 °C causes injury to sympathetic nerves and blood vessels, particularly in the extremities. In the early vasospastic phase, the tissue is cold to the touch and is essentially insensate. Approximately 24–48 h after the initial exposure and rewarming, the involved tissue becomes hyperemic with blisters, erythema, and ulceration; intense pain also characterizes this vasodilated phase of the injury. Because of the moisture component, nonfreezing cold injury has a particular risk for development of cellulitis and therefore should be monitored closely. An additional phase may occur with a secondary exposure 2–6 weeks following the initial injury in which the tissue becomes cyanotic and the patient has heightened sensitivity to cold in the affected area.

Management recommendations for nonfreezing cold injury include removal from the cold environment and slow, dry rewarming of the affected extremity or extremities. Elevation helps to ameliorate edema formation, and pressure-bearing areas should be padded and protected from secondary injury. The worst sequelae of nonfreezing cold injury derive from the damage to the sympathetic nerves and blood vessels, and include persistent edema and hyperhidrosis, or severe chronic neuropathic pain with ulceration and tissue loss [2]. Almost all patients who sustain nonfreezing cold injury will have long-term increased cold sensitivity.

Frostbite

The key differentiating characteristic between nonfreezing cold injury and freezing cold injury (frostbite) is the development of ice crystals in

A. Cochran, M.D., F.A.C.S. (✉)
Department of Surgery, University of Utah, Healthcare, 30 North 1900 East, SOM 3B110, Salt Lake City, UT 84132, USA
e-mail: amalia.cochran@hsc.utah.edu

D.G. Greenhalgh (ed.), *Burn Care for General Surgeons and General Practitioners*,
DOI 10.1007/978-3-319-29161-1_17

and around the cells of the affected tissues in frostbite. Frostbite may be characterized as superficial, traditionally known as first and second degree, or deep, traditionally described as third or fourth degree; these clinical categorizations are similar to those for burn injuries.

The best means of treatment for frostbite is primary prevention. The homeless and mentally ill are the most persistent population of frostbite patients, with alcohol and drug use exacerbating the risk of frostbite injury [3, 4]. Frostbite has become more common in the USA due to increasing interest in wilderness and adventure activities, particularly extreme sports during inclement weather. Measures to decrease frostbite risk during cold-weather wilderness activity include wearing appropriate dry and wind/water-resistant clothing, seeking appropriate shelter in response to changing conditions, and performing "cold checks" of at-risk or suspect areas [2, 5].

Clinical Presentation of Frostbite

Frostnip is the mildest form of freezing cold injury and is a transient epidermal process with no resulting dermal involvement. Numbness and tingling occurs in the affected body part and the involved skin becomes pale and insensate. The skin is hyperemic upon rewarming and blistering does not occur. Of note, no ice crystal formation occurs to cause residual damage to the tissues if the patient is removed from the cold environment and rewarmed, though it may serve as a harbinger of more severe freezing cold injury if shelter is not sought.

Frostbite is the most severe type of cold tissue injury and may result in tissue necrosis and loss in its most pronounced form. Tissue damage sustained from frostbite is the result of microvascular thrombosis and electrolyte content changes in the frozen tissues, as well as subsequent ischemia–reperfusion injury with rewarming. In superficial frostbite, the characteristic vesicles contain clear fluid and the underlying tissues are characterized by limited, if any, dermal involvement (see Fig. 17.1). Long-term tissue loss should not occur in superficial frostbite with rapid rewarming and appropriate local tissue care. In contrast, deep frostbite vesicles are hemorrhagic due to the presence of subdermal injury (see Fig. 17.2). Even with rapid rewarming and best local wound care, permanent tissue loss will result. Deep frostbite can injure to the level of tendon and bone and typically progresses to thick, black eschar over the weeks following initial injury (see Fig. 17.3).

Management of Frostbite

Initial and Field Management

Systemic cold injury often accompanies local frostbite injury. Since hypothermia is life threatening, it should be managed before formal treatment of frostbite is initiated. Frostbitten tissue is

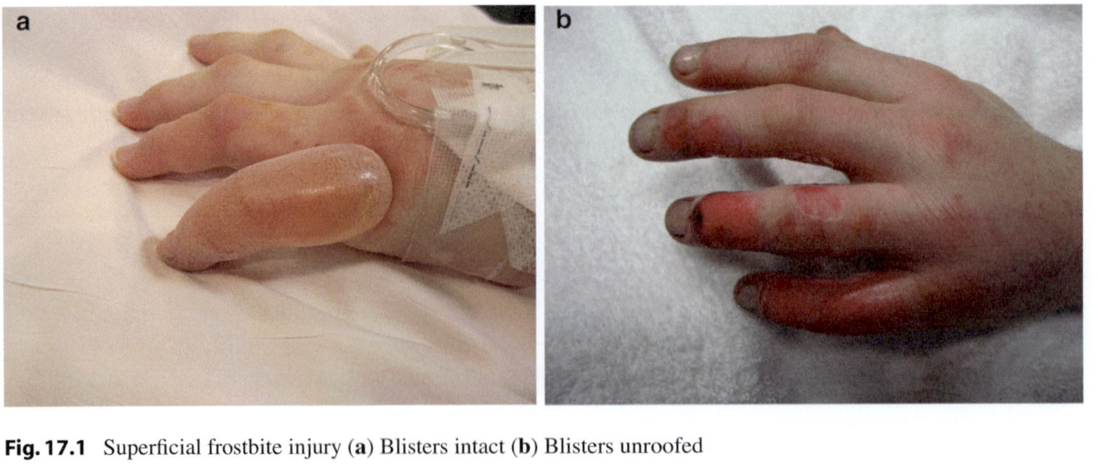

Fig. 17.1 Superficial frostbite injury (**a**) Blisters intact (**b**) Blisters unroofed

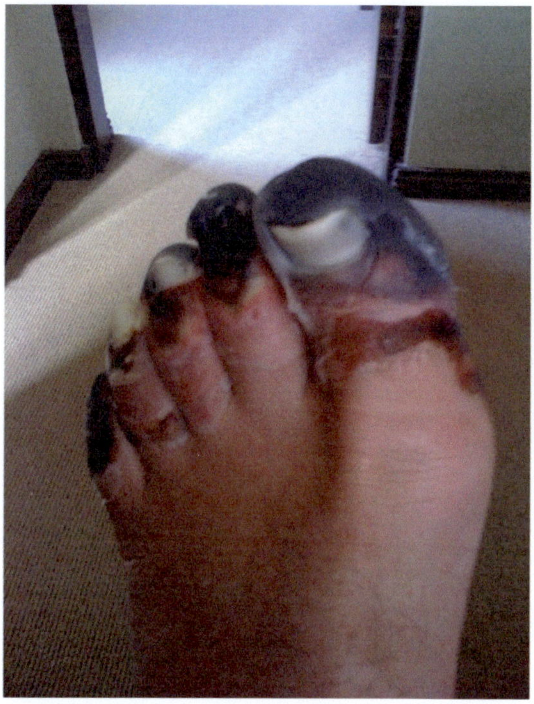

Fig. 17.2 Deep frostbite injury with hemorrhagic vesicles

extremely fragile and is at risk for further damage and therefore it should be handled gently at all times. Historical recommendations for rubbing affected parts in ice and snow are now understood to potentially cause further tissue damage and should be disregarded. If a patient with frostbite is at risk of refreezing the involved tissue in the very short term (e.g., an Alpine expedition in which evacuation may be delayed), it is preferable to not proceed with formal rewarming until the patient can safely reach definitive care; refreezing and rethawing is more damaging to the affected tissue than maintaining it in a frozen state [6]. Injured areas are typically insensate and therefore should also be carefully mechanically protected during transport and during long-term care of frostbite injury.

The current State of Alaska guidelines recommend rewarming of frostbitten extremities in a circulating water bath of 37–39 °C. This temperature range does not substantially increase the time to rewarming from previous recommendations of 40 °C but results in less pain for the patient during the rewarming process [2, 7]. Formal thawing in a water bath usually occurs in about 30 min, but may require as little as 15 min or as long as an hour [2]. Clinical findings that demonstrate rewarming include return of sensation, most often manifested as significant pain in the cold injured extremity, flushing at the distal aspect of involved extremities, and pliability of previously frozen tissues [7]. Because of the pain associated with rewarming, administration of narcotics is appropriate [8]. In addition, because these are tetanus-prone wounds, the patient's tetanus immunization should be verified and updated as appropriate [2, 5, 7, 9].

Post-thaw Management

The timing of patient presentation with frostbite influences the available management options. Patients who arrive at a site for definitive management within 24 h of their thaw time are considered an acute presentation and have a broader range of therapeutic options. Delayed presentations of frostbite occur more than 24 h after tissue thawing, sometimes days to weeks later.

Nonsurgical Therapies

Local care to protect and heal the soft tissues is the top priority once rewarming is complete. Unroofing of blisters is a matter of controversy and current recommendations leave this to provider discretion [5, 9]. The most practical justification for unroofing blisters is the improvement in the clinician's ability to assess the status of the underlying tissues. Heggers' work more than 25 years ago showed that high levels of pro-inflammatory cytokines $PGF_{2\alpha}$ and TXB_2, as well as diminished levels of anti-inflammatory PGE_2, are present in blister fluid following both burns and frostbite [10–12]. This altered chemokine milieu results in vasoconstriction of the involved tissue, increased leukocyte adherence, and increased platelet aggregation, all of which cause progressive dermal ischemia;[11, 13] this scientific work suggests that blister debridement may limit further local tissue damage. Hemorrhagic blisters have a slightly different pathophysiology, with the hemorrhage occurring due to damage to subdermal structures. Therefore,

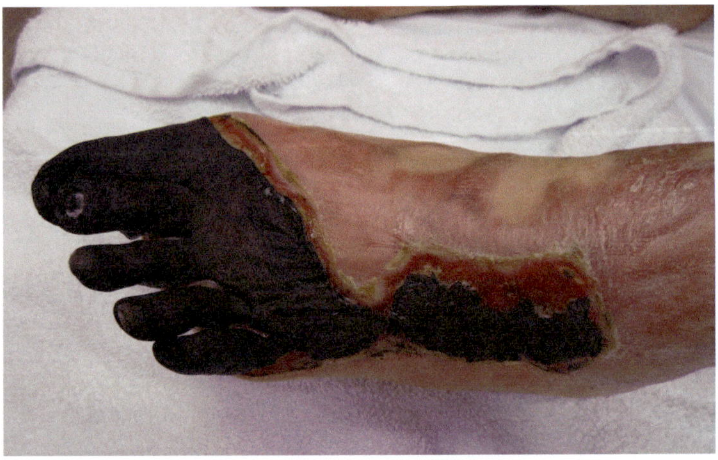

Fig. 17.3 Deep frostbite injury with dry gangrene and mummification, 8 weeks post-injury

debridement of these blisters may worsen the underlying soft tissue injury [14].

Aloe vera counteracts the arachidonic acid cascade and therefore may have value as a topical agent in the care of frostbitten areas. Multimodal therapy using oral NSAIDs, topical aloe vera, and systemic penicillin resulted in less tissue loss, fewer amputations, and decreased hospital stay versus patients managed with traditional topical antimicrobials [15]. Topical aloe vera alone was credited with clinically significant tissue salvage in these patients, and subsequent recommendations have called for the use of aloe vera rather than topical antimicrobials like silver sulfadiazine or mafenide acetate [2, 5, 9, 15]. Local tissue care should include mechanical protection of injured areas by careful padding and splinting, as well as elevation to limit edema formation [5, 7, 9, 14]. Routine antibiotic prophylaxis is not supported by evidence [5]; current recommendations limit systemic antibiotic use to coverage of skin flora in patients who are experiencing significant edema and therefore are at risk of developing soft tissue infection [2, 9].

Pharmacologic management of the frostbite patient includes blockade of the arachidonic acid pathway to counteract the systemic inflammatory response to local cold injury. The use of ibuprofen, which specifically blocks TXA_2, provides the most effective NSAID management in frostbite [2, 5, 7]. Pentoxifylline, a phosphodiesterase inhibitor primarily used in claudication, improves red blood cell flexibility and may decrease blood viscosity, which may limit microvascular sludging and thereby diminish thrombus formation in small vessels. Pentoxifylline has been shown in an animal model to improve tissue viability in conjunction with topical aloe vera [16]. Current recommendations for dosing of pentoxifylline at 400 mg TID for 2–6 weeks following injury are based upon a single study of pedal frostbite [17]. Potential benefit for iloprost, a prostacyclin analogue that also serves as a vasodilator, has been demonstrated, although all data are preliminary and it is not currently available for use in the USA [18]. Studies of both pentoxifylline and iloprost in frostbite are ongoing in Europe and their use should not yet be considered as standard of care, though in time both may provide good pharmacologic options in frostbite.

The most notable clinical advances in the care of frostbite in the last 50 years have centered on thrombolytic therapy. Publications from the two groups in Minneapolis–St. Paul and the Center in Utah have shown significantly improved digit salvage with the use of tissue plasminogen activator (t-PA) [19–21]. Current data indicate that the benefits of t-PA in the management of frostbite are limited because it is only effective within 24 h of thaw, meaning it may not be an option for patients who are injured in austere and remote environments. While digital salvage is improved with the use of TPA, the long-term functional impact of this salvage has not been documented to date.

Imaging and Surgical Management

Scintigraphy may have benefits in shortening the time line for surgical management of frostbite injury, which is historically based upon the adage, "Frostbite in January, amputation in July." Over 20 years ago, Mehta found that perfusion and blood pooling phases demonstrated at-risk tissue and the bone phase showed deep tissue and bone infarction within 4 days of injury [22]. Scintigraphic studies have been shown to correlate with surgical findings in several studies, although the correlation may be best at 7–10 days following injury [23, 24]. Two different protocols have been published using the findings from scintigraphy to direct early surgery following frostbite injury [25, 26]. Greenwald's protocol uses early scintigraphy followed by operative intervention at 7–10 days following injury [25]. Cauchy extends the time frame for early operative intervention to 10–15 days post injury with bone scan, citing the rationale of decreased waiting time for the patient, decreased infection risk, and earlier progression to rehabilitation [26]. Adoption of either protocol has been limited based upon worse historical frostbite outcomes with early surgery, meaning that the prevalent clinical practice remains to time surgery anywhere from 4 weeks to 3 months following injury [8, 9]. This provides time for tissues to clearly demarcate to a clinician experienced in the care of frostbite.

Unintentional Hypothermia

In distinction to the morbid but not mortal nature of tissue-based cold injury, hypothermia is associated with significant mortality. From 2003 to 2013 in the USA, more than 13,000 deaths occurred that were attributable to hypothermia [27]. Death from hypothermia is more likely to occur in older males, and is more common among the mentally ill and in association with intoxication [27]. Primary hypothermia is caused solely by cold environmental exposure. Secondary hypothermia includes an environmental exposure with a mitigating factor that diminishes the patient's ability to thermoregulate [28]. Both types of environmental hypothermia result in a progressive response with loss of adaptation as patient core temperature decreases to below 35 °C. Factors that may exacerbate cold exposure include age, general health, and intoxication; each of these may impair a patient's ability to respond to cold exposure, worsening the severity of hypothermia.

Physiologic Response to Environmental Hypothermia

Because of the characteristic progression of hypothermia, it is commonly classified into a spectrum of mild, moderate, and severe. These

Table 17.1 Physiologic findings based upon severity of hypothermia

Severity	Cardiac	Respiratory	Renal/electrolytes	Neurologic
Mild (32–35 °C)	Tachycardia; normal blood pressure	Tachypnea	No notable changes	Progressive confusion
Moderate (28–32 °C)	Arrhythmias; J wave on EKG; decreased heart rate and blood pressure	Decreased respiratory rate, progressive respiratory acidosis	"Cold diuresis;" hyperkalemia; hyperglycemia	Stupor; muscle rigidity; pupillary dilation
Severe (≤28 °C)	Susceptibility to ventricular fibrillation or asystole; hypotension	Apnea; pulmonary edema	Continued cold diuresis; major acid-base disturbances	Arreflexia with flaccid muscles; loss of consciousness; loss of pupillary response

Table 17.2 Laboratory test findings in hypothermia

Laboratory test	Findings of relevance (severity of hypothermia)
Amylase	Hyperamylasemia (moderate or severe)
Arterial blood gas	Decreased pCO_2 (moderate or severe) Decreased pO_2 (moderate or severe) Decreased pH (moderate or severe)
Coagulation profile	Elevated prothrombin time (moderate) Elevated partial thromboplastin time (moderate) Disseminated intravascular coagulopathy (severe)
Complete blood count	Elevated hemoglobin and hematocrit (moderate) Decreased hemoglobin and hematocrit (severe)
Complete metabolic panel	Hyperkalemia (moderate or severe) Hyperglycemia (moderate or severe) Elevated transaminases (severe)
Creatine kinase	Elevated CK (severe)
Lactic acid	Lactic acidosis (moderate or severe)

categories are clinically meaningful, both for the physiologic responses within each (see Table 17.1) and in terms of the optimal management strategy based upon severity.

In the mild stages of hypothermia (32–35 °C) thermoregulation is still intact and patients will present with shivering as their body attempts to rewarm through an increased metabolic rate. These patients may also have elevations in heart rate and respiratory rate, again associated with physiologic attempts at compensation. Confusion can occur with mild hypothermia, resulting in patients not realizing their need for warmth or in disorientation as they seek an environment for rewarming.

Thermoregulation and shivering both are lost with moderate hypothermia (28–32 °C). In contrast to the hypermetabolic, hyperdynamic physiology observed in mild hypothermia, these patients become bradycardic and typically will have evidence of hypoventilation. The moderately hypothermic patient will show signs of agitation with progression to somnolence—again, a significant danger if patients are isolated in a remote or austere environment.

Severe hypothermia (≤28 °C) is characterized by ongoing rapid cooling; patients can progress quickly from mild to severe hypothermia once they lose their ability to thermoregulate. A characteristic EKG finding in patients with severe hypothermia is the presence of a J (Osborne) wave; the Osborne wave does not have prognostic significance, in contrast to the association of atrial fibrillation and junctional bradycardia with mortality [29]. Because of the severely depressed metabolic rate, patients with severe hypothermia may present in asystole and with apnea. From a neurologic standpoint, these patients are usually comatose.

Evaluation and Management

Initial evaluation of the patient with hypothermia involves determination of the severity of their hypothermia. Many of the traditional methods for determining temperature are inaccurate in this patient population, requiring use of a calibrated low-reading thermometer or by insertion of a thermistor probe into the lower third of the esophagus [30]. Patients with mild hypothermia can be successfully managed in the field with appropriate training and resource availability if there are no associated injuries or medical conditions requiring a higher level of care; patients with moderate to severe hypothermia require transfer to a medical center as soon as safely possible. While in transport, these patients should be handled gently and kept horizontal because of the risk of ventricular fibrillation [7]. Because of the life-threatening nature of hypothermia, patients who have cold injury to their tissues should be systemically warmed before treatment of their tissue injury is initiated.

Several basic laboratory values can be helpful in the initial management of the patient with moderate to severe hypothermia. These values and key findings for each are presented in Table 17.2. Metabolic panel abnormalities are particularly relevant in severe hypothermia because of their impact on patient care strategies. Insulin therapy for hyperglycemia is not recommended because of the potential for rebound hyperglycemia with rewarming. In addition, ongoing clinical treatment of hypothermia in a patient with a serum potassium level greater than 10 mmol per liter is controversial, and greater than 12 mmol per liter is considered futile [30].

Formal evidence for the use of different rewarming techniques for environmental hypothermia is limited; clinical practice is usually driven by physiologic principles. In general, rewarming practices include the use of passive rewarming for mild hypothermia and escalating levels of intensity of active rewarming for more severe hypothermia. Passive warming is noninvasive and involves the patient's removal from the cold environment, coupled with placement of blankets or other insulative materials. In order for passive warming to be effective, the patient's ability to thermoregulate must still be intact, meaning that it is only effective in mild hypothermia.

In contrast, active warming may be external or internal, and involves direct transfer of heat to the patient. The use of active techniques for moderate to severe hypothermia is driven by the loss of thermoregulation in these patients and their risks of cardiac arrhythmias. Active external rewarming includes the use of warming blankets or forced air blankets, heating pads, overhead heaters, or immersion in warm water. A key caution with most external rewarming techniques is the potential for thermal injury to the hypoperfused skin. Active internal, or core, rewarming is often used in conjunction with active external techniques and may be the central focus for rewarming of a severely hypothermic patients. Active core measures include heated intravenous fluids, peritoneal or thoracic lavage with warm fluids, and heating of air for ventilated patients. Extracorporeal rewarming is typically reserved for the most severe cases of hypothermia, including patients in full cardiac arrest, and has shown reasonable survival results in this population [31]. Multiple techniques exist for extracorporeal blood rewarming, including creation of a venovenous circuit, use of a hemodialysis or arteriovenous circuit, or cardiopulmonary bypass. The key disadvantage of cardiopulmonary bypass lies in the need for systemic anticoagulation in a patient population with a preexisting coagulopathy resulting from hypothermia.

References

1. Golant A, Nord RM, Paksima N, Posner MA. Cold exposure injuries to the extremities. J Am Acad Orthop Surg. 2008;16(12):704–15.
2. Imray C, Grieve A, Dhillon S. Cold damage to the extremities: frostbite and non-freezing cold injuries. Postgr Med J. 2009;85(1007):481–8.
3. Kowal-Vern A, Latenser BA. Demographics of the homeless in an urban burn unit. J Burn Care Res. 2007;28(1):105–10.
4. Pinzur MS, Weaver FM. Is urban frostbite a psychiatric disorder? Orthopedics. 1997;20(1):43–5.
5. McIntosh SE, Opacic M, Freer L, Grissom CK, Auerbach PS, Rodway GW, et al. Wilderness Medical Society practice guidelines for the prevention and treatment of frostbite: 2014 update. Wilderness Environ Med. 2014;25(4 Suppl):S43–54.
6. Mills WJ, Whaley R. Frostbite: experience with rapid re-warming and ultrasonic therapy. Alaska Med. 1960;35(6).
7. Mills WJ, Medical EMS. State of Alaska cold injuries guidelines. 2014. http://dhss.alaska.gov/dph/Emergency/Documents/ems/documents/Alaska%20DHSS%20EMS%20Cold%20Injuries%20Guidelines%20June%202014.pdf. Accessed March 15, 2015.
8. Jurkovich GJ. Environmental cold-induced injury. Surg Clin North Am. 2007;87(1):247–67. viii.
9. Mohr WJ, Jenabzadeh K, Ahrenholz DH. Cold injury. Hand Clin. 2009;25(4):481–96.
10. Heggers JP, Ko F, Robson MC, Heggers R, Craft KE. Evaluation of burn blister fluid. Plast Reconstr Surg. 1980;65(6):798–804.
11. Robson MC, Heggers JP. Evaluation of hand frostbite blister fluid as a clue to pathogenesis. J Hand Surg Am. 1981;6(1):43–7.
12. Heggers JP, Loy GL, Robson MC, Del Beccaro EJ. Histological demonstration of prostaglandins and thromboxanes in burned tissue. J Surg Res. 1980; 28(2):110–7.
13. Robson MC, Del Beccaro EJ, Heggers JP. The effect of prostaglandins on the dermal microcirculation after

burning, and the inhibition of the effect by specific pharmacological agents. Plast Reconstr Surg. 1979;63(6):781–7.

14. McCauley RL, Hing DN, Robson MC, Heggers JP. Frostbite injuries: a rational approach based on the pathophysiology. J Trauma. 1983;23(2):143–7.
15. Heggers JP, Robson MC, Manavalen K, Weingarten MD, Carethers JM, Boertman JA, et al. Experimental and clinical observations on frostbite. Ann Emerg Med. 1987;16(9):1056–62.
16. Miller MB, Koltai PJ. Treatment of experimental frostbite with pentoxifylline and aloe vera cream. Arch Otolaryngol Head Neck Surg. 1995;121(6):678–80.
17. Hayes Jr DW, Mandracchia VJ, Considine C, Webb GE. Pentoxifylline. Adjunctive therapy in the treatment of pedal frostbite. Clin Pod Med Surg. 2000;17(4):715–22.
18. Cauchy E, Cheguillaume B, Chetaille E. A controlled trial of a prostacyclin and rt-PA in the treatment of severe frostbite. N Engl J Med. 2011;364(2):189–90.
19. Twomey JA, Peltier GL, Zera RT. An open-label study to evaluate the safety and efficacy of tissue plasminogen activator in treatment of severe frostbite. J Trauma. 2005;59(6):1350–5.
20. Bruen KJ, Ballard JR, Morris SE, Cochran A, Edelman LS, Saffle JR. Reduction of the incidence of amputation in frostbite injury with thrombolytic therapy. Arch Surg. 2007;142(6):543–6.
21. Gonzaga T, Jenabzadeh K, Anderson CP, Mohr WJ, Endorf FW, Ahrenholz DH. Use of intraarterial thrombolytic therapy for acute treatment of frostbite in 62 patients with review of thrombolytic therapy in frostbite. J Burn Care Res. 2015;24.
22. Mehta RC, Wilson MA. Frostbite injury: prediction of tissue viability with triple-phase bone scanning. Radiology. 1989;170(2):511–4.
23. Cauchy E, Chetaille E, Lefevre M, Kerelou E, Marsigny B. The role of bone scanning in severe frostbite of the extremities: a retrospective study of 88 cases. Eur J Nucl Med. 2000;27(5):497–502.
24. Cauchy E, Marsigny B, Allamel G, Verhellen R, Chetaille E. The value of technetium 99 scintigraphy in the prognosis of amputation in severe frostbite injuries of the extremities: a retrospective study of 92 severe frostbite injuries. J Hand Surg Am. 2000;25(5): 969–78.
25. Greenwald D, Cooper B, Gottlieb L. An algorithm for early aggressive treatment of frostbite with limb salvage directed by triple-phase scanning. Plast Reconstr Surg. 1998;102(4):1069–74.
26. Cauchy E, Chetaille E, Marchand V, Marsigny B. Retrospective study of 70 cases of severe frostbite lesions: a proposed new classification scheme. Wilderness Env Med. 2001;12(4):248–55.
27. Hypothermia-related deaths – Wisconsin, 2014, and United States, 2003–2013 Accessed 9 Jun, 2015 from http://www.cdc.gov/mmwr/preview/mmwrhtml/mm6406a2.htm.
28. Jurkovich GJ. Environmental injuries. In: Mulholland MW, Lillemoe KD, Doherty GM, Maier RV, Simeone DM, Upchurch GR, editors. Greenfield's surgery: scientific principles and practice. 5th ed. Philadelphia, PA: Lippincott Williams and Wilkins; 2010. p. 466–85.
29. Graham CA, McNaughton GW, Wyatt JP. The electrocardiogram in hypothermia. Wilderness Environ Med. 2001;12(4):232–5.
30. Brown DJA, Brugger H, Boyd J, Paal P. Accidental hypothermia. N Engl J Med. 2012;367(20):1930–8.
31. Walpoth BH, Walpoth-Aslan BN, Mattle HP, Radanov BP, Schroth G, Schaeffler L, et al. Outcome of survivors of accidental deep hypothermia and circulatory arrest treated with extracorporeal blood warming. N Engl J Med. 1997;337(21):1500–5.

Exfoliating and Necrotizing Soft Tissue Diseases

18

Kevin N. Foster

Introduction

Burn centers often manage skin diseases other than acute thermal injuries. These skin diseases are typically categorized as exfoliating and necrotizing soft tissue diseases, and include toxic epidermal necrolysis (TENS) or Stevens–Johnson syndrome (SJS), necrotizing soft tissue infections (NSTI), and purpura fulminans (PF). The severity of these diseases may vary from mild and local with minimal systemic manifestations to 100 % total body surface area (TBSA) involvement with severe, multisystem dysfunction. The unifying characteristic of these diseases is skin and soft tissue compromise and thus these patients are best managed in burn centers with expertise in wound care.

K.N. Foster, M.D., M.B.A., F.A.C.S. (✉)
Department of Surgery, The Arizona Burn Center at Maricopa Integrated Health System, 2601 E Roosevelt, Phoenix, AZ 85008, USA
e-mail: kevin_foster@dmgaz.org

Toxic Epidermal Necrolysis and Stevens–Johnson Syndrome

Definitions

TENS and SJS represent different points on a severity spectrum of exfoliating skin diseases [1–3]. There are multiple classification schemes for these diseases. A simple and useful classification stratifies the disease into two entities based on the degree of cutaneous involvement. Consensus publications usually define SJS when the skin involvement is less than 10 % TBSA and TENS when the skin involvement is greater than 30 % TBSA. When the skin lesions are between 10 and 30 % TBSA, this is labeled as SJS-TENS overlap [4]. However, in the USA, it is common to refer the disease as SJS when the skin disease is less than 30 % and TENS when it is greater than 30 % [5]. This simple convention will be followed here. Both SJS and TENS also manifest additional mucosal surface lesions (e.g., eye, mouth, and gastrointestinal tract). The lack of additional mucosal involvement should bring the diagnosis of either SJS or TENS into question. For simplicity sake, the following manuscript uses the term TENS/SJS to refer to this spectrum of exfoliating skin diseases.

D.G. Greenhalgh (ed.), *Burn Care for General Surgeons and General Practitioners*,
DOI 10.1007/978-3-319-29161-1_18

Etiology and Pathogenesis

Most cases of TENS/SJS are caused by a reaction to a newly administered medication [4, 6–8]. Many causative medications and groups of medications have been described but the most frequently implicated drugs can be grouped as follows:

- Antibiotics, particularly sulfonamides, β lactams, and quinolones.
- Anticonvulsants, such as phenytoin, carbamazepine, and phenobarbital.
- Nonsteroidal anti-inflammatory drugs (NSAIDS).

Additionally, upper respiratory infections, acute pharyngitis, otitis media, *Mycoplasma pneumonia* infections, and viral infections, including HIV, have been associated with the development of TENS/SJS [9]. It is not unusual for a patient with TENS/SJS to report no new medications or preceding illness. There is sound evidence that TENS/SJS may have a genetic component [10, 11].

The pathogenesis of TENS/SJS involves a medication-induced immune reaction against keratinocyte and mucosal epithelial cells resulting in apoptotic-type death in these cells followed by subsequent widespread epithelial necrosis and sloughing. The precise mechanisms of this process remain elusive. The immune reaction appears to be a T-cell mediated process similar to graft versus host disease. Pro-apoptotic signals such as tumor necrosis factor alpha (TNF-α), Fas-FasL, and granzyme B are also overexpressed and elevated in TENS/SJS patients. Perforin, a cytotoxin produced by killer lymphocytes, is elevated early [4, 5]. Interleukins 6 and 10 are also elevated [12, 13].

Clinical Features and Diagnosis

TENS/SJS often begins with fever, lethargy, and myalgia. This may be accompanied by cough, dysphagia, vomiting, and/or diarrhea. It is not unusual for the rash to present either before or without these generalized symptoms.

The rash is erythematous and macular with lesions of differing sizes. The rash tends to begin on the trunk symmetrically and progress centrifugally. The lesions tend to expand in size and then coalesce. As fluid accumulates within the individual maculae, they begin to appear as target lesions with a dark center and lighter periphery. At this time, the lesions may spontaneously slough. Alternately, manual pressure on the blistered lesions may cause sloughing. This is referred to a Nikolsky's sign. Nikolsky's sign is not pathognomonic for this disease, and lack of the sign does not rule out the disease. Once blistering and sloughing as started, it typically progresses rapidly and may advance to total epidermal loss (see Figs. 18.1, 18.2, 18.3, and 18.4).

Histologic examination reveals sloughing at the epidermal–dermal junction and keratinocyte necrosis. There may be a slight inflammatory infiltrate of lymphocytes and mononuclear cells, but the inflammation is rarely extensive.

Involvement of the blistering and sloughing process involves other mucosal surface with stratified epithelial surfaces. The mouth and upper gastrointestinal tracts are often involved

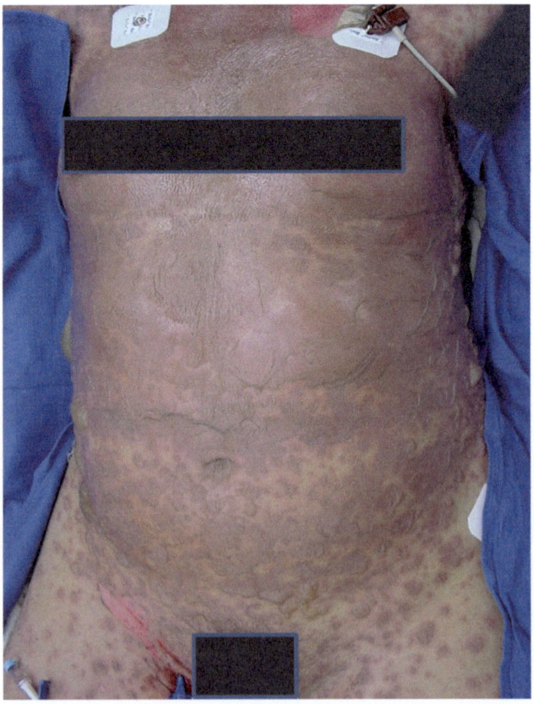

Fig. 18.1 TENS/SJS target lesions and blisters

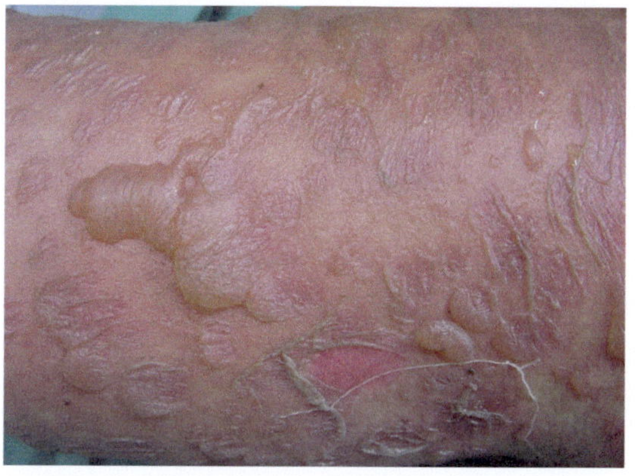

Fig. 18.2 TENS/SJS Nikolsy's sign

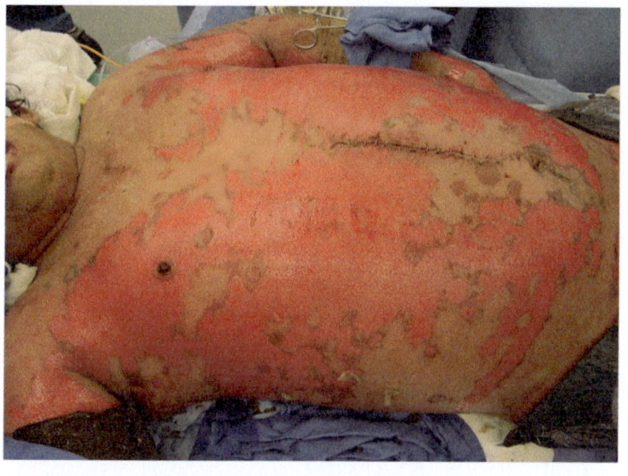

Fig. 18.3 TEN/SJS desquamating lesions

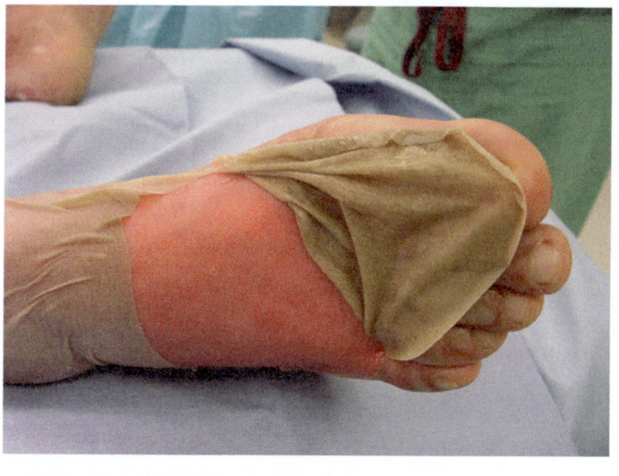

Fig. 18.4 TEN/SJS desquamating lesions

leading to dysphagia and inability to eat and drink normally. Involvement of the upper respiratory tract may cause cough and shortness of breath. Patients often require intubation. Ocular involvement can cause conjunctivitis and subsequent bacterial superinfection. Finally, the vagina and anus can also be affected [14, 15].

The diagnosis can often be made based on history and physical examination alone. However, if the diagnosis is unclear, it can be confirmed with skin biopsy at the border of one of the lesions followed by histology [16]. The differential diagnosis of TENS/SJS includes staphylococcal scalded skin syndrome, erythema multiforme, pemphigus vulgaris or bullous pemphigoid, and impetigo or other infectious skin disorders.

Treatment

Treatment of TENS/SJS includes supportive care, wound management, and specific pharmacologic or immune therapies and interventions. Patients should be cared for in or transferred to a burn center or wound care center staffed with health care professionals who have experience in treating this disease process and caring for complex wounds [17, 18].

Supportive care begins with prompt discontinuation of any possible inciting medications. Fluid and electrolyte repletion is performed with intravenous fluid resuscitation. The volume of fluid replacement is dictated subsequent urinary output [19]. Analgesia and anxiolysis using intravenous medications are initiated. Nutrition is important for wound healing and must be pursued aggressively. If patients are able to tolerate PO intake, they should be allowed to do so. Often the oral and/or gastrointestinal involvement precludes this. Under these circumstances and feeding tube is placed and enteral nutrition provided. It is rare for patients to require total parenteral nutrition. Venous thromboembolism and stress ulcer prophylaxis are provided. Prophylactic antibiotics are not indicated. Antibiotics should be administered for strongly suspected or documented infectious complications only. Patients should have physical and occupational therapy as tolerated.

The primary goals in wound management in TENS/SJS are to provide a moist healing environment and to prevent infection. Once the sloughing process has begun, gentle debridement and removal of the nonviable and exfoliated epidermis is indicted. Debrided wounds must be dressed to facilitate healing and to prevent infection. The ideal wound dressing will not impede the normal healing process, will protect the wound from desiccation and absorb exudate thus avoiding maceration, will prevent infection, be easy to apply and comfortable. Numerous dressings meet the above criteria and have been used successfully. These include topical antibiotics such as silver sulfadiazine or sulfamylon cream, bismuth impregnated gauze, calcium alginate, biologic materials such as xenograft (pig skin) or allograft (cadaver skin), or a synthetic bilaminar membrane. Recently, silver dressings have been used successfully. These include silver impregnated hydrofiber or silver impregnated foam dressings [20–25].

Specific pharmacological or immune therapies have not been shown to have definitive benefit in TENS/SJS [26]. Nevertheless, several of these therapies are still routinely used in some centers. Probably the most common intervention used in TENS/SJS is the administration of corticosteroids. For many years corticosteroids were used because of the potential effect on blunting the immune system and thus hopefully alleviating TENS/SJS symptoms. Today there is no evidence that corticosteroids have any utility in TENS/SJS; indeed, some investigators think corticosteroids may be detrimental because of the possibility of increased infectious complications. Other immunosuppressive agents such as cyclophosphamide, cyclosporine, and infliximab have also not been shown to have definitive benefit.

Plasmapheresis is a process where plasma, the acellular liquid component of blood is separated and removed from the cellular component. The plasma component contains antibodies and presumably its removal will also remove the pathogenic antibodies responsible for causing TENS/SJS. There are multiple reports of successful use of plasmapheresis in TENS/SJS, but there currently is no consensus on the routine use of this treatment in TENS/SJS [4, 5, 27].

Human intravenous immunoglobulin (IVIG) is a fairly new treatment modality for TENS/SJS. IVIG is pooled human immunoglobulin that is mostly IgG. The mechanism of action of IVIG is to block the cell surface receptor that is involved in the immune complex initiation of keratinocyte apoptosis. Initial reports utilizing IVIG in the treatment of TENS/SJS demonstrated reduced mortality. Subsequent studies have shown no benefit or even worse mortality. And IVIG has potential adverse side effects. It represents a significant colloid load, it may cause renal failure and it may be associated with thromboembolic events. So at the present time it is unclear whether the efficacy and risk–benefit ratio of IVIG warrant its use in TENS/SJS [4, 5, 28].

Complications and Prognosis

Most young, healthy patients who experience uncomplicated TENS/SJS will recover completely and uneventfully within 10–14 days. Usually there are no long-term adverse sequelae. Even a large %TBSA desquamation will heal without scarring. Patients with comorbidities or patients who develop complications may have long-term adverse effects. Cutaneous events are unusual and include hypertrophic scarring, skin discoloration and nail dystrophies. Ocular complications may be the most common and serious complications following TENS/SJS. To avoid complications, early ophthalmologic consultation is recommended. Complications include dry eye, entropion, synechiae, and symblepharon. These may lead to visual impairment and even blindness [29–31]. Other gastrointestinal and urogenital complications such as tongue tethering and vaginal scarring may also occur.

SJS tends to have a better prognosis lower mortality than TENS (1–5 % compared to 25–50 %). Additionally, increasing age, multiple and/or serious comorbidity(ies), and increasing %TBSA involvement tend to confer a worse prognosis. Bastuji-Garin et al. validated a scoring system specific for TENS/SJS, which they called SCORTEN. This score assigns one point to each of seven independent variables. The mortality is based on the sum of each of these variables. This is demonstrated in Table 18.1. Several studies have validated this scoring system but other studies have demonstrated contradictory results [32–36].

Table 18.1 SCORTEN (Bastuji-Garin)

Prognostic parameter	Score
Age >40 years	1
>10 % TBSA involved	1
Malignancy	1
Heart rate > 120 BPM	1
Serum urea >28 mg/dl	1
Serum glucose >252 mg/dl	1
Serum bicarbonate <20 mEq/l	1
SCORTEN (sum)	Mortality (%)
0–1	3.2
2	12.2
3	35.3
4	58.3
≥5	90.0

Summary

- TENS/SJS is a medication-related exfoliating skin disease with necrosis of keratinocytes and sloughing of skin at the epidermal–dermal junction.
- Patients generally present with a progressive desquamating rash with or without systemic symptoms.
- The diagnosis can usually be made by history and physical examination but skin biopsy can confirm the diagnosis in equivocal cases.
- Treatment is largely supportive with meticulous wound care; specific treatments such as corticosteroids, plasmapheresis and IVIG are of unknown benefit.
- Patients should be cared for in burn centers or other centers of excellence with experience with TENS/SJS and in advanced wound care.

Necrotizing Soft Tissue Infections

Definitions

Necrotizing soft tissue infections (NSTI) are characterized by bacterial infection of the subcutaneous tissues and muscle fascia causing necrosis of these tissues. The skin is often involved, and the infection can spread to underlying muscle and, and involve underlying neurovascular structures, and even bone. These infections have previously also been grouped under the term necrotizing fasciitis in testament to the ease at which the infection can infect and spread along the muscle facial plane. However, the infection affects tissue other than the fascia and the term NSTI is preferred.

Etiology and Pathogenesis

NSTIs are caused by bacteria that colonize and then infect the subcutaneous tissue and muscle fascia. This infection then spreads through the subcutaneous tissue and muscle fascia. The most devastating from of NSTI is cause by group A bet-hemolytic *Streptococcus*, a skin bacterium that is part of the normal flora of human skin and typically is innocuous and nonpathogenic [37]. Under certain circumstances, the bacterium causes widespread and rapidly progressive necrosis of subcutaneous tissue, fascia, and skin, often leading to death in a matter of hours. Mortality for group A beta-hemolytic streptococcal NSTI is 80–100 % [38].

A second type of particularly virulent NSTI is cause by *Clostridia* species. This type of NSTI is called gas gangrene and is leads to progressive necrosis of involved tissues and a high mortality rate. Fortunately, these two forms of NSTI are fairly rare.

NSTIs are most frequently polymicrobial infections, and are combinations of gram-positive, gram-negative and anaerobic bacteria. Causative microorganisms include *Staphylococcus*, *Streptococcus*, *Enterococcus*, *Bacteroides*, and gram-negative enteric species such and *E. coli* and *Klebsiella* [39].

Three patient factors predispose to the development of NSTI. First, there is often a history of trauma or prior infection (abscess, carbuncle, furuncle, etc) that introduces bacteria into the subcutaneous spaces. This history is not always present and its lack does not exclude NSTI. Secondly, patients tend to have systemic disease that result in immunosuppression of inability to fight infection. This includes conditions such as diabetes mellitus, chronic immunosuppressive medication use, obesity, malnutrition, or intravenous drug use. Thirdly, patients may have peripheral vascular disease or poor blood supply to the infected areas.

Risk factors for the development of NSTI include: immunosuppression, diabetes mellitus, alcoholism, peripheral vascular disease, intravenous drug use, corticosteroids, HIV infection, malignancy, major trauma, and surgery. Events that precede the development of NSTI include *Varicella* infection, bone fractures, liposuction, insect bites, childbirth, and thermal injury [40].

It is noted that NSTI can occur in otherwise healthy individuals with no predisposing factors whatsoever. Regardless of bacterial type and risk factors, the bacteria gain access to the subcutaneous space, colonize and then infect the local area, and then spread locally and distally.

Clinical Features and Diagnosis

The presenting signs and symptoms and clinical features of NSTI are highly variable depending upon the causative bacteria, site of initial infection, and patient comorbidities. Typically, NSTIs begin as a localized cellulitis or abscess. The first indication that the infection may be a NSTI is failure to respond to appropriate treatment (e.g., antibiotics, drainage). NSTI should be suspected when a patient presents with a local infection that is not improving with treatment or is worsening with treatment. It is not uncommon for patients to present with a fulminant NSTI never having sought medical attention [41–43].

Patients with NSTI tend to have systemic manifestations of an infectious process and are usually toxic appearing, and have signs and symptoms of the systemic inflammatory response syndrome (SIRS). They are typically febrile, tachycardic, and tachypneic. They may be hypotensive and have mental status changes. Blood chemistry analysis typically demonstrates leukocytosis often with immature leukocytes, and possibly elevated creatinine, acidosis with a negative base excess, and elevated lactate levels.

Examination of the involved skin and soft tissues may reveal deceptively benign findings that do not herald the serious nature of the underlying infectious process. The involved skin is usually erythematous, swollen, warm, and painful. It may be difficult to differentiate an active NSTI from simple cellulitis on physical examination. Patients with NSTIs tend to be systemically much sicker than patients with uncomplicated cellulitis. Additional findings, which suggest NSTI, include the presence of crepitus, induration of overlying skin, a bluish discoloration to overlying skin, the presence of blisters or bullae, especially hemorrhagic bullae, and purulence (see Figs. 18.5 and 18.6)

Plain radiographs of the involved extremities or computed tomography of involved areas may show subcutaneous air characteristic of NSTIs, and may suggest the presence and extent of necrosis especially myonecrosis. However, radiographic studies have relatively low sensitivity and specificity and take time to perform. A biopsy may show necrosis and the presence of bacteria.

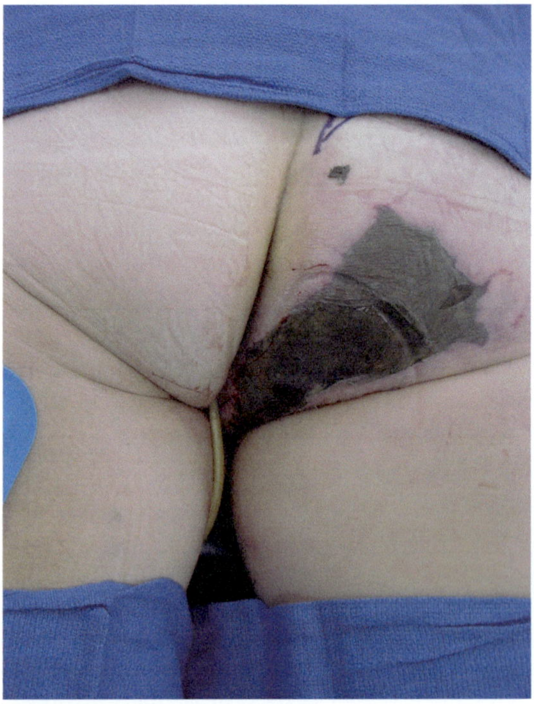

Fig. 18.5 NSTI necrotic skin lesion

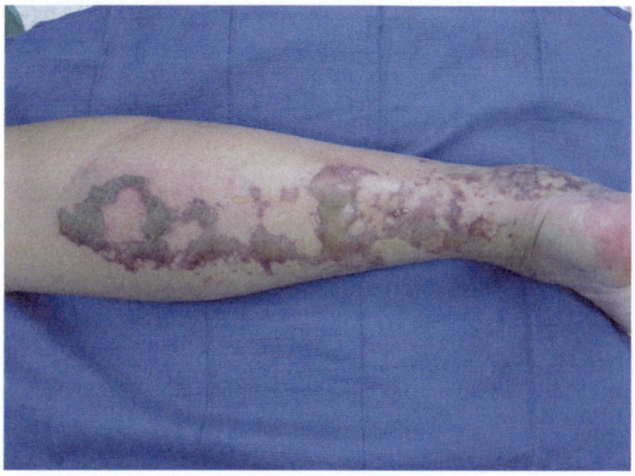

Fig. 18.6 NSTI hemorrhagic blisters

A subsequent Gram's staining may indicate whether the infection is gram-positive or gram-negative.

The diagnosis of NSTI is a clinical diagnosis and must be made on the skin and soft tissue findings on physical examination and the systemic toxicity of the patient. The ultimate diagnosis is made at the time of surgical exploration. If the diagnosis is unclear, the safest clinical course is to take the patient to the operating room for exploration. Surgical exploration in these circumstances can truly be considered an extension of a diagnostic physical examination. An exploration that demonstrates no NSTI exposes the patient to a general anesthetic and local wound exploration. Failure to explore a patient with a NSTI will likely result in that patient's death.

Treatment

The most important factors in successful management of NSTIs are rapid diagnosis and early surgical exploration with radical resection of infected tissues [44]. Once the diagnosis of NSTI is considered, the patient should have rapid and aggressive fluid resuscitation. A bladder catheter should be placed to monitor urine output as an indication of resuscitation. Broad-spectrum antibiotics should be initiated immediately, and should be chosen to cover gram-positive, gram-negative, and anaerobic bacteria. Fluid resuscitation, antibiotic administration, and diagnostic studies such as radiographs or CT scans should not delay surgery.

The initial incision is at or over the most severely infected area. The incision is carried down through skin and subcutaneous tissue to the level of the muscle fascia. If there is any concern of myonecrosis, the fascia is incised to examine muscle. All necrotic and grossly infected tissue is excised and removed. This usually requires excision of skin, subcutaneous tissue and fascia. Occasionally, necrotic or infected muscle must also be excised. Tissue is sent to microbiology for quantitative culture. The excision is continued proximally and distally until all abnormal tissue is excised. Tissue of questionable viability is excised until obviously normal tissue is reached. There is a tendency to attempt to preserve tissue of questionable viability and this is to be avoided. The best chance for successful outcome is excision of all infected, dead tissue at the time of the first surgery. Adequate excision of an extremity may necessitate emergent amputation of that extremity. Attempts to preserve an extremity that will ultimately be nonfunctional because of the extent of resection are not warranted.

Following adequate excision the patient is placed in topical antibiotic solutions, continues to receive aggressive fluid resuscitation, and continues to receive antibiotics that ultimately are tailored to quantitative culture and sensitivity testing. The patient is schedule for second look surgery in 12–24 h. Repeat surgeries are performed every 12–24 h until the wound is completely free of nonviable tissue. Adjuvant therapy in addition to surgery, fluid resuscitation, and intravenous antibiotic therapy remains of questionable benefit. The use of plasmapheresis, IVIG, and hyperbaric oxygen has been reported. Results have been equivocal, and these treatments cannot be recommended and standard therapy [45]. Reconstruction is initiated once the wound is completely clean and the patient is nontoxic. Reconstruction typically consists of a combination of negative pressure wound therapy, local flap advancement, and skin grafting.

As with TENS/SJS, because of the complexity of wound management and the need for aggressive surgical resection, NSTI patients are best cared for in burn centers. However, transfer should not delay the initial operative debridement [46].

Complications and Prognosis

The radical resection necessitated by this disease process often presents challenges for rehabilitation and recovery. However, even following amputation and/or radical soft tissue debridements most patients are able to reach a level of functioning at or close to their premorbid condition [47, 48]. Prognostic factors for NSTI include: diabetes mellitus, intravenous drug use, age great than 50, hypertension, and malnutrition/obesity. The presence of three or more of these risk factors confers a mortality of greater than 50 % [49].

Summary

- NSTI is a polymicrobial infection of skin and soft tissues with many predisposing factors and high mortality with inadequate treatment.
- The diagnosis is clinical based on wound appearance and systemic toxicity.
- The primary management is immediate and aggressive surgical resection.
- Patients should be cared for in burn centers or other centers of excellence with experience with NSTI and in advanced wound care.

Purpura Fulminans

Purpura fulminans is a rare, acute necrotizing infection characterized by patchy, full-thickness hemorrhagic necrosis of skin and soft tissue usually necessitating radical resection and reconstruction. The disease usually is preceded by an uncomplicated viral or bacterial infection. It has been most commonly associated with systemic *Meningococcal* infections, but has also been seen following *Staphylococcal*, *Streptococcal*, and gram-negative enteric, and viral infections. The disease is also associated with a relative or absolute deficiency and/or dysfunction of protein C anticoagulant. However, the disease can manifest without obvious prior infection or without any signs of protein C deficiency or hypercoagulability.

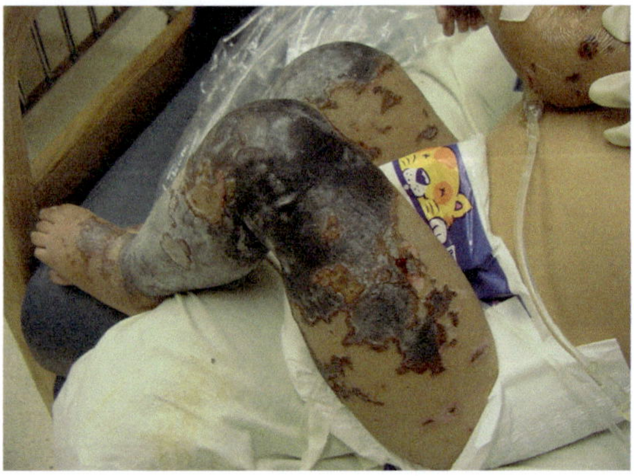

Fig. 18.7 Purpura fulminans skin lesions

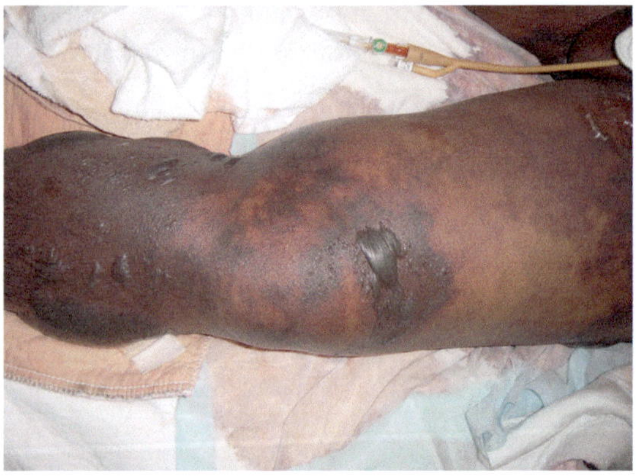

Fig. 18.8 Purpura fulminans skin lesions

The skin and soft tissue lesions usually begin as petechiae, followed by bullae, which coalesce and become hemorrhagic. This progresses to full-thickness hemorrhagic and ischemic skin necrosis. The lesions are patchy and involve the distal extremities and face preferentially. Often the patient has clinical manifestations of sepsis and/or disseminated intravascular coagulopathy (DIC) (see Figs. 18.7 and 18.8)

Treatment is aimed initially at the underlying infectious etiology. The coagulopathy may be treated by anticoagulants such as heparin, and may halt progression of the skin lesions. Once infection and coagulopathy are under control, then the skin lesions are resected and reconstructed. Mortality is typically 20–40 % [50–52].

References

1. Stevens AMJ, Johnson FC. A new eruptive fever associated with stomatitis and ophthalmia: a report of two cases in children. Am J Dis Child. 1922;24:526–33.
2. Lyell A. Toxic epidermal necrolysis: an eruption resembling scalding of the skin. Br J Dermatol. 1956;68(11):355–61.
3. Roujeau JC et al. Medication use and the risk of Stevens-Johnson syndrome or toxic epidermal necrolysis. New Engl J Med. 1995;333(24):1600–7.
4. Lissia M et al. Toxic epidermal necrolysis (Lyell's disease). Burns. 2010;36(2):152–63.
5. Endorf FW, Cancio LC, Gibran NS. Toxic epidermal necrolysis clinical guidelines. J Burn Care Res. 2008;29(5):706–12.
6. Khalili B, Bahna SL. Pathogenesis and recent therapeutic trends in Stevens-Johnson syndrome and toxic epidermal necrolysis. Ann Allergy Asthma, Immunol. 2006;97(3):272–80. quiz 281–3.
7. Letko E et al. Stevens-Johnson syndrome and toxic epidermal necrolysis: a review of the literature. Ann Allergy Asthma Immunol. 2005;94(4):419–36. quiz 436–8.
8. Weinand C et al. 27 years of a single burn centre experience with Stevens-Johnson syndrome and toxic epidermal necrolysis: analysis of mortality risk for causative agents. Burns. 2013;39(7):1449–55.
9. Peppercorn AF et al. High-level human herpesvirus-6 viremia associated with onset of Stevens-Johnson syndrome: report of two cases. J Burn Care Res. 2010;31(2):365–8.
10. Hung S-I et al. Genetic susceptibility to carbamazepine-induced cutaneous adverse drug reactions. Pharmacogenet Genomics. 2006;16(4):297–306.
11. Hung SI et al. HLA-B*5801 allele as a genetic marker for severe cutaneous adverse reactions caused by allopurinol. Proc Natl Acad Sci U S A. 2005;102(11):4134–9. Erratum appears in Proc Natl Acad Sci U S A. 2005 Apr 26;102(17):6237.
12. Borchers AT et al. Stevens-Johnson syndrome and toxic epidermal necrolysis. Autoimmun Rev. 2008;7(8):598–605.
13. Correia O et al. Increased interleukin 10, tumor necrosis factor alpha, and interleukin 6 levels in blister fluid of toxic epidermal necrolysis. J Am Acad Dermatol. 2002;47(1):58–62.
14. Chave TA et al. Toxic epidermal necrolysis: current evidence, practical management and future directions. Br J Dermatol. 2005;153(2):241–53.
15. Pereira FA, Mudgil AV, Rosmarin DM. Toxic epidermal necrolysis. J Am Acad Dermatol. 2007;56(2):181–200.
16. Mofid MZ et al. Drug-induced linear immunoglobulin A bullous disease that clinically mimics toxic epidermal necrolysis. J Burn Care Rehabil. 2000;21(3):246–7.
17. Goyal S et al. Toxic epidermal necrolysis in children: medical, surgical, and ophthalmologic considerations. J Burn Care Res. 2009;30(3):437–49.
18. Palmieri TL et al. A multicenter review of toxic epidermal necrolysis treated in U.S. burn centers at the end of the twentieth century. J Burn Care Rehabil. 2002;23(2):87–96.
19. Shiga S, Cartotto R. What are the fluid requirements in toxic epidermal necrolysis? J Burn Care Res. 2010;31(1):100–4.
20. Coban YK, Erbatur S, Aytekin AH. A useful combination in the treatment of toxic epidermal necrolysis: octenoidine dihydrocholoride solution and Aquacel-Ag. Burns. 2011;37(3):545–6.
21. Lindford AJ et al. Comparison of Suprathel and allograft skin in the treatment of a severe case of toxic epidermal necrolysis. Burns. 2011;37(7):e67–72.
22. Ng RWM, Cheng YL. Calcium alginate dressing-related hypercalcemia. J Burn Care Res. 2007;28(1):203–4.
23. Boorboor P et al. Toxic epidermal necrolysis: use of Biobrane or skin coverage reduces pain, improves mobilisation and decreases infection in elderly patients. Burns. 2008;34(4):487–92.
24. Huang S-H et al. AQUACEL Ag in the treatment of toxic epidermal necrolysis (TEN). Burns. 2008;34(1):63–6.
25. Huang S-H et al. Aquacel Ag with Vaseline gauze in the management of toxic epidermal necrolysis (TEN). Burns. 2010;36(1):121–6.
26. Abood GJ, Nickoloff BJ, Gamelli RL. Treatment strategies in toxic epidermal necrolysis syndrome: where are we at? J Burn Care Res. 2008;29(1):269–76.
27. Mosier MJ, DeChristopher PJ, Gamelli RL. Use of therapeutic plasma exchange in the burn unit: a review of the literature. J Burn Care Res. 2013;34(3):289–98.
28. Stella M et al. Toxic epidermal necrolysis (TEN) and Stevens-Johnson syndrome (SJS): experience with high-dose intravenous immunoglobulins and topical conservative approach. A retrospective analysis. Burns. 2007;33(4):452–9.
29. Lin A et al. Management of ocular conditions in the burn unit: thermal and chemical burns and Stevens-Johnson syndrome/toxic epidermal necrolysis. J Burn Care Res. 2011;32(5):547–60.
30. Oplatek A et al. Long-term follow-up of patients treated for toxic epidermal necrolysis. J Burn Care Res. 2006;27(1):26–33.
31. Hii BW et al. Hospital management and clinical factors associated with ophthalmic involvement in toxic epidermal necrolysis. Burns. 2014;40(5):903–8.
32. Bastuji-Garin S et al. Clinical classification of cases of toxic epidermal necrolysis, Stevens-Johnson syndrome, and erythema multiforme. Arch Dermatol. 1993;129(1):92–6.
33. Zhu QY et al. Toxic epidermal necrolysis: performance of SCORTEN and the score-based comparison of the efficacy of corticosteroid therapy and intravenous immunoglobulin combined therapy in China. J Burn Care Res. 2012;33(6):e295–308.
34. Sekula P et al. Evaluation of SCORTEN on a cohort of patients with Stevens-Johnson syndrome and toxic epidermal necrolysis included in the RegiSCAR study. J Burn Care Res. 2011;32(2):237–45.

35. Cartotto R et al. SCORTEN accurately predicts mortality among toxic epidermal necrolysis patients treated in a burn center. J Burn Care Res. 2008;29(1):141–6.
36. Imahara SD et al. SCORTEN overestimates mortality in the setting of a standardized treatment protocol. J Burn Care Res. 2006;27(3):270–5.
37. Haywood CT, McGeer A, Low DE. Clinical experience with 20 cases of group A streptococcus necrotizing fasciitis and myonecrosis: 1995 to 1997. Plast Reconstr Surg. 1999;103(6):1567–73.
38. Patino JF, Castro D. Necrotizing lesions of soft tissues: a review. World J Surg. 1991;15(2):235–9.
39. Caruso DM, Foster KN, Chellappan A. Burn center treatment of necrotizing soft tissue infections: necrotizing fasciitis, Fournier's gangrene, and purpura fulminans. Probl Gen Surg. 2003;20(1):138–45.
40. Endorf FW, Cancio LC, Klein MB. Necrotizing soft-tissue infections: clinical guidelines. J Burn Care Res. 2009;30(5):769–75.
41. Wall DB et al. A simple model to help distinguish necrotizing fasciitis from nonnecrotizing soft tissue infection. J Am Coll Surg. 2000;191(3):227–31.
42. Wong C-H et al. Necrotizing fasciitis: clinical presentation, microbiology, and determinants of mortality. J Bone Joint Surg. 2003;85-A(8):1454–60.
43. Wong C-H, Wang Y-S. The diagnosis of necrotizing fasciitis. Curr Opin Infect Dis. 2005;18(2):101–6.
44. Endorf FW et al. Necrotizing soft-tissue infections: differences in patients treated at burn centers and non-burn centers. J Burn Care Res. 2008;29(6):933–8.
45. Endorf FW, Supple KG, Gamelli RL. The evolving characteristics and care of necrotizing soft-tissue infections. Burns. 2005;31(3):269–73.
46. Bernal NP et al. Trends in 393 necrotizing acute soft tissue infection patients 2000-2008. Burns. 2012; 38(2):252–60.
47. Pham TN et al. Assessment of functional limitation after necrotizing soft tissue infection. J Burn Care Res. 2009;30(2):301–6.
48. Pikturnaite J, Soldin M. Impact of necrotising fasciitis on quality of life: a qualitative analysis. Burns. 2014;40(5):848–51.
49. Francis KR et al. Implications of risk factors in necrotizing fasciitis. Am Surg. 1993;59(5):304–8.
50. Adcock DM, Brozna J, Marlar RA. Proposed classification and pathologic mechanisms of purpura fulminans and skin necrosis. Semin Thromb Hemost. 1990;16(4):333–40.
51. Chasan PE, Hansbrough JF, Cooper ML. Management of cutaneous manifestations of extensive purpura fulminans in a burn unit. J Burn Care Rehabil. 1992;13(4):410–3.
52. Adcock DM, Hicks MJ. Dermatopathology of skin necrosis associated with purpura fulminans. Semin Thromb Hemost. 1990;16(4):283–92.

Pain Management

19

Damien Wilson Carter, Gretchen J. Carrougher, and Tam N. Pham

Introduction

Pain in burn patients is multifaceted and can be challenging to manage. However, optimal pain control is a hallmark of quality burn care and should be the goal with each burn patient. Patients with burn injuries experience significant pain and discomfort that are unique when compared to other types of trauma [1]. Although most acknowledge the importance of pain control as an aspect of complete burn care, burn pain has been historically undertreated [2]. The importance of adequate pain control in the acute phase must be underscored. Poor pain control leads to both short and long-term complications [3, 4]. Notably, poor pain control is linked to increased incidence of depression and post-traumatic stress disorder (PTSD). Recent evidence indicates a link between patient discomfort and risk of burn infection, increased suicidal ideation and attempts as well as longer hospitalizations [3]. Furthermore, there is considerable evidence that poor pain control in the acute phase of burn care may predispose to the development of chronic pain and pruritic syndromes [3]. We aim to provide a framework to understand the types of acute pain and appropriate pain assessment instruments in the burn patient as well as broad strategies to consider in managing this complex entity.

D.W. Carter, M.D.
Department of Surgery, Maine Medical Center, Tufts University, Portland, ME, USA

G.J. Carrougher, R.N., M.N.
T.N. Pham, M.D., F.A.C.S. (✉)
Department of Surgery, University of Washington Regional Burn Center, Harborview Medical Center University of Washington, 325 9th Avenue, Seattle, WA 98104, USA
e-mail: tpham94@uw.edu

Acute Pain Types

Pain experienced by the individual burn patient varies greatly with respect to burn size, cultural/religious background and will also depend on coexisting non-burn trauma [2]. Whereas partial-thickness burns are extremely painful due to preserved dermal nerve endings, full-thickness burns will be less sensate, at least initially. During the healing phase, patients often experience increased pain when devitalized tissues are lifted and replaced by new skin epithelium. If the patient has a history of chronic pain, this aspect will add another layer of complexity to the management. The first task in managing pain in the burn patient is to recognize the type and quality of pain the patient is experiencing.

Acute burn injury usually presents with a basal level of pain referred to as **background pain**. Background pain is of dull, persistent character with exacerbations when the wound(s) are

D.G. Greenhalgh (ed.), *Burn Care for General Surgeons and General Practitioners*,
DOI 10.1007/978-3-319-29161-1_19

exposed. Pain secondary to needle sticks, line insertion, debridement, dressing changes, etc. is referred to as **procedural pain** and is typically characterized as intense, and of short duration. This type of pain—when ineffectively controlled—is thought to lead to long-term sequelae as stated above [5]. Notably, in anticipation of procedures, anxiety and psychological stress need to be addressed in order to minimize the impact of actual pain produced by the procedure. There are also periods of unanticipated bursts of moderate intensity pain referred to as **breakthrough pain**. Development of significant breakthrough pain is thought to be related to inadequate control of background pain [6]. Specifically, a common error is to prescribe "PRN" (as needed) opioid medications. As such, these medications are not administered at scheduled intervals—this practice delays treatment of background pain, leads to episodes of breakthrough pain and should be avoided [7]. Background pain management should be titrated in the acute phase to eliminate breakthrough pain as well.

As wound healing progresses during a hospitalization, patients often develop **neuropathic pain**. Neuropathic pain in this context is a manifestation of afferent sensory nerve dysfunction in a healing burn wound. The pain or discomfort is often described as intense itching, burning, "pins and needles," shooting, and/or electric shock like sensations. It is not unusual for this type of pain sequelae to dominate a patients overall level of discomfort [7, 8]. A discussion of chronic pain and its management is beyond the scope of this chapter.

Acute Pain Assessment

To manage pain effectively, it is critical to be able to assess pain levels as well as response to initiated therapies. An important aspect of pain assessment is to set goals for effective pain control. Often, this requires a discussion with the patient about pain expectations. It is useful to explain that complete pain relief (i.e., no pain at all) is not practical with this type of injury in a conscious, awake patient. We are attempting to control pain and manage it effectively, not eliminate it completely. A primary aspect of pain assessment is to determine a pain level goal that is acceptable to the patient/family and deemed reasonable by the care team. We need to balance the effect that different medications may have on a patient's overall comfort as well as determine where non-pharmacologic strategies may assist in a comprehensive pain management plan. For young children, infants, and altered or intubated patients, the care provider is forced to rely more heavily on observational pain assessment instruments to determine adequacy of treatment. Even with the pain assessment tools available, pain management as opposed to pain elimination remains the goal. Notably, use of higher doses and/or more frequent administration of opioids (levels discussed below) may be reasonable during procedures, but does require frequent assessment to achieve a steady range of acceptable pain relief.

Several scoring systems and pain measurement tools are available that have been validated in the literature (see Table 19.1). These include measurement tools specifically designed for pediatric burn patients and patients who are preverbal. Pain assessment in children is challenging and requires frequent and diligent assessment to titrate dosage. There is no single tool appropriate for assessment of all age groups, thus the care provider must select one that is age and developmentally appropriate. The Wong–Baker FACES Scale© is the most validated tool available for ages 4–15 years. A new revised Faces Pain Scale (FPS-R) was developed to improve the original FACES scale and is validated for ages 4–16 years. The Oucher™ Pain scale is useful in the preschool age group and is currently available in five versions (White or Caucasian; Black or African-American; Hispanic; First Nations (boy and girl); Asian (boy and girl)). There are also rating scales designed specifically for developmentally delayed children and adults as well as for anxiety and itching. The International Association for the Study of Pain (http://www.iasp-pain.org) is a good resource for selecting pain assessment tools.

Table 19.1 Recommended pain assessment instruments by age/cognition ability

Group delineation	Behavioral-observational instruments	Self-reporting instruments
Preverbal children (e.g., infants and toddlers)	FLACC	–
School-age children	FLACC (validated in children up to age 7 years)	Wong–Baker FACES Scale Oucher Pain Scale (photo portion of scale) R-FPS
Adolescents		Oucher Pain Scale (numerical portion of scale) NRS for pain VAS for pain
Adults		NRS for pain VAS for pain
Non-communicative adults (e.g., dementia without verbal skills)	Abbey Pain Scale PAINAD	–

FLACC faces, legs, activity, cry and consolability
R-FPS revised faces pain scale
VAS visual analog scale
NRS numerical rating scale
PAINAD pain assessment in advanced dementia

Strategies for Acute Pain Management

We advocate a multimodal approach to pain management, including incorporation of non-pharmacological therapies. The acute phase is best divided into three periods: Early (<96 h after injury), acute (96 h until wound closure), and a rehabilitative phase (wound closure to scar maturation). The rehabilitative phase may persist for as long as 3 years and involves outpatient management.

There is a common misconception that patients with full-thickness burns do not experience significant pain. Multiple studies have demonstrated significant pain requirements in patients with full-thickness burns [9]. As discussed above, while full-thickness burns are initially less sensate, pain increases as devitalized tissue is lifted from the wound bed. In the early period, pain in full-thickness injuries can be curtailed by burn wound excision. Even temporary coverage with xenograft or allograft skin can significantly reduce burn pain [10]. In second-degree burns—which can be exquisitely painful—patients should be treated with dressings to allow for healing and demarcation of areas that may have prolonged healing. Recently, silver impregnated dressings have gained popularity as they are changed less frequently after initial application [11]. At our center, we have maintained extended dressings in place for up to 1 week given their sustained antibacterial properties.

Pharmacologic treatment of background pain in the early period after injury centers on the use opioid analgesics. The use of nonsteroidal anti-inflammatory drugs (NSAIDs) is often impractical given the potential bleeding complications associated with their use [12]. However, if non-operative management is decided early or if patients have completed operative management, NSAIDs should be included in the treatment of background pain. Routine acetaminophen doses are also scheduled on all burn patients that do not have a specific contraindication. Again, it is wise to titrate opioid and non-opioid pain medications on a scheduled regimen and avoid relying on "PRN" demands.

Procedural pain in the early period must take into account the anxiety provoked by these activities. The use of distracting non-pharmacologic adjunctive therapies is useful. These options are discussed later in the chapter. Benzodiazepines are the pharmacologic mainstay for anxiolytics in the early and acute periods. Opioid analgesics and benzodiazepines can be given orally and intravenously as dictated by the clinical situation.

Intravenous administration is common in this group. Postoperative pain is a type of procedural pain that ensues after general anesthesia has worn off. It is managed with a temporary escalation of background pain medication and increased breakthrough pain analgesia allotments. For instance, pain in donor sites is most acute in the first 3–4 days after a skin graft operation, and is a common cause for increased pain requirements in the postoperative period.

For management of procedural pain in the early and acute periods, Fig. 19.1 illustrates options for escalation of pharmacotherapy from local analgesia, oral opioids, and benzodiazepines to general anesthesia when needed (see Fig. 19.1). Benzodiazepines are most effective for anxiolysis in the periprocedural period and should be avoided for the relief of baseline or chronic anxiety (except in those patients who were prescribed these medications prior to burn injury) [13]. Several mood altering and antipsychotic medications are very effective for non-procedural anxiety (e.g., quetiapine, olanzapine, citalopram, and haldol) [14]. In the non-intubated patient, care must be taken when escalating to levels of deep sedation. Specifically, the patient must be in an appropriately monitored situation with trained personnel and standardized procedures and protocols in place [15]. Practice varies widely and depends on institutional experience.

As the patient moves into the acute period (i.e., greater than 4 days from injury), we advocate adding methadone as an effective remedy to background pain that may intensify in the first 1–3 weeks [16]. Though methadone use outside of drug addiction management and chronic pain is unusual, it is well suited to treat burn related background pain. We avoid the use of other long-acting opioids (e.g., OxyContin, Roxicodone, or MS Contin) as we have found that the use of methadone is associated with a lower incidence of dependency and drug seeking behavior as well as a lower frequency of over-sedation in our patients. The observation of QTc prolongation with the use of methadone is common. However, even with observed QT prolongation (>500 ms),

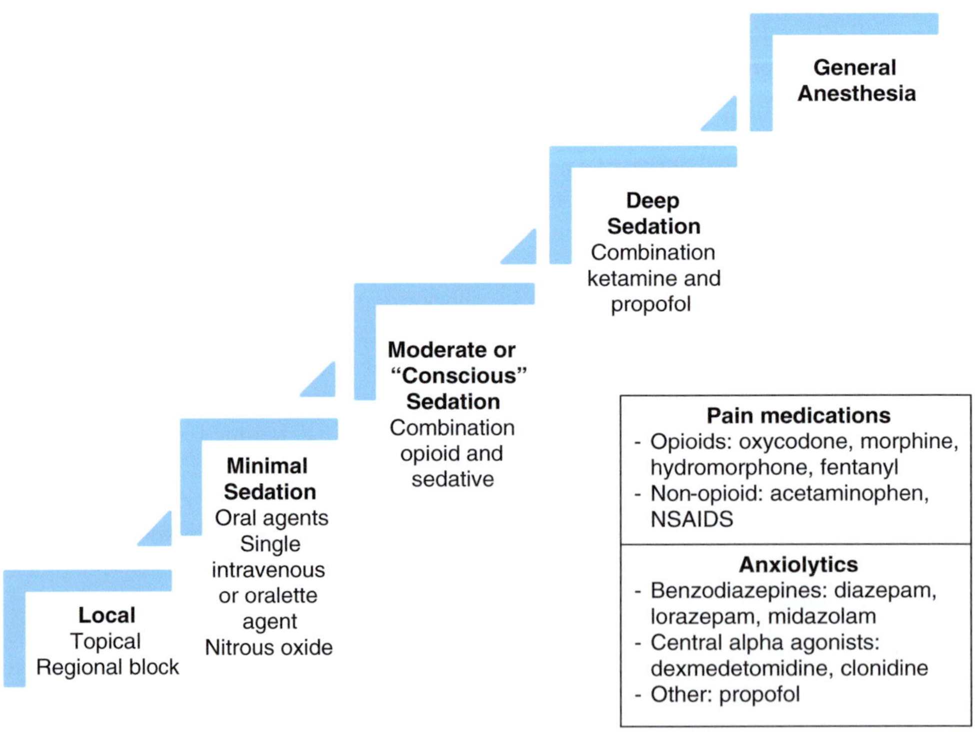

Fig. 19.1 Procedure pain and sedation escalation, with examples

significant cardiac arrhythmias are exceedingly rare [17]. Recent evidence from the electrophysiology community has challenged the clinical significance of medication induced QT prolongation. While still controversial, a consensus is building in the electrophysiology community that only patients with certain genetic "channelopathies" are at risk for fatal arrhythmias [18]. Further discussion of this data is beyond the scope of this chapter. Nonetheless, methadone remains a safe pain medication in the care of burn patients and is widely used for this purpose in burn centers across North America and worldwide [19].

As wound closure approaches, pain associated with healing donor sites and partial thickness injuries can increase significantly. Many patients will temporarily require higher doses of opioid medication to control pain in these healing wounds. As the patient transitions to the rehabilitative phase, transitioning to NSAIDs as the predominant medication strategy can help to wean overall opioid usage [7, 20]. The practitioner begins the process of weaning opioid medications as wounds are epithelializing. This process starts during inpatient, and continued in outpatient care.

For severe burns, the rehabilitative phase may begin while hospitalized. Background pain will likely wane over time, but many burn patients begin to manifest neuropathic type pain symptoms several weeks after closure of the wound. Many will have neuropathic pain even during the acute phase [21].

New onset neuropathic pain is difficult to manage. Pruritus specifically can lead to scratching that is destructive to grafts and delays wound healing. Some evidence points to long acting NSAIDs and ibuprofen as effective in reducing the severity of itching [22], Opioids should be used with new neuropathic pain as they can depress abnormal afferent signaling in the nervous system and may effectively control this type of pain [23]. If one particular opioid is ineffective, it is useful to try others as all have varying effects (i.e., some improve, others worsen, whereas some have no effect). Additionally, the use of antihistamines such as diphenhydramine and cetirizine for neuropathic itch is common. Despite providing good anecdotal itch relief, several large studies have demonstrated limited usefulness for these medications [24]. Nevertheless, diphenhydramine and cetirizine remain part of many routine itch treatment protocols, including at our institution.

Tricyclic antidepressants may have a role in acute neuropathic pain and are clearly effective in a subset of patients [25]. North American burn centers also prescribe gabapentin and pregabalin off label for neuropathic pain. Typical dosing is often two to four times the usual doses for other indications. However, evidence to support this practice remains scant with recent research challenging their efficacy as an evidenced-based therapy [26, 27]. Neuropathic pain may ultimately depend on scar formation and maturation. Effective management is complex and requires titration among different combinations. Non-pharmacologic therapies may improve neuropathic pain as well and should be incorporated in the treatment plan.

Strategies for Outpatient Pain Management

Several retrospective studies indicate that greater than 80 % of burn patients are discharged on opioid medications [6, 28]. In one retrospective study, investigators found that the median daily prescribed amount was 114 mg morphine equivalents (ME) for control of pain [28]. Given the recent rise in overdose related mortality from compliant use of prescription drugs at ME levels less than the typical burn patient, these data may cause some alarm. Nonetheless, one study showed essentially no mortality that could be attributed to these high levels of opioid use in burn patients at a single verified burn center [28]. Despite the burn patients clear need for high levels of analgesia to function and participate in therapy, there is consensus that the burn care community should look to strategies to decrease reliance on these potent drugs [28]. With each outpatient visit, reduction in opioid medications in a stepwise fashion with increases in other analgesics (e.g., NSAIDs, Tramadol) and non-pharmacologic therapies (i.e., operant conditioning, exercise) should be employed. There is some evidence that codeine—particularly in combination with ibuprofen—gives good synergistic opioid/NSAID effects in the outpatient and postoperative setting without the side effects typically associated with the use of codeine with or without acetaminophen. We have traditionally avoided use of this medication due to a significant side effect profiles experienced by our patients; however, significant evidence supports its use (ibuprofen/codeine combination) in postoperative patients [29]. Codeine is a prodrug that must be metabolized to acquire an opioid effect. Whatever medication combination is used, we recommend protocolized opioid medication weaning be part of the routine care of burn patients.

Non-pharmacologic Therapies

There is a strong psychological factor associated with pain and anxiety in the care of injured patients. Periprocedural anxiety is particularly associated with burn patients and is known to intensify the acute pain experienced by this patient population [30]. Given the nature of burn injuries, the clinician caring for burn patients should incorporate non-drug strategies and therapies when managing all levels of periprocedural pain in the conscious patient. These strategies should also be employed with physical therapy activities [31]. To use psychological interventions in pain management, it is important to understand the psychological principles of classical conditioning and operant conditioning as well as different coping behaviors.

In classical conditioning, a patient will develop a conditioned response (i.e., anxiousness) to certain environmental and behavioral stimuli that precede a painful procedure. An often quoted example in the literature has shown that healthcare workers merely wearing scrubs during wound care was sufficient to elicit fear in burn injured children [32]. Logically, environmental interventions can be effective in mitigating this effect. With adults and adolescents, enhancing patient control of the environment is particularly effective. In general, when an adult feels like they have no control, anxiety increases. Suggestions to mitigate this would include providing a choice of music during wound care, scheduling meal times, offering food choices and timing of procedures such as wound care. Another approach is to prepare the patient using a procedure-based approach (i.e., explaining the mechanics of the procedure step by step allowing the patient to prepare) or sensory-based approach (i.e., you will likely feel a tugging sensation as I pull off your dressings). With children, classic conditioning is more involved and requires creating a comforting environment. As such, it is preferable to perform wound care in a separate procedure room, as opposed to their hospital room, which is considered a safe place. One strategy employed by many burn centers turns hydrotherapy into "bath tub—play time" with requisite floating toys and games. Allowing comforting items like play toys (must be able to be cleaned and disinfected) to accompany the child to the procedure room can reduce anxiety. Another technique that is often employed with children is to increase their sense of control with forced choices. For example, "Do you want to have lunch before or after wound care" and "Do you want to take your medication with chocolate milk or orange juice"? The idea is to give two choices that are acceptable to the healthcare team and still achieve the primary goal(s). Increasing children's perception of control during procedures can reduce the incidence of learned helplessness and improves pain tolerance [33].

Another useful classical conditioning approach is relaxation training. Several studies have demonstrated that adults and children receiving massage therapy to non-burned areas prior to wound care reported lower pain scores with as little as 15 min of treatment [34]. Other non-pharmacologic strategies—particularly for adults—are the use of meditation, prayer, and exercise. Teaching skills in meditation and stretching can relax patients and dampen the pain response as well as improve compliance with physical therapy [35].

With operant conditioning, patients perceive a sense of support or reinforcement to escape or avoid painful procedures. This could be achieved by screaming loudly or becoming excessively combative during a procedure, particularly if stopping the procedure or therapeutic intervention reinforces it. When staff members allow patients to terminate procedures or therapies, they can inadvertently increase escape behavior. If allowed to continue, this type of conditioning can devolve into a combative unpleasant experience for everyone and impede therapeutic progress.

This type of behavior should first prompt a reassessment of the adequacy of pain control and suggests escalation of management (see Fig. 19.1). However, if pharmacologic management is deemed appropriate, there are some effective "limit setting" interventions. Allowing rest between stages of wound care—perhaps with additional pain and anxiolytic medications—is a successful technique to minimize undesirable and destructive behavior. Also useful with adults and adolescents is a quota system [3, 31]. Often used to obtain physical therapy goals, the quota system involves an initial baseline assessment. For example, a patient needs to walk on the soles of their feet. They are encouraged to walk until tired for four sessions and the distance achieved is documented (i.e., ambulated 50 ft/day without stopping). This distance becomes the baseline and daily ambulation goal is increased by 5 % for each subsequent day. This approach is particularly useful with patients who lack motivation or are easily overwhelmed by multiple therapies [3, 31]. This approach also addresses appropriate pacing and reduces over-fatigue in burn patients.

Employing operant principles in children, such as "time out passes" and "alternative economies" are two very effective approaches. With time-out passes, the child gets a certain number of cards that allow a 1-min break or rest. They can present it anytime during the procedure until they run out of cards. This approach also employs classical principles in that it allows a perception of greater control over the procedure and introduces an element of gamesmanship. Similarly, token economies are arranged to "reward" a child for completing wound care or other procedures with stars, buttons, stickers or other prizes. A few burn centers give color beads for particularly painful procedures that are applied to a necklace or bracelet [36]. Children—both boys and girls—often wear these necklaces as a badge of honor and may interpret wound care procedures as a personal challenge [3, 37]. With older children (10–13 years old), accumulation of points to purchase a desired award is effective as well. When using token economy strategies, it is important to reward for completion of the procedure or activity and not bravery. Rewarding (or not rewarding) bravery can be interpreted as a form of punishment to young children (4–8 years old) and should be avoided [3, 33].

Lastly, coping strategies are often very unique to individuals and are influenced by cultural, environmental and possibly genetic influences that precede a burn injury [38]. This variation needs to be recognized in order to employ the various cognitive interventions in an effective manner. Simply stated, both adults and children are thought to have coping styles that are on a continuum from approach oriented to avoidant [3, 39]. The avoidant coping style prefers to be distracted or "removed" during a painful procedure. Logically, distraction techniques (e.g., meditation, virtual reality, hypnosis, massage) are most effective with this type of coping. At the other end of the spectrum, the approach oriented style desires to be involved as much as possible in all aspects of their care. Techniques that enhance control and involve the patient in each step (e.g., psychological preparation, involvement in the actual wound care, selection of music during wound care) of the procedure as well as maximizing communication of information are most effective with this style. Using distraction techniques with a patient who has an approach oriented coping style will likely increase anxiety and pain perception.

Certain non-pharmacologic therapies described above require significant investment in trained personnel and specialized equipment that is likely impractical for centers treating a small number of burn patients annually. Nonetheless, understanding the basic principles of procedural pain psychology as outlined above, provides a toolbox of "low tech" minimal resource interventions that any burn care team can and should provide to their patients (see Tables 19.2 and 19.3).

Table 19.2 Non-pharmacologic strategies

Principle	Techniques/strategies/treatment
Classical conditioning	Enhanced patient control; psychological preparation; create "comforting" environment; relaxation training, forced choices (children); pre-procedure massage therapy; meditation training; exercise; music and art therapy; aromatherapy
Operant (reinforcement) conditioning	Planned rest stages with wound care/procedures; quota system; time-out passes; alternative/token economies
Approach coping style	Enhanced control of setting/environment; psychological preparation; involvement in procedure/wound care; maximize communication of information and each step of wound care/procedure
Avoidant coping style	Massage therapy; meditation training; hypnosis; virtual reality technology (VR); virtual reality hypnosis (VH)

Table 19.3 Distraction modalities

Technique	Advantages	Disadvantages
Massage Meditation therapy	• Effective classical conditioning approach • Shown to decrease periprocedural pain scores over time	• Less useful with approach coping style • Cost for trained therapists/instructors
Hypnosis	• Involves blend of imagery, meditation and relaxation • >75 anecdotal reports of efficacy—most included burns • Two RCTs have shown decreased affective pain scores and PTSD	• Can generate increased anxiety with approach type coping styles • Not effective with certain individuals for unclear reasons • Cost of access to a trained hypnotist
Virtual reality (VR)	• Immersion in computer generated world with engagement in that world • Only partly passive, making it an effective distraction technique • Excellent therapy for avoidant coping type • Strong evidence of pain reduction when combined with pharmacotherapy vs. pharmacotherapy alone	• Equivocal evidence for an effect on patient anxiety with procedures • May be disconcerting to some with approach type coping • Cost of equipment, maintenance and staff training
VR Hypnosis (VRH)	• Combines effectiveness of both therapies without need for trained hypnotist at each session	• Cost of equipment and staff training

Summary

Effective pain management in the burn patient requires active assessment, continuous reassessment, and flexibility with treatment options. This chapter outlines broad strategies and given specific recommendations on the management of pain in burn patients through progressive phases of care. The acknowledgement of the different types of pain, how they are assessed, and the varied treatment options—both pharmacologic and non-pharmacologic—are the basis of optimal pain management in burn patients.

Flexibility in managing the pain and anxiety of each burn patient in a personalized and tailored fashion tends to result in improved cooperation from the patient in their own care. The success of operative and nonoperative burn care hinges on effective management of patient comfort. Many of our patients will experience prolonged hospitalizations with repeated interventions, wound care, improvements in function and setbacks over weeks, months and potentially years. Attention to detail in the management of pain and discomfort facilitates effective overall recovery and long-term functionality.

We must reiterate that managing pain expectations with each patient is as important as the specific medications and non-pharmacologic therapy employed. Burn patients commonly experience significant anxiety with prolonged treatments and therapy that is unusual in other forms of trauma or illness. Thus, managing these complex patients may not be suitable in certain practice environments. The burn practitioner should consider transfer to a burn center if pain and/or behavior and anxiety management is beyond the resources of their care setting.

References

1. Choiniere M, Melzack R, Rondeau J, Girard N, Paquin MJ. The pain of burns: characteristics and correlates. J Trauma. 1989;29:1531–9.
2. Retrouvey H, Shahrokhi S. Pain and the thermally injured patient—a review of current therapies. J Burn Care Res. 2015;36(2):315–23.
3. Meyer W, Wiechman S. Management of pain and other discomfort. In: Herndon DN, editor. Total burn care. 4th ed. Philadelphia, PA: Saunders; 2012.
4. Patterson DR, Tininenko J, Ptacek JT. Pain during burn hospitalization predicts long-term outcome. J Burn Care Res. 2006;27(5):719–26.
5. Richardson PM, Mustard L. The management of pain in the burns unit. Burns. 2009;35:921–36.
6. Browne AL, Andrews R, Schug SA, Wood F. Persistent pain outcomes and patient satisfaction with pain management after burn injury. Clin J Pain. 2011;27:136–45.
7. Pal SK, Cortiella J, Herndon DN. Adjunctive methods of pain control in burns. Burns. 1997;23:404–12.
8. Kukkar A, Bali A, Singh N, Jaggi AS. Implications and mechanism of action of gabapentin in neuropathic pain. Arch Pharm Res. 2013;36:237–51.
9. Zor F, Ozturk S, Bilgin F, Isik S, Cosar A. Pain relief during dressing changes of major adult burns: ideal analgesic combination with ketamine. Burns. 2010;36:501–5.
10. Gerding RL, Imbembo AL, Fratianne RB. Biosynthetic skin substitute vs. 1% silver sulfadiazine for treatment of inpatient partial-thickness burns. J Trauma. 1988; 28:1265–9.
11. Varas RP, O'Keeffe T, Namias N. A prospective, randomized trial of Acticoat versus silver sulfadiazine in the treatment of partial thickness burns: which method is less painful? J Burn Care Rehabil. 2005;26:344–7.
12. Cashman JN. The mechanisms of action of NSAIDs in analgesia. Drugs. 1996;52 Suppl 5:13–23.
13. Patterson DR, Ptacek J, Carrougher GJ, Sharar SR. Lorazepam as an adjunct to opioid analgesics in the treatment of burn pain. Pain. 1997;72(3):367–74.
14. Stoddard FJ, Sheridan RL, Saxe GN. Treatment of pain in acutely burned children. J Burn Care Rehabil. 2002;23:135–56.
15. Tosun Z, Esmaoglu A, Coruh A. Propofol-ketamine vs. propofol-fentanyl combinations for deep sedation and analgesia in pediatric patients undergoing burn dressing changes. Paediatr Anaesth. 2008;18:43–7.
16. Jones GM, Porter K, Coffey R. Impact of early methadone initiation in critically injured burn patients: a pilot study. J Burn Care Res. 2013;34:342–8.
17. Chowdhury M, Wong J, Cheng A, Khilkin M, Palma E. Methadone therapy in underserved urban community: QTc prolongation and life-threatening ventricular arrhythmias. Cardiovascul Ther. 2015;33(3): 127–33.
18. Mujtaba S, Romero J, Taub C. Methadone QTc prolongation & Torsade: current concepts, managemetn and a hidden twist in the tail? J Cardiovasc Dis Res. 2013; 4(4):229–35.
19. Berde CB, Beyer JE, Bournaki MC. Comparison of morphine and methadone for prevention of postoperative pain in 3 to 7 year old children. J Pediatr. 1994;119:136–41.
20. Christie MJ, Connor M, Vaughan CW, Ingram SL, Bagley EE. Cellular actions of opioids and other analgesics: implications for synergism in pain relief. Clin Exp Pharmacol Physiol. 2000;27:520–3.
21. Schneider JC, Harris NL, El Shami A, Sheridan RL, Schulz JT, Bilodeau M, et al. A descriptive review of neuropathic-like pain after burn injury. J Burn Care Res. 2006;27(4):524–8.
22. Tauben D. Non-opioid medications for pain. Phys Med Rehabil Clin N Am. 2015;26(2):219–48.
23. Schug S, Goddard C. Recent advances in the pharmacologic management of acute and chronic pain. Ann Palliat Med. 2014;3(4):263–75.
24. Goutos I. Neuropathic mechanisms in the pathophysiology of burns pruritus: redefining directions for therapy and research. J Burn Care Res. 2013;34(1): 82–93.
25. Bernstein JE, Whitney DH, Keyoumars S. Inhibition of histamine-induced pruritus by topical tricyclic antidepressants. J Am Acad Dermatol. 1981;5:582–5.
26. Goutos I, Eldardiri M, Khan AA, Dziewulski P, Richardson PM. Comparative evaluation of antipruritic protocols in acute burns. The emerging value of gabapentin in the treatment of burns pruritus. J Burn Care Res. 2010;31:57–63.
27. Goutos I, Clarke M, Upson C, Richardson PM, Ghosh SJ. Review of therapeutic agents for burns pruritus and protocols for management in adult and paediatric patients using the GRADE classification. Ind J Plastic Surg. 2010;43(Suppl):S51–62.
28. Wibbenmeyer L, Oltrogge K, Kluesner K, Zimmerman MB, Kealey PG. An evaluation of discharge opioid prescribing practices in a burn population. J Burn Care Res. 2015;36(2):329–35.
29. Derry S, Karlin S. Single dose oral ibuprofen plus codeine for acute postoperative pain. Cochrane Database Syst Rev. 2015;2:CD010107.

30. Patterson D, Sharar S. Burn pain. In: Loeser J, editor. Bonica's management of pain. London: Lippincott; 2003. p. 778–87.
31. Ehde DM, Patterson DR, Fordyce WE. The quota system in burn rehabilitation. J Burn Care Rehabil. 1998;19:436–40.
32. Meyer D. Children's responses to nursing attire. Pediatr Nurs. 1992;18:157–60.
33. Kavanaugh CK, Lasoft E, Eide Y. Learned helplessness and the pediatric burn patient: dressing change behavior and serum cortisol and beta endorphins. Adv Pediatr. 1991;38:335–63.
34. Field T, Peck M, Hernandez-Reif M. Post-burn itching, pain, and psychological symptoms are reduced with massage therapy. J Burn Care Rehabil. 2000;21: 189–93.
35. Knudson-Cooper MS. Relaxation and biofeedback training in the treatment of severely burned children. J Burn Care Rehabil. 1981;2(2):102–10.
36. Martin-Herz SP, Thurber CA, Patterson DR. Psychological principles of burn wound pain in children: part II: treatment applications. J Burn Care Rehabil. 2000;21(5):458–74.
37. Thurber CA, Martin-Herz SP, Patterson DR. Psychological principles of burn wound pain in children: part I: theoretical framework. J Burn Care Rehabil. 2000;21(4):376–87.
38. Wernick RL, Jaremko ME, Taylor PW. Pain management in severely burned adults: a test of stress inoculation. J Behav Med. 1981;4:103–9.
39. Sharar S, Carrougher G, Nakamura D. Factors influencing the efficacy of virtual reality distraction analgesia during postburn physical therapy: preliminary results from 3 ongoing studies. Arch Phys Med Rehabil. 2007;88:S43–9.

Important Developments in the Management of Fibroproliferative Scars and Contractures After Burn Injury

20

Kevin Mowbrey, Geneviève Ferland-Caron, and Edward E. Tredget

Introduction

Scar formation is a natural response to injury to restore tissue integrity and strength [1]. For burn patients recovering from injury, scars may present functional, cosmetic, and psychological problems that impair quality of life and interfere with activities of daily living. At 1 year post-burn, 23–45 % of patients reported PTSD related to their injury and the residual deformities [2], which emphasizes the importance of optimal scar management to improve the quality of life for the patients suffering thermal injury.

Clinical Features of Hypertrophic Scar After Burn Injury

Hypertrophic scar (HTS) is a red, raised hyperemic and rigid scar that remains within the original boundaries of the original wound which causes pain, erythema, heat intolerance, and pruritus (Fig. 20.1). HTS is a fibroproliferative disorder that complicates up to 80 % of burn injuries requiring hospitalization and imposes functional and cosmetic complications that often require extensive rehabilitation leading to prolonged delay in return to work or school following injury [3].

Although risk factors including age, ethnicity, gender, wound morphology, and location are etiologically implicated in pathologic scarring, it is the prolonged inflammation of a slow healing burn wound that best predicts its occurrence (Fig. 20.2) [1, 4]. Moreover, children are at higher risk of HTS because of their rapid cellular turnover. HTS seems to display a proclivity to develop in patients of African, Hispanic, and Asian descent [4]. A fundamental etiological factor in HTS is thought to be excessive tension across the wound, producing a firm, red, raised scar within the first month of injury. HTS most commonly develops in wounds across flexion surfaces such as the extremities, neck, sternum, and breast [5]. HTS is often the result of an aberration in one of the healing phases: inflammation, proliferation, or remodeling. In some cases, the natural history of HTS includes remodeling leading to slow improvement in appearance over the first 6 months post-injury, followed by a plateau in improvement. HTS is a self-limited process following injury and will regress in height and color naturally, however, if left unabated this process can take several years. HTS post-burn may

K. Mowbrey, B.M.Sc., M.D.
G. Ferland-Caron, M.D., F.R.C.S.C.
Division of Plastic and Reconstructive Surgery, University of Alberta, 2D2.31 WMC, 8440-112 Street, Edmonton, AB, Canada, T6G 2B7
e-mail: kmowbrey@ualberta.ca

E.E. Tredget, M.D., M.Sc., F.R.C.S.C. (✉)
Division of Plastic and Reconstructive Surgery and Critical Care, Department of Surgery, University of Alberta, 2D2.31 WMC, 8440-112 Street, Edmonton, AB, Canada, T6G 2B7
e-mail: etredget@ualberta.ca

D.G. Greenhalgh (ed.), *Burn Care for General Surgeons and General Practitioners*, DOI 10.1007/978-3-319-29161-1_20

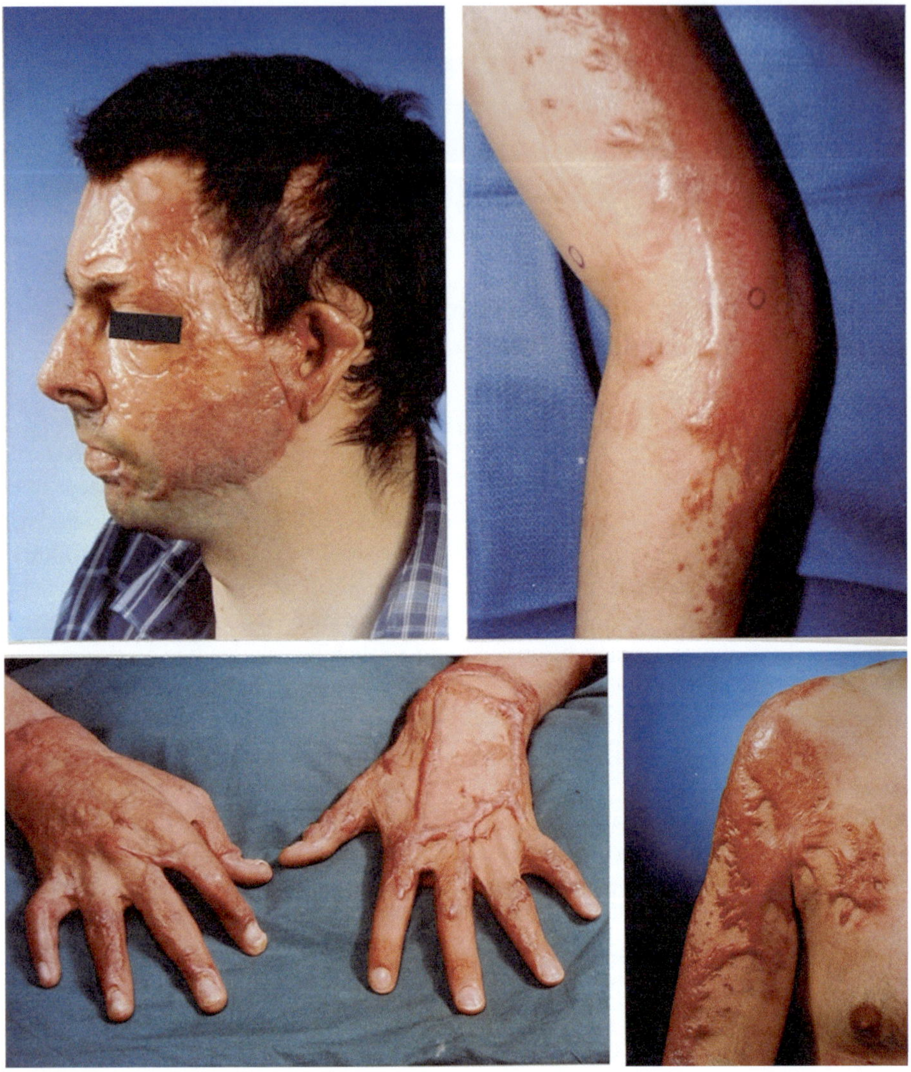

Fig. 20.1 Hypertrophic scarring developed on a 34-year-old Caucasian male 8 months after a burn involving 60 % of his total body surface area. (Reprinted from Scott, PF et al. Biological Basis of Hypertrophic Scarring. In: Malhotra, SK, editor. Advances in Structural Biology, Vol. 3. Greenwich, CT. JAI Press; 1994. [66])

also progress to contracture development secondary to reorganization of collagen in the dermal matrix [6].

Scar Contractures Following Thermal Injury to the Skin

A contracture presents when scar tissue has undergone the process of contraction resulting in a functional problem such as a limitation in ROM or instability with repetitive wound breakdown (Fig. 20.3). Despite increasing attempts to prevent burn contractures in the acute phase, the development of burn contracture is often difficult to avoid [7]. Contractures may result in severe morbidity for the patient, especially if they involve a free margin such as the lip or eyelid. Under normal circumstances, burn contractures remain limited to scar or graft and a layer of superficial connective tissue typically displacing underlying structures such as fat, breast gland, or orbital tissue.

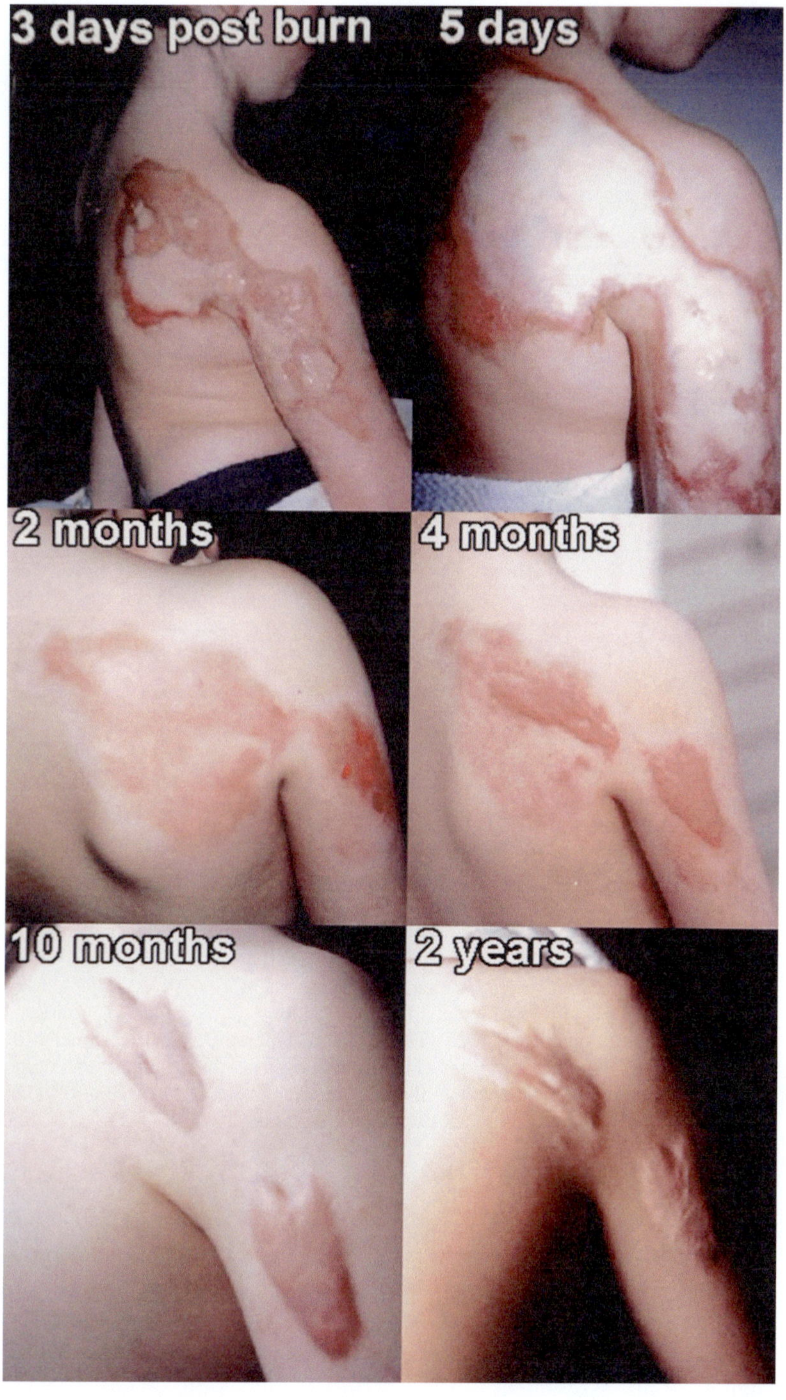

Fig. 20.2 Hypertrophic burn scars after delayed healing of deep dermal burns. Ten old patient with deep scald burn which developed HTS in the deeper regions of the burn but not in the superficial burn which healed over shorter periods of time

Contractures are classified as linear and well-defined, versus broad and diffuse with further subdivision as simple or complex [8]. A simple contracture involves skin only, whereas a complex contracture extends deeper to entrap underlying tissue such as fascia, or muscle. Linear contractures have a well-defined band with pliable skin on one or both sides. Conversely, diffuse contractures are extensive, broad, and surrounded by scarred skin with no single identifiable band (Fig. 20.3).

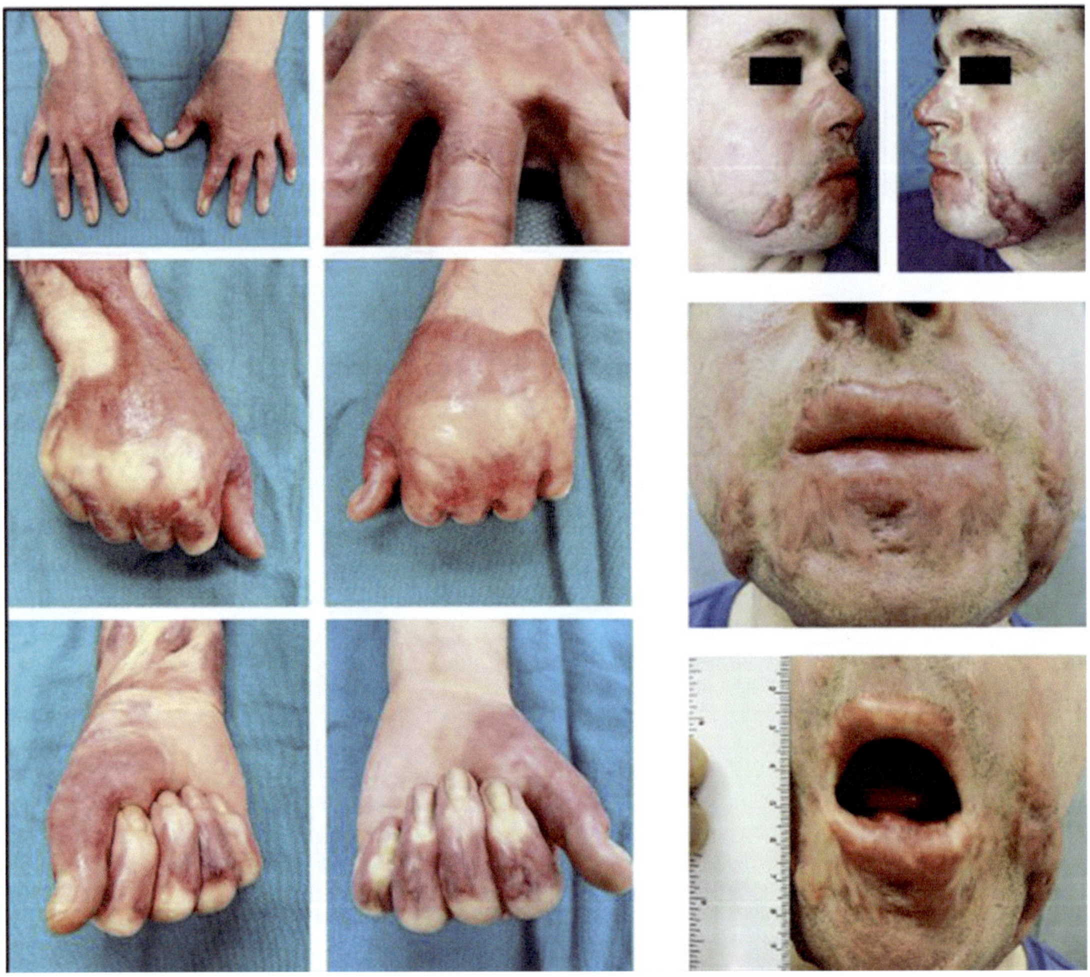

Fig. 20.3 A 24-year-old white male, 11 months following a 21 % total body surface area (TBSA) burn. This patient developed hypertrophic scars (HTS) resulting in cosmetic and functional problems that included restricted opening of mouth and tight web spaces of fingers that limited range of motion on hands. (Reprinted from Tredget EE, Levi B, Donelan MB. Biology and principles of scar management and burn reconstruction. Surg Clin N Am 94(2014); 793–814 [13] with permission from Elsevier.)

Burn Scar Assessment

Whether treating HTS or burn contractures, successful reconstructive planning relies on thorough, serial assessment. The history and progression of the scar must be documented. The exact etiology, history of infection, and symptoms such as pruritus and ROM restriction, of a scar must be documented. Additional information regarding radiation and steroid exposure, especially of tissue adjacent to the scar, is also very helpful. Physical exam should focus on characterizing the scar in terms of color, dimension, relationship to normal structures, tethering, and contracture, as well as changes with movement and rest. Disturbances of pigmentation are classified as hyperpigmentation/hypopigmentation, or mixed, whereas redness is characterized as hyperemic or plethoric [9]. Scar bulk and contour can be described as regular, irregular, or cobblestone. An evaluation of any preexisting scars can be helpful to identify predispositions to aberrant wound healing and anticipate pathologic scarring. Importantly, the transition from a physiologically maturing wound to pathologic scar may not be abundantly apparent, therefore, frequent serial exams with early preventative measures are essential.

Multiple assessment tools have been devised to subjectively and objectively characterize pathologic scars. One of the most frequently used subjective assessment tool is the *Burn Scar Index*, also known as the *Vancouver Scar Scale* or VSS (Fig. 20.4). Originally published in 1990, the VSS was designed to assess the maturation of burn scars in response to treatment correlating to a score based on four variables: height, pliability, vascularity, and pigmentation [10]. Scores ranging from 0 to 14 are assigned relative to the scar's variance from normal skin (score 0), and has proven a useful aid in prognosis and evaluation of treatment effectiveness. Several instruments designed to objectively assess scars are available including skin elasticity meters, laser Doppler, and spectrometry for color analysis [11, 12]. The evaluation of pliability is done by durometry, the vascularity by spectrophotometry (dermaspectrometer or chromameter), the perfusion by laser Doppler ultrasound flowmeter, the area by photography and the thickness by histological micrometer or tissue ultrasound palpation system (TUPS) [11].

Pathophysiology of Hypertrophic Scarring (HTS) After Thermal Injury

The Role of Dermal Fibroblasts (Fig. 20.5)

Fibroblasts from HTS as compared normal dermal tissues from the same patient, display a series of unique features including an increase in fibroblast density in HTS as compared to fibroblast cell numbers in normal dermal tissues. More consistently HTS fibroblasts have reduced collagenase (MMP-1) activity, nitric oxide, and decorin production, which is a small dermatan sulfate proteoglycan that restores collagen fibrillogenesis and binds TGF-β [1, 7, 13].

Increased numbers of myofibroblasts constitute a persistent component of the hypercellular matrix in HTS and contain microfilament bundles and stress fibers. The development of myofibroblasts appears to be induced by TGF-β and strongly correlates with the severity of burn injury (TBSA). Myofibroblasts appear to differentiate not only from regional fibroblasts in the wound under the influence of TGF-β, but also from bone marrow-derived blood borne sources [13].

Toll-Like Receptors Signaling in Fibroblasts

Toll-like receptors are a group of highly conserved molecules that allow the immune system to sense molecules commonly present in bacteria and viruses termed pathogen associated molecular patterns, (PAMPs) or endogenous molecules that are released from necrotic tissue termed damage associated molecular patterns (DAMPs) [14]. They function as activators of the innate immune system but most recently, have increasingly been implicated in the switch from normal wound healing responses to fibrosis in many different organs and tissues. Recently, HTS fibroblasts have been found to have increased expression of TLR4 mRNA and surface receptors implicating the Toll receptor system in the activation of dermal fibroblasts in HTS. Aberrant TLR activation by endogenous molecules released by necrotic or activated cells and extracellular matrix molecules upregulated upon injury or degraded following tissue damage DAMPs, have been implicated in a number of diseases where inappropriate, pathogenic inflammation is at the basis of pathology. Although fibroblasts play an important structural role in wound healing, emerging evidence suggests fibroblasts modify the healing microenvironment by inducing inflammation through activation of the TLRs, signaling through NF-κB that leads to both the recruitment of monocytes and immune cells and subsequent production of inflammatory cytokines [1, 7, 13, 14].

Thus, fibroblasts appear capable of stimulating inflammation via TLR activation, likely via NFκB and mitogen-activated protein kinase (MAPK) which upregulates infiltration of inflammatory cells. In addition, activated deep dermal fibroblasts which appear very important in the development of severe FDP of the skin and future investigation of these profibrotic cells may be improved by the understanding of the role of

Modified Vancouver Scar Scale (VSS) Form

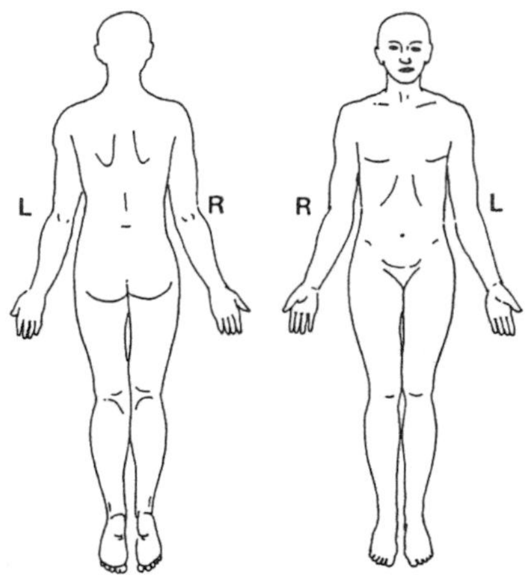

TSSA ____ % normal skin color______

Pliability	0	normal
	1	supple
	2	yielding
	3	firm
	4	adherent
Height	0	normal
	1	1-2 mm
	2	3-4 mm
	3	5-6 mm
	4	>6 mm
Vascularity	0	normal
	1	pink
	2	red
	3	purple
Pigmentation	0	normal
	1	slightly ↑/↓
	2	moderately ↑/↓
	3	severely ↑/↓

no pain ____ worse pain ever experienced

no itchiness ____ worse itchiness ever experienced

Date	Scar #	Pliability	Height	Total	Vascularity	Pigment		Pain	Itchiness	Medication	Initials
						hypo	hyper				

Fig. 20.4 Vancouver burn scar scale. (Reprinted from Nedelec B, Shankowsky H, Tredget E. Rating the Resolving Hypertorphic Scar: Comparison of the Vancouver Scar Scale and Scar Volume. Journal of Burn Care and Research 2000; 21(3) [67] with permission from Wolters Kluwer Health, Inc.)

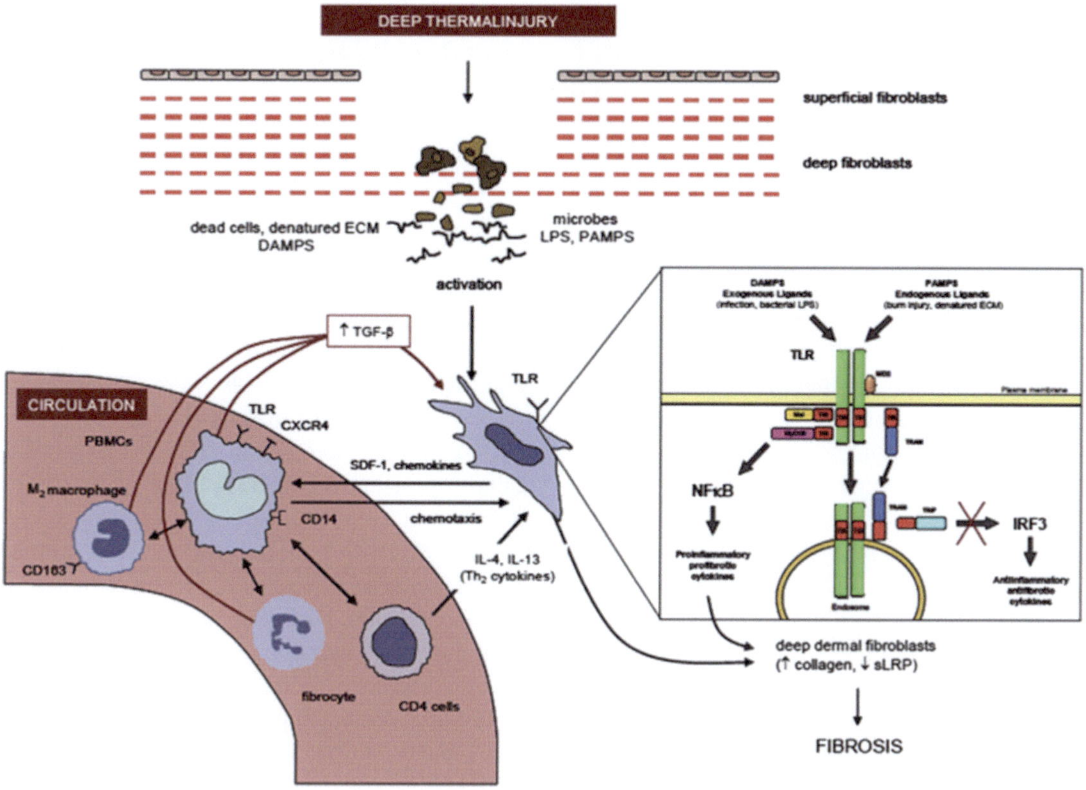

Fig. 20.5 Hypothetical Cellular Mechanism of HTS Formation. It is our hypothesis that burn injury activates fibroblasts in the deep dermis by using PAMPs (i.e., LPS) and DAMPs (i.e., Biglycan) to stimulate the Toll receptors/NFκB pathway on fibroblasts, which in turn release chemokines and growth factors (i.e., TGF-β) recruiting bone marrow-derived monocytes precursors to further activate the production of ECM proteins in deep dermal fibroblasts and subsequently HTS. (Reprinted from Ding J et al. Deep dermal fibroblast profibrotic characteristics are enhanced by bone marrow-derived mesenchymal stem cells. Wound Repair and Regeneration 2013 [68] with permission from John Wiley & Sons)

TLRs in fibrosis and lead to novel therapeutic options to antagonize abnormal activation of fibroblasts by inflammation.

Bone Marrow-Derived Cells in Hypertrophic Scarring

Previously, fibrocytes, a bone marrow derived cell with a fibroblast-like morphology that co-express collagen I and III, CD13, CD34, and the bone-marrow derived surface marker CD 45 make up 0.5 % of peripheral blood leukocytes, but can constitute 10 % of cells infiltrating acute wounds. They are capable of synthesizing ECM proteins, proteases including collagenase, and growth factors including TGF-β1, TNF-α, IL-6, and IL-10, but can also present antigens and thereby prime naïve T lymphocytes [15, 16].

Fibrocytes in burn patients are derived from peripheral blood mononuclear cells (PBMC), where the percentage of type I collagen-positive fibrocytes was significantly higher (up to 10 % of PBMC) than for control individuals (normal level <0.5 %), which correlated with serum levels of TGF-β [15]. Fibrocytes are located in HTS tissue after burn injury primarily in deeper layers of the dermis in increased numbers compared to mature scar and normal skin [16]. Quantitatively, fibrocytes produce modest amounts collagen compared to HSc fibroblasts; however, fibrocytes appear to stimulate dermal fibroblasts to proliferate, produce, and contract ECM, as well as producing TGF-β and connective tissues growth factor (CTGF) [15, 16]. Thus, the principal source of collagen in HTS appears to be local fibroblasts, but fibrocytes have an important paracrine function in HTS. It is possible to antagonize many of these fibrogenic effects of fibrocytes in vitro with IFNα where significantly decreased numbers of fibrocytes were found in the tissues of burn patients in response to systemic IFN treatment in vivo, associated with fibrosis resolution and scar remodeling as well as a reduction in angiogenesis [17].

Heterotopic ossification (HO) is a clinical condition where mature lamellar bone is formed in damaged tissues such as muscle, tendon and fascia particularly after burns and traumatic injuries that leads to skin breakdown, significant soft tissue deformity, joint ankylosis, and chronic pain substantially prolonging rehabilitation. In burn patients, the incidence of HO varies between 0.2 and 4 %, and is more frequent in patients with extensive burns (>20 % total body surface area) [13, 18]. Although HO may occur in joints unrelated to burn injuries, lesions usually develop under areas of deep burns complicated by HTS, especially in the elbow and is associated with prolonged loss of consciousness (i.e., mechanical ventilation), long-term immobilization, burn wound infection and/or delayed closure, loss of skin grafts, and recurring local trauma including passive range of motion. Fibrocytes have been identified in heterotopic ossification (HO), where mature lamellar bone is formed in damaged tissues such as muscle, tendon and fascia particularly after burns and traumatic injuries, where they traffic to injured areas and interact with resident cells and lead to skin breakdown, significant soft tissue deformity, joint ankylosis, and chronic pain. HO and hypertrophic scar have common features and appear to be causally related after significant initial local tissue injury which leads to a systemic inflammatory response, where unique PBMCs, including fibrocytes contribute the fibrotic and osteogenic matrix in as yet unidentified ways [13, 18].

The Th_1/Th_2 Immune Response After Burn Injury

In burn patients with HTS, a deficiency of circulating interferon-producing Th_1 lymphocytes and increased lymphocytes which produce Th_2 cytokines (IL-4, 5, 10, 13) exists within 3 months after burn injury, which persists for up to 1 year after injury, i.e., a polarized Th_2 response [18]. Similar elevations in systemic IL-10 protein levels in the first 2 months post-injury persist until 1 year, whereas IL-12 levels were significantly lower and inversely related to IL-10. IFN-γ mRNA was not detected in HTS tissues until 6 months post-injury, whereas IL-4 increased in HTS within 2 months post-injury.

CD4+/TGF-β^+ lymphocytes are also present in an increased frequency in the circulating immune cells of burn patients as compared to normal control individuals. These cells secrete increased levels of TGF-β, which promotes proliferation of dermal fibroblasts, as well as α-SMA and wound contraction. The development of $CD4^+$TGF-β^+ cells may contribute to the suppression of Th_1 immunity similar to trauma patients, where increased T regulatory $CD4^+CD25^+$ cells which produce TGF-β, have been found systemically. Thus, these findings suggest that after thermal injury, a polarized Th_2 environment favors the subsequent development of increased Th_3^+ cells and fibrocytes, which can induce fibrosis in a paracrine fashion [13, 19].

Like lymphocytes, macrophages respond to Th_2 cytokines and numerous studies have shown that macrophages exposed to IL-4 develop an alternate activation state termed "alternatively activated macrophages" or M_2 macrophages, and their role may be equal to if not more important than the type of $CD4^+$ T-helper cell response in many different types of fibroses. M_1 macrophages can induce MMP-1 secretion and promote ECM degradation while M_2 macrophages can secret large amount of TGF-β1, which can stimulate myofibroblast transformation and lead to ECM deposition [20, 21].

Stromal cell-derived factor 1 (SDF-1) is a potent chemokine that attracts lymphocytes and monocytes by binding exclusively to its receptor,

CXCR4 [12, 21]. SDF-1 expression is increased in HTS tissue and serum of the burn patients with increased number of CD14+ CXCR4+ peripheral blood mononuclear cells, which suggested SDF-1/CXCR4 signaling recruits cells such as monocytes to sites of prolonged inflammation, where they contribute to HTS formation. Using a CXCR4 antagonist, CTCE-9908, to inhibit the SDF-1/CXCR4 signaling in nude mouse model of HTS, significant attenuation of scar formation and contraction with reduced number of CXCR4 expressing monocytes in the circulation and differentiated macrophages in the HTS tissue was found supporting a role of SDF-1/CXCR4 chemoattracted monocytes and macrophages in HTS formation [22].

Fibroblast Heterogeneity and the Profibrotic Microenvironment

Sorrell and Caplan have found that normal adult human skin contains at least three separate subpopulations of fibroblasts, which occupy unique niches depending on the depth in the dermis and exhibit distinctive differences when isolated by limited dilution cloning [23]. Fibroblasts associated with hair follicles show distinctive characteristics from cells in the papillary and reticular dermis. Papillary dermal fibroblasts, which reside in the superficial dermis, are heterogeneous in terms of morphology and proliferation kinetics, whereas reticular fibroblasts in the deep dermis possess myofibroblast-like characteristics by greater collagen lattice contraction and α-SMA expression.

Fibroblasts that arise from the deeper layers proliferate at a slower rate, but are significantly larger morphologically, and collagenase mRNA is significantly lower in deep dermal fibroblasts [23, 24]. Fibroblasts from the deeper layers produce more TGF-β, CTGF, and heat shock protein 47 (HSP47), a human chaperon protein for type I collagen, compared to those from superficial layers [1, 13, 24]. Fibroblasts from the deeper layer produced more α-SMA protein and contracted collagen gels more efficiently. Fibroblasts from the deeper layer also produced more collagen, but had less collagenase activity and produced more of the fibrocartilaginous proteoglycan versican, but less decorin. Decorin and other members of the sLRP family, fibromodulin and lumican, function to bind type I collagen in the extracellular matrix regulating the kinetics of collagen fibrillogenesis and the diameter and distance between fibrils [25]. Decorin and fibromodulin can also bind to and inhibit TGF-β_1 activity in vitro and in vivo. A low level of growth factor production by fetal cells, especially TGF-β_1, is a major factor in the absence of excess collagen deposition and scar formation [24–26]. Fibroblasts isolated from the deep dermis produce less decorin and more large cartilage-like proteoglycans, including versican and aggrecan that can account for the ultrastructural abnormalities in HTS (Fig. 20.5). Fibrocytes have also been described to produce less small leucine rich proteoglycans (sLRPs) and more versican, hyaluronan, perlecan, and biglycan in the ECM [24, 25]. These features of hypertrophic scar fibroblasts are very consistently found in fibroblasts located in the deeper layers of the skin or reticular dermis as compared to superficial papillary fibroblasts.

Recently, two different groups have reaffirmed and identified distinct lineages of fibroblasts in the deep dermal regions of the skin which possess intrinsic fibrogenic potential and determine the ultimate dermal architecture in the skin after wound healing [27, 28]. Dunkin et al. quantified the association between scarring and the depth of dermal injury in 113 human volunteers using a novel jig to create a human dermal scratch model with HTS and normotrophic scar within the same lesion [29]. They found a threshold depth of dermal injury of 0.56±0.03 mm or 33 % of the lateral hip thickness, beyond which scarring develops. In patients with thermal injury and we found that the superficial 1/3 of this scratch wound healed normally with minimal scar, whereas the deep dermal end region healed with a thickened wider scar typical of HTS and contained significantly greater numbers of fibrocytes [25, 26] (Fig. 20.5). These data strongly demonstrate that fibroblasts from the deeper layers resemble HTS fibroblasts, suggesting that the activated deeper layer fibroblasts may play a critical role in the formation of HTS.

Treatment of HTS Following Burn Injury

Prevention of Abnormal Scarring

Multiple studies have demonstrated that HTS will spontaneously resolve to varying degrees [30, 31]. This natural history entails remodeling of the ECM, a phenomenon that has proven a fruitful therapeutic target. Based on the pathophysiology of HTS, early recognition of deep dermal burns and subsequent resurfacing improves the quality of wound healing based on several features of HTS that have been illustrated by in vivo and in vitro studies [1, 13].

Therefore, successful prevention of HTS is facilitated through diagnostic accuracy of burn depth. Tools such as thermography and scanning laser Doppler assist prediction of deep burns in need of excision and grafting that would otherwise be left to heal secondarily [11, 12]. Regardless of the assessment tool used to identify deep dermal wounds, studies suggest that clinical observation and subjective judgment have limitations in the surgical decision-making of modern burn centers.

Novel Therapies for Scar Management

Novel and emerging therapeutic options including interferon-α (IFN-α), chemokine and CXCR4 inhibitors, and TGF-β modulators have shown great promise in controlling abnormal scar progression [1, 13, 17]. Interferon treatment has been suggested for prevention of scar hypertrophy recurrence post-excision but has not demonstrated the same efficacy in treatment of established HTS. The action of interferon results in a modification of fibroblast behavior. Recent studies on chemokines, CXCR4 inhibitors and TGF-β antagonists, have shown potential therapeutic value for the treatment of HTS, but further clinical studies are needed [15, 22].

Nonoperative Treatment for HTS Post-burn Injury

Traditionally, conservative measures for the management of HTS have relied on pressure garments and silicone gel therapy; both considered long-term treatments (Fig. 20.6). Although the exact mechanism of compression treatments is not fully understood, remodeling of the ECM occurs. Various in vitro studies have proposed specific mechanisms such as increased MMP-9 activity, α-SMA inhibition, and generalized ischemia leading to cell damage with reduced collagen production [13, 31, 32]. Potential complications of compression garments include skin breakdown, obstructive sleep apnea, bony deformity, discomfort, dento-alveolar deformation, and cost, which may hinder compliance. Potential benefits identified in a 12-year prospective trial included an overall improvement in clinical appearance, regardless of ethnicity, as evidenced by a decrease in scar thickness, height, and softening of pigmentation [32].

Similar to compression garments, the mechanism of action of silicone gel therapy is poorly understood. In vitro studies correlate silicone gel with decreased TGF-β levels and reduced fibroblast-mediated collagen contraction, functioning to enhance hydration of the stratum corneum, O_2 delivery to tissues, surface skin temperature, and reduce tissue turgor. This may manifest clinically as improved scar elasticity, softness, and overall appearance. Although conflicting results regarding the efficacy of silicone sheeting abound in the literature, a number of meta-analyses and large scale reviews support their use [33–36].

Other nonsurgical techniques of HTS management include intralesional corticosteroids, topical retinoic acid, intralesional 5-fluorouracil, cryosurgery, and radiotherapy. Scar massage also represents a treatment modality for HTS which maintains or improves joint mobility and softening fibrous bands or contractures. Massage has also been proven to decrease itching and to be part of the desensitization process and is performed two to five times a day for 5 min [36].

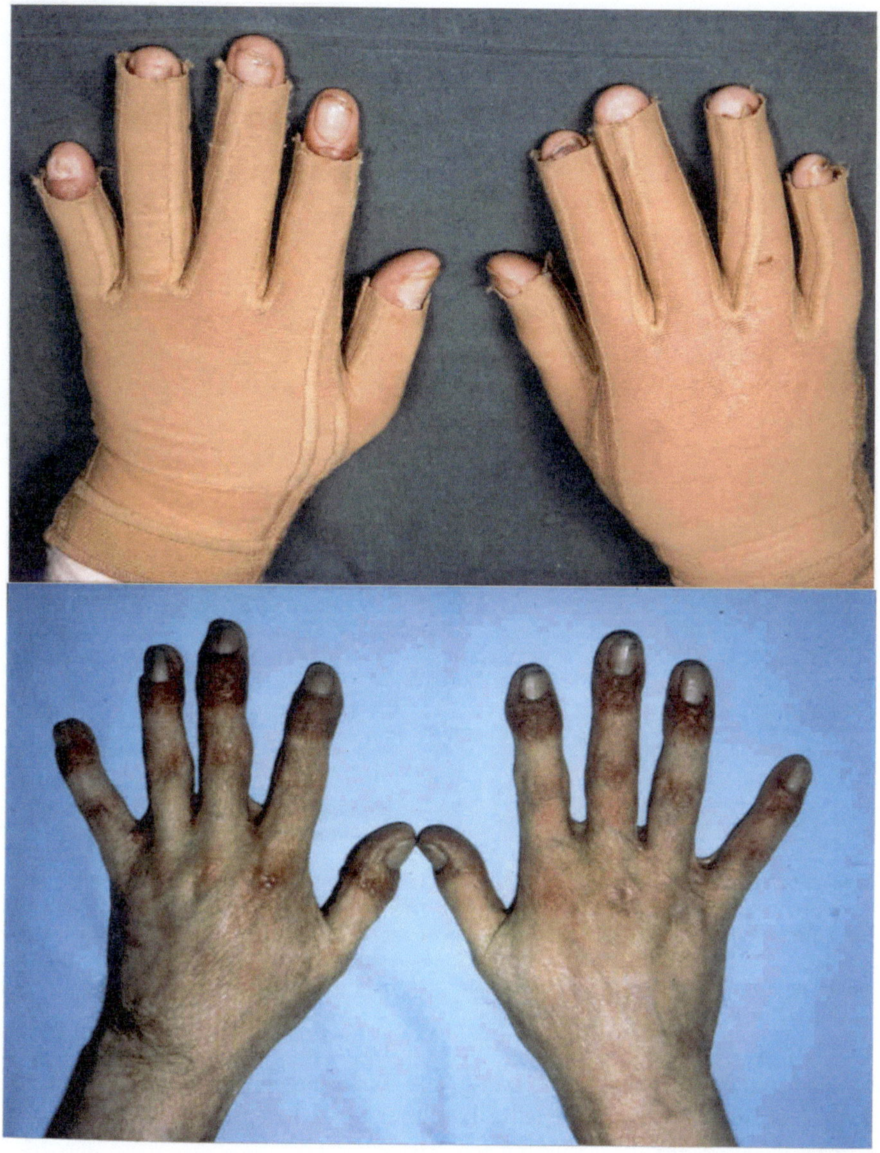

Fig. 20.6 Pressure garment used to remodel HTS post-burn injury. Note the differences in scar remodeling in the fingertips where the garments had been cut out

Surgical Management of HTS and Burn Contractures

Chapter 11 is a well-written, complete review of the surgical approach that is applicable to reconstruction of acute burn deformities and includes an approach to specific deformities in different region of the body. However, for management of burn scars a surgical procedure requires an understanding of appropriate timing and the range of techniques available as discussed and illustrated below in a much more limited fashion.

Operative scar management involves the excision of scar followed by replacement with healthy transplanted tissue whenever possible (Fig. 20.7). The operative approach to scar management needs to invoke principles of tissue

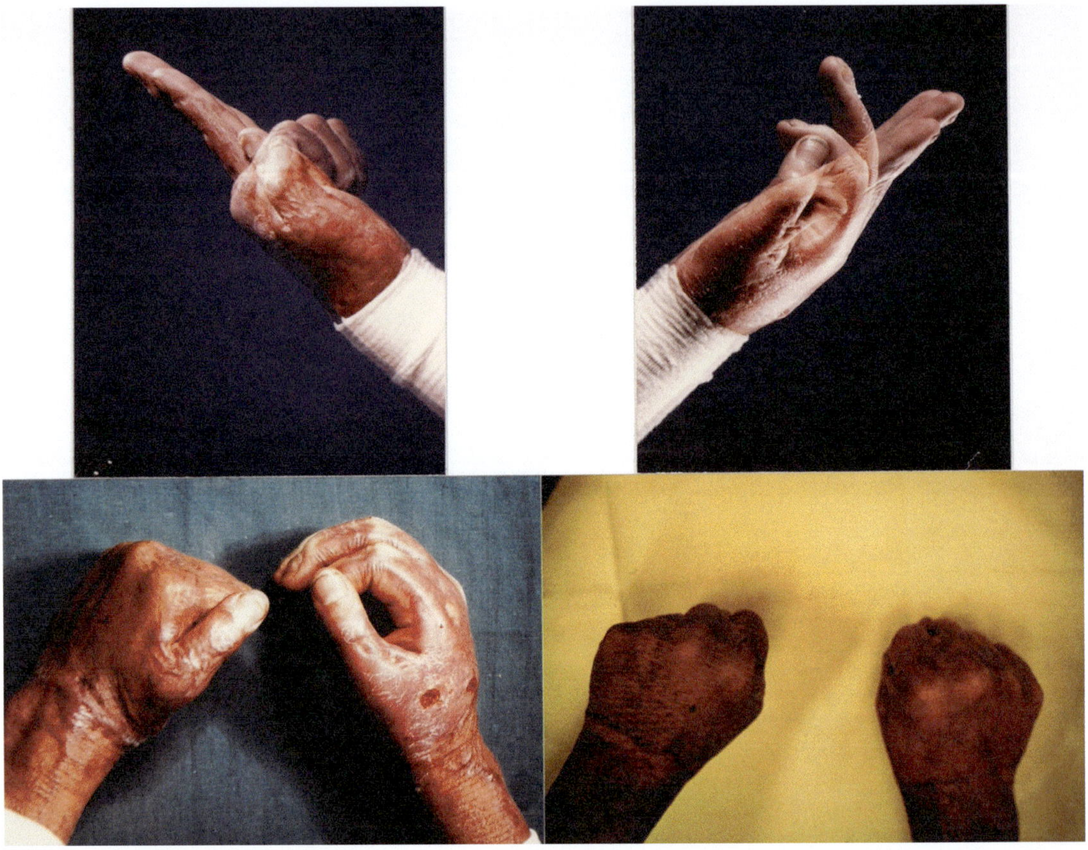

Fig. 20.7 Restoration of hand function with excision of HTS and split thickness skin graft. Burn scar contracture of the right hand after spontaneous wound healing over 3 weeks due to a lack of available skin graft donors. This 18-year-old man with a 70 % TBSA burn who underwent split thickness skin grafting of the clinically deeper burned left hand restoring function at 1 month post-burn (*bottom left*) but required excision of the HTS and skin grafting at 6 months post burn to the right hand which was less deep and allowed to heal spontaneously to restore function (*bottom right*)

replacement and rehabilitation with a multimodal strategy that includes surgical release of tension followed by replacement of missing tissue, vascular laser treatment of erythematous scars, and fractional ablative laser treatment of hypertrophic scar. Because all burn patients present with some degree of tissue deficit, tension is always a factor the burn surgeon must contend with, therefore, HTS is always a risk. Fortunately, surgical release of tension across a scar usually results in the improvement of hypertrophy, after which treating scar depigmentation, and pruritus may be approached with laser therapy. Typically, scar management can be categorized temporally into acute, intermediate, and late reconstruction [37–39].

Burn surgeons need to be involved in patient care immediately to assess for cases requiring urgent reconstruction. Acute surgery should be performed for cases such as threatened airway from cervical contracture, eating difficulties secondary to severe microstomia, exposure keratitis from severe eyelid injury, and exposure of vital structures (Fig. 20.3). Upon initial assessment, functionally and cosmetically sensitive areas like the hands and face need special consideration. For example, meshed grafts will yield abnormal appearance after healing and should be avoided especially on the face and hands [38]. Furthermore, HTS is a potential even at donor sites, and therefore, areas of tissue harvest should be chosen strategically to leave inconspicuous scars. Where possible, accurate and objective assessment of burn depth should dictate which wounds are superficial and should be given time to heal, avoiding aggressive excision and grafting.

Once the graft and donor sites exhibit healing in the acute phase, aim can be taken at optimizing scar in the intermediate phase. Evidence suggests physiologic wound healing benefits from hydration through modalities including silicone sheeting, water-based moisturizers, and occlusive dressing [38, 39]. Although evidence is still emerging, tension off-loading by means of compression garments is often utilized in an effort to decrease the incidence and severity of HTS [5, 38, 39].

Several methods of scar management in the late phase have been described, ranging from various contracture releases and skin grafting to the use of laser therapy. When planning to release a scar contracture, the location, width, extensiveness, and geometry must be carefully considered. There is no substitute for a carefully executed contracture release to alleviate the tension across a burn scar. However, a meta-analysis by Ogawa et al. demonstrated an absence of standardized treatment algorithms for managing scar contracture based on a paucity of randomized-controlled trials [40]. Although no consensus exists as to when to employ a given technique for contracture release, operative interventions can be divided into four categories: skin grafts, random pattern flaps (V-Y, Z-plasty), defined vascular pattern flaps (perforator flaps, free flaps), and dermal substitutes such as *Alloderm*™ [LifeCell Corporation, Bridgewater, N.J.], *or Integra*™ [Integra LifeSciences, Cincinnati, O.H.]). Regardless of the specific treatment employed, the goal of surgery remains the same; achieve optimal mobility of the underlying structures [5, 37–42].

A fundamental principle in scar management is the timing of operative intervention. In general, surgery should be delayed until scar maturity has been reached, which may range between 12 and 24 months post-burn [41]. Corrective efforts performed on immature scar prove more technically demanding and may be met with more aggressive scar formation postoperatively. Furthermore, conservative measures such as pressure garments and silicone sheeting are often utilized to allow scars to mature nonoperatively. Indications for intervention prior to scar maturity include wounds with exposed vital structures, risk for invasive infection, severe contractures causing significant functional deficits or growth disturbance in children [5, 41, 42].

As discussed in Chap. 11, z-plasty functions to decrease longitudinal tension of a scar by lengthening its central limb and medial transposition of lateral flaps serves to reduce the width of the scarred area, ultimately improving collagen remodeling through tension off-loading (Fig. 20.8) [43, 44]. In the context of burn scar contractures, releasing incisions should be limited to superficial planes enabling deep underlying structures to relax and expand into their original architecture [45]. Due to the frequency with which scar excision results in significant tissue deficits, a carefully considered plan for closure must always be included in preoperative planning. Where persistent tissue deficit persists, variable thicknesses of skin grafts can be utilized with wound bed contact maximized through the use of bolsters, splints, and wraps. Full-thickness skin grafts (FTSGs) prove more resistant to contracture recurrence, but the defect size may limit their use, in which case a thick split-thickness skin graft STSG can be considered. If healthy local tissue is present, a regional transposition flap may be the best option and in select cases, a free flap may be indicated for large defects or exposed vital structures. When assessing the success of contracture release, outcome measures may include functional improvement, VSS rating, surface area measurements, and patient satisfaction [46].

Soft Tissue Expansion for Burn Scar Reconstruction

Scar management often entails surgical excision that leaves a tissue deficit not immediately amenable to primary closure with graft, or local flap coverage. In such cases, tissue expansion becomes invaluable for reconstruction of adjacent soft tissue defects. The core advantages of tissue expansion are its reliability and ability to replace defects with tissue that is an excellent

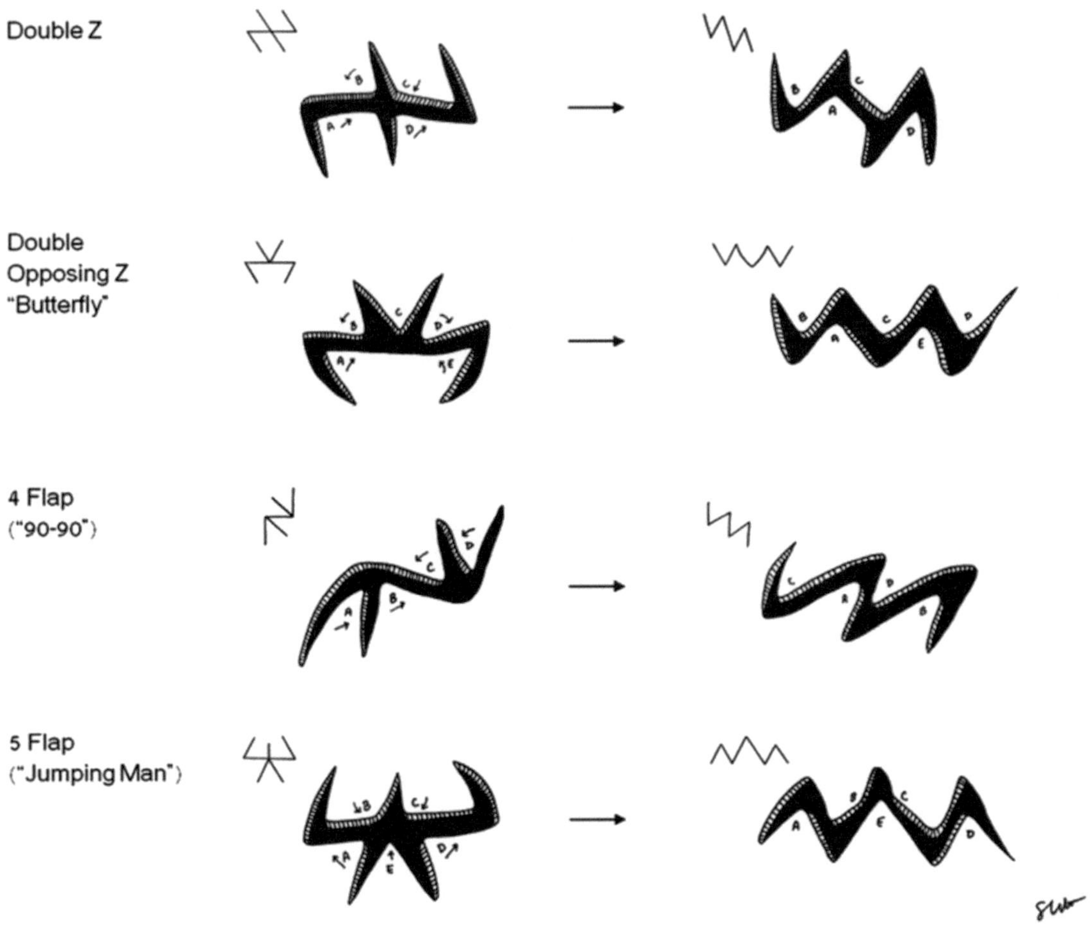

Fig. 20.8 Diagram of a number of z-plasty variations useful for burn scar release and reconstruction. (Reprinted from Tredget EE, Levi B, Donelan MB. Biology and principles of scar management and burn reconstruction. Surg Clin N Am 94(2014); 793–814 [13] with permission from Elsevier)

color, texture, thickness, and hair-bearing pattern match [47–49]. Caution must be exercised when performing tissue expansion in patients with connective tissue disease, poorly controlled diabetes or peripheral vascular disease, in regions of irradiated tissue and the young child's scalp. At the cellular level, tissue expansion relies on a robust angiogenic response similar to that of the incisional delay phenomena.

A typical tissue expander consists of a silicone elastomer reservoir placed beneath donor tissue, which is subsequently filled with saline at scheduled intervals (Fig. 20.9). Filling of the expander results in a net increase in surface area per unit volume of the overlying soft tissue envelope. Filling ports may be remote, connected to the expander through silastic tubing, or integrated within the expander. Integrated filling ports carry the risk of inadvertent puncture of the expander during filling, whereas subcutaneous placement of remote ports must be carefully located to avoid filling difficulty [48].

An expander should be chosen with a base two to three times the diameter of the expected soft-tissue deficit, with a rigid backing to direct expansion perpendicular to the wound bed. Expander shape varies, and should be chosen based on anatomic location. Rectangular expanders, most commonly used in the trunk and extremities, yield the greatest theoretical gain in tissue (40 %), whereas round expanders used in breast reconstruction provide the least (25 %).

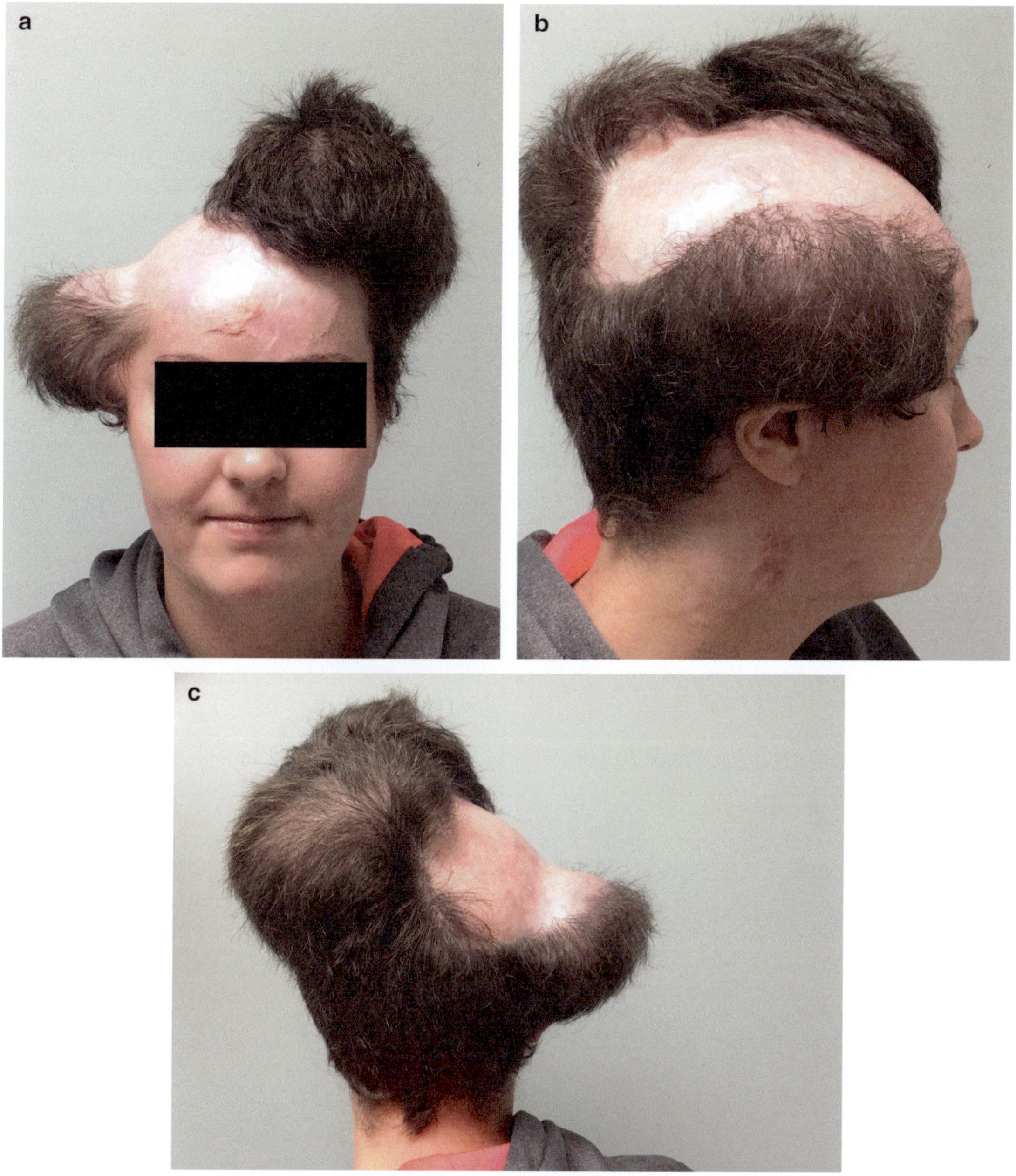

Fig. 20.9 (**a–c**) Soft tissue expansion for burn scar reconstruction. This 30-year-old female suffered burn injury from a campfire after suffering a seizure who is undergoing soft tissue expansion and reconstruction of the non-hair bearing region of the scalp after placement of three crescent shaped expanders inflated biweekly for 3 months to a total of 400 cc prior to second stage scalp reconstruction

Crescent expanders gain more tissue centrally than peripherally and are useful in scalp defects. Perhaps the most important considerations in successful expansion are placement of incisions and positioning of the expander. Incisions for expander placement should be designed radially to the pocket in order to minimize tension and, therefore, risk of extrusion. Placement should be away from joints and parallel to the long-axis of the prospective defect, deep to well-vascularized

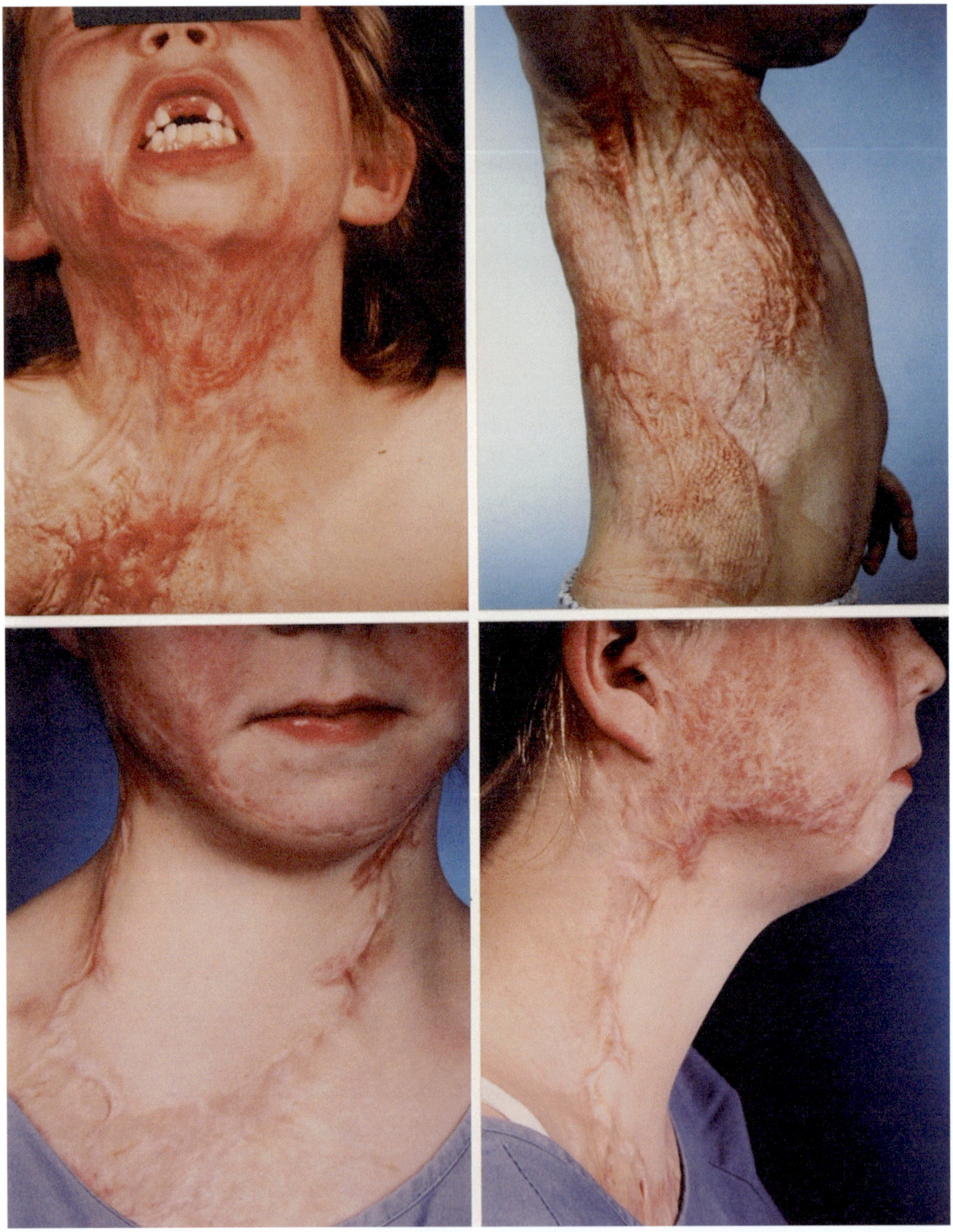

Fig. 20.10 A 7-year old child with burn scar contractures of the neck and axilla who underwent burn scar release of the neck region using microsurgical soft tissue transfer of a pre-expanded radial forearm free flap

tissue that is free of unstable scar [49, 50]. The risk of extrusion can be decreased further by avoidance of excessive dissection, meticulous hemostasis, and designing the pocket to allow the expander to sit completely flat without wrinkling. Pockets for the expander can be developed in the submuscular, subgaleal, or subcutaneous plane depending on reconstructive demands.

Laser Therapy of Burn Scars

Since introduction in the 1980s by Castro et al. and Apfelberg et al., therapy using *l*ight *a*mplification by *s*timulated *e*mission of *r*adiation, or *laser* has undergone rapid expansion in scar management [50, 51]. Although high-level evidence regarding efficacy for scar tension, pruritus, and appearance is lacking, laser therapy is viewed by many as a substantial development in the treatment of HTS. Following surgical release, many surgeons view the next stage in scar management to involve laser. Laser interaction with scar tissue is based on three different effects including thermal, chemical, and mechanical. Four key variables are involved in laser treatment: energy, power, fluency, and irradiance. Energy, measured in joules, is proportional to the number of photons released by excited electrons as they return to a resting state. Power, quantified in watts, is a measure of energy per unit time (J/s), whereas fluency is energy per unit area (J/cm^2). Irradiance is a measure of power per unit area (W/cm^2). Theoretically, laser therapy causes controlled damage of targeted tissue, which, in turn, induces favorable scar remodeling. Proposed mechanisms on a histological scale include induction of acute inflammation, MMP-mediated turnover of ECM proteins, and orderly production of collagens I and III, and elastin [52].

Laser therapy proves beneficial for HTS through a process first described in 1983 by Anderson and Parish termed selective photothermolysis [53]. As light encounters a medium such as skin, it can be absorbed, scattered, transmitted, or reflected. The stratum corneum of the epidermis reflects 4–7 % of light, whereas the dermis largely scatters laser light [54]. Selective photothermolysis relies on light of specific wavelengths being absorbed by chromophores such as melanin, water, hemoglobin, and oxyhemoglobin. Upon absorption by chromophores, thermal effects ranging from protein denaturation to vaporization occur as well as chemical effects due to photon emissions. Tissue can be targeted for focused damage by lasers with specific wavelengths, pulse durations, and fluencies. The effects of laser regarding burns scar remains controversial. Parameters such as the laser type and the time between treatments have not been conclusively determined. In order to achieve the desired effect, two parameters must be met. The pulse duration of the absorbed light must be greater than the thermal relaxation time of the target tissue, defined as the time for the tissue to cool to 50 % of the initial temperature achieved [54]. Secondly, the fluency of the laser must be greater than the threshold fluency of the target tissue. Based on its mechanism of action, different lasers with specific parameters can be used to target certain symptoms.

Pulsed-dye lasers (PDL), are indicated for the treatment of scar erythema. At wavelengths of 585 or 598 nm PDLs are absorbed by oxyhemoglobin with millisecond domains that target small blood vessels. This type of laser seems more efficient for red or immature scar. Pulses of 0.4–20 ms at fluencies of 4–7 J/cm^2 induce focal damage in vascular endothelium and platelet thrombi, which correlates with improved scar pain, pruritus, and erythema [55]. Potential complications include erythema, purpura, hyperpigmentation and hypopigmentation, and thermal injury. The most frequent complication is purpura for few days to 1 week; however, cryogenic cooling can bolster epidermal protection. Despite its effectiveness for improving scar erythema, PDL proves minimally beneficial in addressing scar contour or thickness.

Ablation laser therapy, which describes the total removal of target tissue by vaporization, is capable of treating deep thickness scars through reduction of scar mass and the spontaneous release of tension on restrictive scars. With water as its chromophore, ablational lasers cause tissue damage with a wavelength of 10,600 nm through nonspecific vaporization [56]. Fractional CO_2

ablative lasers are adjusted to target specific columns of epidermis and dermis, which causes thermal damage in microthermal treatment zones. The tiny laser columns drill multiple holes into the tissue. Around each of the tunnels there is injured scar from heat, which is caused by vaporization. Due to those injuries, the process of healing and scar maturation starts over again with new remodeling phase. Disorganized collagen fibrils are disrupted within these zones while concurrently allowing untreated adjacent areas to function as collagen reservoirs for healthy tissue regeneration. As with other lasers, the stimulation of fibroblast activity and new collagen expedite the healing process. Ablated microchannels have a diameter of 60–250 μm surrounded by a 50–150 μm thick rim of thermal coagulation. The key strength of ablative lasers is their depth of penetration (0.08–4 mm) and thus their ability to treat thick scars [56, 57]. Pulse energy can be adjusted based on scar thickness as judged through palpation; however, consensus is lacking with regards to penetration beyond the depth of scar. Normal skin treated with these lasers rapidly heals without scar; however, caution should be exercised at higher energies.

Other types of lasers such as fractional non-ablative (NAFL) 1540/1550 nm has been studied and showed promising therapeutic potential with a decrease in residual thermal dermal damage and faster healing. The Alexandrite laser has also been used to destroy growing hair follicles and obstructed sweat glands that can be symptomatic for burn patients [57].

General consensus appears to dictate the delay of laser therapy until at least 3 months post-injury, with most starting at 6–12 months after healing, at which point scar maturation is progressed. The risks of premature treatment lay in the marginal gain secondary to unstable epidermal coverage, and less tolerance of younger scars to rigorous treatment at the necessary settings [58–60]. Early intervention has been suggested by an international panel of experts to be effective in preventive of HTS [60]. The surface area commonly involved in laser therapy often mandates its performance under some form of sedation, typically a general anesthetic; however, relatively small areas may be treated under local anesthesia. An interval of 1–3 months between treatments is common, with multiple treatments often necessary until benefit has plateaued as judged by patient and surgeon. Scar remodeling has been reported as early as 1–2 weeks post-laser; however, beneficial changes may progress over several months. No consensus has been reached, nor data presented, to definitively illustrate a relationship between laser efficacy and the location or age of scar. Early research does demonstrate that outcomes are stable at 2-years after the last laser treatment. A study by Hultman et al. concluded that the greatest clinical gains from laser therapy occurred when treatment was initiated before the 18-months post-burn, and with an average of 5.3 sessions per patient, a mean reduction in the VSS score from 10.43 to 3.29 was achieved [56].

Despite the potential benefits, laser therapy is not without risk or complication. Most commonly, hypopigmentation, erythema, temporary hyperpigmentation, infection, scarring, and pain have been reported [60]. Thermal injury is always a risk, but can be mitigated by vigilant selection of laser settings, minimizing redundant passes, adjusting the density at each new treatment interval, wearing protective eyewear, and judicious use of concurrent therapies. Preoperatively, patients with a history of herpes simplex infection should receive antiviral prophylaxis. Normal activity can be resumed immediately, with the exception of sun exposure, and immersion in water. Petroleum-based ointment and light dressings are typically applied postoperatively, with dressing removal at the 48-h mark, and continued application of ointment until reepithelialization between postoperative days 3 and 4. Adjunctive steroid therapy in the form of intralesional injections, or topical application has been described [60]. Distribution of the steroid throughout the scar is facilitated by the micropores created by the laser. Adjunctive steroids should be discontinued at the first sign of tissue atrophy, telangiectasias, or hypopigmentation. Other adjunctive therapies described include 5-fluorouracil, and hydroquinones which may also improve erythema through decreased pigmentation of the epidermis [60–62].

Microvascular Free Tissue Transfer in Burn Reconstruction

Microvascular free flaps may be beneficial in the acute phase of thermal or electrical burn for coverage of exposed structures as vessels, nerves, tendons, and bone and in some cases represent the only option for limb salvage [63, 64]. Free flaps allows the transfer of large area of healthy tissue with an intact vascular supply but also can be used as composite reconstruction with bone, nerves, tendon, or cartilage. The types of flaps can be fasciocutaneous, muscular, fascial, combined, prefabricated or prelaminated. Commonly used flaps include the anterior lateral thigh flap, latissimus dorsi myocutaneous flap, scapular/parascapular, lateral arm, and radial forearm free flaps as well as others. Fasciocutaneous flap can provide thin and pliable tissue coverage as suited for reconstruction of burn scar contractures of the neck region (Fig. 20.9). Muscle free flaps are useful when a larger volume of tissue is necessary to obliterate a dead space or for functional muscular transfer.

However, physiological instability, damage to surrounding tissue, restriction of donor site and recipient vessels can limit the use of free tissue transfer for burn patients. Free flaps for burns patients may imply additional challenges such as cardiovascular and respiratory instability, availability and quality of recipient vessels, limited donor site options and a possible increased infection risk. Preoperative planning is essential for those patients. Modalities such as angiography or Doppler can be a useful tool to assess the vascular anatomy of the flap and recipient site. Inadequate debridement of dead tissue has been reported as an important risk factor of flap failure. Free flaps in burn patients are recognized to have a higher risk of complications; however, careful patient selection and monitoring post operatively have improved outcomes [63–65].

Microvascular allotransplantation of composite tissue including face or upper extremity has promising cosmetic and functional benefits to burn patients but must be balanced with the risks of immunosuppression and rejection making patient selection complex [65].

Conclusions

Scar management after burn injury involves the assessment and long-term multimodal treatment of hypertrophic scarring, contractures, and disturbances in pigmentation. As our understanding of the molecular basis for pathological scarring advances, novel targets will lead to specific therapeutic interventions. Currently effective burn surgery requires a sound foundation of skills in the prevention, conservative treatment, and operative reconstruction of pathologic scars in order to deliver a high quality of care to patients burdened with the severe functional and cosmetic complications of thermal injury.

Acknowledgements This work was supported by the Firefighters' Burn Trust Fund of the University of Alberta Hospital, the Canadian Institutes for Health Research, and the Alberta Heritage Trust Fund for Medical Research.

References

1. Kwan P, Desmouliere A, Tredget EE. Chapter 45—molecular and cellular basis of hypertrophic scarring. In: Herndon DN, editor. Total burn care. 3rd ed. Philadelphia: Saunders Elsevier; 2012. p. 495–505.e5.
2. Bombaro KM, Engrav LH, Carrougher GJ, et al. What is the prevalence of hypertrophic scarring following burns? Burns. 2003;29:299–302.
3. Engrav LH, Covey MH, Dutcher KD, et al. Impairment, time out of school, and time off from work after burns. Plast Reconstr Surg. 1987;79:927–34.
4. Brown JJ, Bayat A. Genetic susceptibility to raised dermal scarring. Br J Dermatol. 2009;161(1):8–18.
5. Gauglitz GG, Korting HC, Pavicic T, Ruzicka T, et al. Hypertrophic scarring and keloids: pathomechanisms and current and emerging treatment strategies. Mol Med. 2011;17:113.
6. Jaskille AD, Shupp JW, Jordan MH, et al. Critical review of burn depth assessment techniques: part I. Historical review. J Burn Care Res. 2009;30(6):937–47.
7. Kwan P, Hori K, Ding J, et al. Scar and contracture: biological principles. Hand Clin. 2009;25(4):511–28.
8. Ketchum L, Cohen IK, Masters FW. Hypertrophic scars and keloids—a collective review. Plast Reconstr Surg. 1974;53:140–54.
9. Vercelli S, Ferriero G, Sartorio F, et al. How to assess postsurgical scars: a review of outcome measures. Disabil Rehabil. 2009;31:2055–63.
10. Sullivan T, Smith J, Kermode J, et al. Rating the burn scar. J Burn Care Rehabil. 1990;11:256–60.

11. Stewart TL, Ball B, Schembri PJ, et al. The use of laser Doppler imaging as a predictor of burn depth and hypertrophic scar post-burn injury. J Burn Care Res. 2012;33(6):764–71.
12. Perry DM, McGrouther DA, Bayat A. Current tools for the noninvasive objective assessment of skin scars. Plast Reconstr Surg. 2010;126:912.
13. Tredget EE, Levi B, Donelan MB. Biology and principles of scar management and burn reconstruction. Surg Clin N Am. 2014;94:793–814.
14. Wang J, Hori K, Ding J, Huang Y, Kwan P, Ladak A, et al. Toll-like receptors expressed by dermal fibroblasts contribute to hypertrophic scarring. J Cell Physiol. 2011;226(5):1265–73. doi:10.1002/jcp.22454.
15. Yang L, Shankowsky HA, Scott PG, Tredget EE. Peripheral blood fibrocytes from burn patients: identification and quantification of fibrocytes in adherent cells cultured from peripheral blood mononuclear cells. Lab Invest. 2002;82:1183–92.
16. Wang JF, Jiao H, Stewart TL, Shankowsky HA, Scott PG, Tredget EE. Fibrocytes from burn patients regulate the activities of fibroblasts. Wound Repair Regen. 2007;15(1):113–21.
17. Wang J, Stewart TL, Chen H, Shankowsky H, Scott PG, Tredget EE. Improved scar in post-burn patients following interferon alpha 2b treatment is associated with decreased angiogenesis mediated by vascular endothelial cell growth factor. J Interferon Cytokine Res. 2008;28(7):423–34.
18. Medina A, Shankowsky H, Tredget EE, et al. Characterization of heterotopic ossification in burn patients. J Burn Care Res. 2014;35(30):251–6.
19. Tredget EE, Yang L, Delehanty M, Shankowsky H, Scott PG, Polarized T. Helper Cells Th_2 cytokine production in patients with hypertrophic scar following thermal injury. J Interferon Cytokine Res. 2005;26: 179–89.
20. Wang J, Jiao H, Stewart TL, Shankowsky HA, Scott PG, Tredget EE. Increased TGF-beta-producing CD4+ T lymphocytes in post-burn patients and their potential interaction with dermal fibroblasts in hypertrophic scarring. Wound Repair Regen. 2007;15(4):530–9.
21. Wynn TA, Barron L. Macrophages: master regulators of inflammation and fibrosis. Semin Liver Dis. 2010;30(3):245–57.
22. Ding J, Ma Z, Liu H, Kwan P, Iwashina T, Shankowsky HA, et al. The therapeutic potential of a C-X-C chemokine receptor type 4 (CXCR-4) antagonist on hypertrophic scarring in vivo. Wound Repair Regen. 2014;22(5):622–30.
23. Sorrell JM, Baber MA, Caplan AI. Clonal characterization of fibroblasts in the superficial layer of the adult human dermis. Cell Tissue Res. 2007;327: 499–510.
24. Wang J, Dodd C, Shankowsky H, Scott PG, Tredget EE. Deep dermal fibroblast may dictate hypertrophic scarring. Lab Invest. 2008;88(12):1278–90.
25. Honardoust D, Varkey M, Hori K, Ding L, Shankowsky HA, Tredget EE. Small leucine-rich proteoglycans, decorin and fibromodulin, are reduced in post-burn hypertrophic scar. Wound Healing Regen. 2011;19(3):368–78.
26. Honardoust D, Varkey M, Hori K, Ding L, Shankowsky HA, Tredget EE. Reduced decorin, fibromodulin and TGF-β3 in deep dermis lead to hypertrophic scar. J Burn Care Res. 2012 Mar-Apr; 33(2):218–27.
27. Rinkevich Y, Walmsley GG, Hu MS et al. Identification and isolation of a dermal lineage with intrinsic fibrogenic potential. Science. 2015;348(6232): aaa2151-1-aaa2151.
28. Driskell RR, Lichtenberger BM, Hoste E et al. Nature. 504(7479):277–281. doi: 10.1038/nature12783. Accessed 12 Dec 2013.
29. Dunkin CS, Pleat JM, Gillespie PH, et al. Scarring occurs at a critical depth of skin injury: precise measurement in a graduated dermal scratch in human volunteers. Plast Reconstr Surg. 2007;119(6):1722–33.
30. Wainwright DJ. Burn reconstruction: the problems, techniques, and the applications. Clin Plast Surg. 2009;36:687–700.
31. Anzarut A, Olson J, Singh P, et al. The effectiveness of pressure garment therapy for the prevention of abnormal scarring after burn injury: a meta-analysis. J Plast Reconstr Aesthet Surg. 2009;62(1):77–84.
32. Engrav LH, Heimbach DH, Rivara FP, et al. 12-year within-wound study of the effectiveness of pressure garment therapy. Burns. 2010;36:975–83.
33. Harte D, Gordon J, Shaw M, et al. The use of pressure and silicone in hypertrophic scar management in burn patients: a pilot randomized controlled trial. J Burn Care Res. 2009;30(4):632–42. 29.
34. Nedelec B, Carter A, Forbes L, et al. Practice guidelines for the application of non-silicone or silicone gels and gel sheets after burn injury. J Burn Care Res. 2014;35:207–11.
35. O'Brien L, Pandit A. Silicone gel sheeting for preventing and treating hypertrophicand keloid scars. Cochrane Database Syst Rev 2006;(1):CD003826. Review. Update in: Cochrane Database Syst Rev 2013;(9):CD003826.
36. Costa AM, Peyrol S, Porto LC, et al. Mechanical forces induce scar remodeling. Study in non-pressure-treated versus pressure-treated hypertrophic scars. Am J Pathol. 1999;155(5):1671–9.
37. Longacre JJ, Berry HK, Basom CR, et al. The effects of Z plasty on hypertrophic scars. Scand J Plast Reconstr Surg. 1976;10:113.
38. Cartotto R, Cicuto BJ, Kiwanuka HN, et al. Common postburn deformities and their management. Surg Clin N Am. 2014;94(4):817–37.
39. Steinstraesser L, Flak E, Witte B, et al. Pressure garment therapy alone and in combination with silicone for the prevention of hypertrophic scarring: randomized controlled trial with intra-individual comparison. Plast Reconstr Surg. 2011;128:306e.
40. Huang C, Murphy GF, Akaishi S, Ogawa R. Keloids and hypertrophic scars: update and future directions. Plast Reconstr Surg. 2013;115(4):621–8.

41. Berman B, Viera MH, Amini S, et al. Prevention and management of hypertrophic scars and keloids after burns in children. J Craniofac Surg. 2008;19(4): 989–1006.
42. Davis JS. The relaxation of scar contractures by means of the Z-, or reversed Z-type incision: stressing the use of scar infiltrated tissues. Ann Surg. 1931;94:871.
43. Furnas DW, Fischer GW. The Z-plasty: biomechanics and mathematics. Br J Plast Surg. 1971;24:144–60.
44. Rohrich RJ, Zbar RI. A simplified algorithm for the use of Z-plasty. Plast Reconstr Surg. 1999;103:1513–7.
45. Stekelenburg CM, Marck RE, Tuinebreijer WE, De Vet HCW, et al. A systematic review on burn scar contracture treatment: searching for evidence. J Burn Care Res. 2015;36(3):e155.
46. DraaiJers LJ, Tempelman FR, Botman YA, et al. The patient and observer scar assessment scale: a reliable and feasible tool for scar evaluation. Plast Reconstr Surg. 2004;113:1960–5.
47. Baker SR. Fundamentals of expanded tissue. J Head Neck Surg. 1991;13:321–7.
48. Jackson IT, Sharpe DT, Polley J, et al. Use of external reservoirs in tissue expansion. Plast Reconstr Surg. 1987;80:266–73.
49. Manders EK, Schenden MJ, Hetzler PT, et al. Soft-tissue expansion: concepts and complications. Plast Reconstr Surg. 1984;74:493–507.
50. Apfelberg DB, Maser MR, Lash H, et al. Preliminary results of argon and carbon dioxide laser treatment of keloid scars. Lasers Surg Med. 1984;4:283–90.
51. Castro DJ, Abergel RP, Meeker C, et al. Effects of the Nd:YAG laser on DNA synthesis and collagen production in human skin fibroblast cultures. Ann Plast Surg. 1983;11:214–22.
52. Manuskiatti W, Wanitphakdeedecha R, Fitzpatrick RE. Effect of pulse width of 595-nm flashlamp-pumped pulsed dye laser on the treatment response keloidal and hypertrophic sternotomy scars. Dermatol Surg. 2007;33:152.
53. Anderson RR, Parrish JA. Selective photothermolysis: precise microsurgery by selective absorption of pulsed radiation. Science. 1983;220:524.
54. Manstein D, Herron GS, Sink RK, et al. Fractional photothermolysis: a new concept for cutaneous remodeling using microscopic patterns of thermal injury. Lasers Surg Med. 2004;34:426.
55. Donelan MB, Parrett BM, Sheridan RL. Pulsed dye laser therapy and z-plasty for facial burn scars: the alternative to excision. Ann Plast Surg. 2008;60:480.
56. Hultman CS, Friedsat JS, Edkins RE, et al. Laser resurfacing and remodeling of hypertrophic burn scars. Ann Surg. 2014;260:519–32.
57. Waibel J, Beer K. Fractional laser resurfacing for thermal burns. J Drugs Dermatol. 2008;7:59.
58. Brewin MP, Lister TS. Prevention or treatment of hypertrophic burn scarring: a review of when and how to treat with the pulsed dye laser. Burns. 2014;40:797–804.
59. Niessen FB, Spauwen PH, Schalkwijk J, Kon M. On the nature of hypertrophic scars and keloids: a review. Plast Reconstr Surg. 1999;104:1435–58.
60. Waibel J, Beer K. Ablative fractional laser resurfacing for the treatment of a third degree burn. J Drugs Dermatol. 2009;8:294.
61. Garden JM, Tan OT, Kerschmann R, et al. Effect of dye laser pulse duration on selective cutaneous vascular injury. J Invest Dermatol. 1986;87:653.
62. Tierney EP, Hanke CW. Fractionated carbon dioxide laser treatment of photoaging: a prospective study in 45 patients and review of the literature. Dermatol Surg. 2011;37:1279.
63. Jabir S, Quentin F, et al. A systematic review of the application of free tissue transfer in burns. Burns. 2014;40:1059–70.
64. Jabir S et al. Microvascular free tissue transfer in acute and secondary burn reconstruction. Injury. 2015;46(9):1821–7.
65. Oni G, Saint-Cyr M, Mojallal A. Free tissue transfer in acute burns. J Reconstr Microsurg. 2012;28(2):77–84.
66. Scott PF et al. Biological basis of hypertrophic scarring. In: Malhotra SK, editor. Advances in structural biology, vol. 3. Greenwich, CT: JAI Press; 1994.
67. Nedelec B, Shankowsky H, Tredget E. Rating the resolving hypertorphic scar: comparison of the Vancouver scar scale and scar volume. J Burn Care Res. 2000;21(3):205–12.
68. Ding J et al. Deep dermal fibroblast profibrotic characteristics are enhanced by bone marrow-derived mesenchymal stem cells. Wound Repair Regen. 2013;21(3):448–55.

Psychosocial Recovery

21

Radha K. Holavanahalli, Amy Acton, and Shelley Wiechman

Introduction

With the advances in resuscitation over the last couple of decades, people are surviving larger burns and can live long lives. As a result, psychosocial recovery and long-term quality of life warrant more attention. Research has shown that controllable factors early in the hospitalization, such as social support, pain control, anxiety, and delirium, can have long-term effects on a person's recovery and should be addressed [1–7]. Essentially, achieving long-term quality of life starts in the intensive care unit (ICU). For new burn team members the significance of the psychological and social impact of a traumatic burn injury is not hard to imagine. The traumatic nature of the injury accompanied by the long and painful treatment will test the most resilient patient and family. Research supporting the challenges of psychosocial adjustment after a burn injury continues to grow but less documented is the evidence of successful interventions to support and improve psychosocial outcomes. The persistent difficulties in psychological and social adjustment are often under-recognized and hence undertreated [8]. There is no systematic effort to address these critical social and psychological rehabilitation needs leaving patients to cope on their own [8, 9]. The family and patient each process the loss and fears associated with the burn injury in different ways and at their own pace. A significant percentage of those impacted experience psychological distress long after discharge from the hospital and clinic setting. This chapter will highlight the potential psychosocial diagnosis related to burn trauma, and examine the psychosocial needs of a patient at each phase of recovery with an emphasis on setting the patient up for success long after the burn has healed. We will also recommend how and when to screen for common psychiatric issues and provide suggestions on when to intervene.

R.K. Holavanahalli, Ph.D. (✉)
Department of Physical Medicine and Rehabilitation, University of Texas Southwestern Medical Center, 5323 Harry Hines Blvd., Dallas, TX 75390-9136, USA
e-mail: radha.holavanahalli@utsouthwestern.edu

A. Acton, R.N., B.S.N.
Phoenix Society for Burn Survivors, 1835 RW Berends Dr. SW, Grand Rapids, MI 49519-4955, USA
e-mail: amy@phoenix-society.org

S. Wiechman, Ph.D., A.B.P.P.
Department of Rehabilitation Medicine, University of Washington School of Medicine, Seattle, WA, USA
e-mail: wiechman@u.washington.edu

Preparing Yourself

The impact of your compassionate and empathetic communication with patient and family throughout all phases of the care continuum cannot be overstated in helping to set the stage for

D.G. Greenhalgh (ed.), *Burn Care for General Surgeons and General Practitioners*,
DOI 10.1007/978-3-319-29161-1_21

the best possible outcomes. However, a very important first step is to learn about the potential long-term outcomes of those with severe burn injuries. It is important to understand the potential of a patient who is recovering from a significant burn trauma. Listening to training videos of burn survivors sharing their story will help in self-awareness of beliefs and judgments regarding the quality of life of someone with severe disfigurement. This greater understanding of what to expect will also help in conveying a hope for the future at the bedside. The ongoing psychological distress including a sense of hopelessness, fear of the unknown, loss of control, and body image concerns are just a few of the challenges patients mention at the outset. Information and tools to help families understand the recovery process from a burn injury is critical and must be offered throughout the hospital stay and at a pace that they can absorb. Just because patients do not ask about their appearance does not mean they are not feeling stress and anxiety about this and other areas of their life. Asking open-ended questions to the family and patient will allow them to share their feelings and open the dialog for crucial conversations about their recovery. An example is when looking at a new graft for the first time instead of sharing the excitement about the surgical success and how great the graft looks, the patient can be asked about what they think about the appearance of the graft. This will likely open up a whole different conversation about how they are feeling about their appearance. An empathetic communication style, listening to and acknowledging patient concerns, can lend itself to valuable teaching moments about the process of healing and how the appearance will improve over time. This too can be an opportunity to introduce the available survivor community resources to decrease the feelings of isolation and exploring the psychosocial stressors that are often not a specific diagnosis. As someone new to the burn rotation you may not have all the answers but as long as you show compassion, listen and validate the needs of the patient and family you will help set the stage for emotional as well as the physical healing.

Each step of the recovery from a burn injury is different, just like each burn survivor and family. The journey involves not just healing the body, but also the mind and spirit. Burn care has to support the whole person, while also engaging a survivor's loved ones and support systems. The entire multidisciplinary team needs to be involved at all phases of recovery. For these sections, the social worker, psychologist, and psychiatrist will be referred to as the *mental health team* and the doctors, nurses, physical therapists (PTs), occupational therapists (OTs), and child life specialists will be referred to as the *medical team*. Burn Centers should also consider engaging the Phoenix Society early in a patient's hospitalization. The Phoenix Society for Burn Survivors is a leading national nonprofit organization dedicated to empowering anyone affected by a burn injury through peer support, education, and advocacy. The Phoenix Society works with burn survivors, their loved ones, and medical teams across the country to care for the whole family after a burn injury. The educational programs, peer-to-peer support, online community, in-person events, referrals to local organizations and more provide essential support to the burn survivor community. The Phoenix Society has been serving as the national hub for aftercare activities for nearly 40 years. For the purposes of this chapter, burn recovery is classified into three phases—the intensive care and resuscitation phase, the acute care phase, and the rehabilitation phase, including community reintegration. "Aftercare" reintegration begins at the time of injury (mission statement of the Joint Aftercare Reintegration Committee of the American Burn Association [ABA] and the Phoenix Society for Burn Survivors). Unlike in the past when attention to the rehabilitation of survivors of burn injury was only an afterthought [10], each phase of burn recovery now has the ultimate goal of returning the patient as close as possible to a pre-injury way of life. The psychosocial reentry is the most difficult part of a burn survivor's personal recovery [11]. Long-term psychosocial recovery of burn patients is dependent on successful reintegration into the community [12].

Intensive Care and Resuscitation

During the time of receiving care in the ICU, considerable emphasis will be on providing emotional support to the family. The patient's mental status is likely to fluctuate and their ability to truly process what has happened is limited. The psychosocial needs and considerations during this phase of recovery are given in Table 21.1.

Family Support

Social support can be a contributing factor to a person's well-being, either positive or negative [1]. For example, the number of supporters at the bedside is not as important as the quality of the support. One person present who can provide positive support is more important than a lot of people at the bedside who are in constant conflict and struggling with their own emotional needs. Understanding the needs of family members at this stage can help us to intervene appropriately. A 1999 survey by Thompson and colleagues [13] found that the patient's well-being, medical condition of the patient, having personal needs met (parking, bathrooms, transportation, and food), and the patient's emotional status were primary sources of stress for the family. They also found that family members of pediatric patients worry about the amount of pain the patient is experiencing and the potential need for surgery. The burn team can work together to ensure that the family at the bedside gets their needs met. The medical team can assist by keeping the family informed of the patient's current status and understanding the long-term plan for recovery. Going over the plan or goals of the day, informing them of any changes in condition, and periodically holding family meetings can make this communication smoother. The mental health team can assist by providing support to the family, encouraging the family's own self-care (e.g., giving them permission to leave the hospital to take care of other matters, sleeping and eating regularly, and exercising). The mental health team can also be a sounding board for the family to vent concerns and to solve problems. If necessary, the mental health team may need to intervene with family conflicts to keep the patient's room free of conflict and ease the stress on the medical providers.

Table 21.1 Psychosocial needs and considerations during the intensive care and resuscitation phase of recovery

Provide support and education to
Family members
Patient
Pharmacological and nonpharmacological pain management
Screen for anxiety, acute stress disorder, and delirium

In a study [13] that asked family members what was helping them get through hospitalization, the responses included family and friends, burn center staff, spirituality, optimism, and retaining hope. Further, over 60 % of patients in a survey [14] responded that addressing religious and spiritual needs was important in their recovery and should be a part of medical care. Providing pastoral care visits to patients and family members (unless refused) may be helpful in recovery. Most burn centers have utilized the Phoenix Society's *Survivors Offering Assistance in Recovery* (SOAR) program and those peer visits of survivor and family members who have experienced a similar injury can also be useful at this phase in providing support and hope to the family and establishing a good relationship early in the hospitalization. Providing quality information and a sense of connection for some family members may help decrease stress and the feeling of being out of control. There are a wealth of resources on the Phoenix Society website (http://www.phoenix-society.org/resources/) including moderated Phoenix Society SOAR online chats and forums available to family members who often feel they need to be doing something to help. Self-directed learning about recovery often reinforces what the burn team is already sharing and helps families feel supported while the focus is intensively on the patient.

The relationship that all members of the burn team form with the family at this stage is critical for the long-term partnership that is needed to care for the patient for years to come. When the family trusts the burn team, that trust will transfer to the patient and forms the basis of a solid working relationship [1]. Communication and the need for consistent messages from the burn team are vital to building trust—the words matter. An example—Some survivors talk about what they hear when you say you "don't know," they perceive you may be keeping something from them but when reassured that the type of injury and the healing process outcomes vary and there are things we cannot answer yet.

Patient Support

Oftentimes, the patient is using the defense of denial to minimize the impact of the injury. This is an appropriate and necessary defense at this stage when the focus is on survival. We advocate support of whatever defenses the patient is using to cope with their injury, as long as those defenses are not interfering with participation in care. If the patient is either giving up, or minimizing the severity of the injury to the point of refusing occupational therapy/physical therapy (PT/OT) or wound care, then the mental health team should be consulted for intervention. Again, getting a Phoenix Society SOAR peer visitor involved at this stage can be a tremendous source of hope for the patient.

Pain, Anxiety, Acute Stress Disorder, and Delirium Management

Pain, anxiety, and delirium management are all common complications in the intensive care unit (ICU). Research has shown that ineffective management of these issues early in the hospitalization can lead to negative outcomes for many years following discharge. Specifically, high inpatient pain levels predict higher rates of depression and suicidal ideation up to 2 years following the burn injury [5, 15, 16]. High inpatient pain levels also predict rates of post-traumatic stress disorder (PTSD) following the injury and many patients report that the trauma that they are re-experiencing is not the initial burn trauma, but the subsequent painful wound care.

Both procedural and baseline anxiety can also increase a patient's perception of pain and should be treated as aggressively as we treat pain. Unfortunately, pharmacologic treatment of both pain and anxiety with opiates and benzodiazepines will also lead to delirium. In addition, high pain and anxiety levels can also lead to delirium. Acute Stress Disorder (ASD) occurs between 3 days and 1 month following the injury. The primary diagnostic symptom that differentiates it from PTSD is dissociation, or the feeling of an altered sense of reality or seeing oneself from another's perspective. Untreated ASD can also increase agitation and pain levels [17, 18]. Prolonged periods of delirium increase rates of complications, such as infections, and can lead to longer lengths of stay [6, 7]. Initial research has also shown that inpatient delirium can also lead to decreased cognitive function and increases in rates of depression after discharge.

Screening for these issues is critical. Periodic assessment of patient's pain is now a required part of the nursing assessment and many tools have been recommended in the literature to assess pain either by self- report or by observation in both adults and children [19, 20]. Anxiety can be quickly assessed by asking patients to rate their anxiety on a 0–10 scale. For nonverbal patients or children, a strong indicator of anxiety is whether or not they show pain behaviors or agitation prior to any painful procedures. Screening for Acute Stress Disorder (ASD) can be done by asking patients if they are having any nightmares or flashbacks of the injury, or if they are observed to have disturbed and restless sleep. If so, a consultation from the mental health team is warranted for further assessment.

Delirium is also typically assessed by the bedside nurse. It is important to assess throughout the day (typically once per shift) given that delirium is transient and the medical team needs a sense of the percentage of the day that the patient is delirious to better inform treatment. Common measures to assess delirium are described elsewhere [21] and include the CAM-ICU [22, 23] and the Delirium Rating Scale-Revised-98 [24].

Nonpharmacological interventions are critical adjuncts to medications in treating these three

Table 21.2 Pharmacological and nonpharmacological interventions for delirium management

Minimize medications that can contribute to delirium when possible
Assess medical factors that could contribute to delirium (e.g., infections)
Continuously reorient the patient and place reorientation cues in the room (e.g., calendar, pictures of family)
Announce when you walk into the room and tell the patient what you will be doing
Put the patient on a regularly sleep/wake cycle and differentiate days and nights
Minimize nighttime interruptions
Limit overstimulation (too much light, too many people in the room, TV)
Speak to the patient in a direct, calm manner using easy to understand language and short sentences
Allow the patient extra time to respond to questions
Consider a medication to reduce delirium, such as IV Haldol

complications. Hypnosis, meditation, progressive relaxation, imagery, mindfulness, and environmental interventions have all been shown to be effective in helping to manage pain, anxiety, and delirium [25, 26]. Table 21.2 provides a list of pharmacological and nonpharmacological interventions for delirium management.

Acute Care

As the patient moves out of the ICU and onto the acute care floor, the nature of both the emotional impact and the interventions that can be done changes as they become more alert and oriented to their situation. The patient is able to more actively participate with the mental health provider and more in-depth processing can begin, setting the stage for their long-term adjustment. The same tools as mentioned above can be used to continually screen and monitor pain, anxiety, and delirium. The psychosocial considerations during the acute care phase of recovery are listed in Table 21.3. Post-traumatic Stress Disorder (PTSD) is common after a traumatic injury and symptoms can interfere with care and increase distress. There are many screening tools for PTSD but they are quite lengthy for bedside nurses or social workers. Similarly to the screening of ASD mentioned above, patients can simply be asked if they are having nightmares or flashbacks of the injury or if their sleep is disturbed and restless. If they indicate they are, consult the mental health provider for further assessment. Screening for mood issues such as depression is also important at this phase. The quality consensus committee convened by the ABA has recommended several screening tools for both PTSD and Depression [27]. The Patient Health Questionnaire, either 9-item or 2-item (PHQ-9 or 2) [28], can be easily used by the bedside nurse or social worker and is free of charge. The committee recommends screening for depression at least once prior to discharge and on each subsequent outpatient clinic visit. Screening for depression is only effective once the person's mental status has cleared. A positive screen should lead to consultation with the mental health provider. Pain and anxiety should continue to be managed with nonpharmacological adjuncts as mentioned above.

Table 21.3 Psychosocial needs and considerations during the acute care phase of recovery

Pain management
Screen for anxiety/PTSD, depression
Sleep issues
Adherence to treatment
Adjustment to injury

Sleep issues may also arise as the patient moves out of the ICU. Oftentimes, a patient's days and nights go undifferentiated and they may sleep much of the day and then find it difficult to sleep at night. Anxiety and pain can also interfere with sleep and insufficient sleep can lead to delirium. Behavioral interventions for sleep are highly effective and can include designing a daily schedule for the patient so that they know what to expect throughout the day and evening. Keeping lights on and shades up with activities throughout the day is important, as is turning the TV off and pulling the shades at night when it is time to sleep. Minimizing nighttime interruptions for nursing care is also critical to promoting prolonged sleep. Napping during the day should be discouraged if possible. Pharmacological sleep aides, such as melatonin, should also be considered if behavioral interventions are not adequate. Other medications typically used for sleep may put a patient at risk for delirium, especially in the elderly [29].

Other issues that may arise as a patient's mental status clears include lack of adherence to treatment and more in-depth processing of the impact of their injury. Oftentimes as patients move out of the ICU, they are weaned from opiate medication. This makes for more painful range of motion and therapy. Patients can suddenly "hit a wall" and lose motivation to continue aggressive participation in their physical and occupational therapy, particularly if they have had a long ICU stay. They will be more focused on discharge and getting out of the hospital, despite not being independent enough in wound care and therapies. Strategies to enhance motivation include helping a patient feel more in control of their own care and outcome. The team should engage the patient in setting their own functional goals and having input into their daily routines and discharge planning. Setting up a quota system where the focus is on increasing their performance goals by 10 % every day and working towards that goal versus stopping when there is pain can also be effective [30]. The Phoenix Society SOAR visitors can often exemplify, "the light at the end of the tunnel" and help the patient to overcome these temporary barriers to treatment.

It is also important at this phase to provide supportive counseling so that patients have a safe place to process the impact of their injury and plan for the future. This must be done in a way that is comfortable for the patient and fits into their own pre-injury coping style. Some patients will want to talk about what has happened to them and be more emotional in their processing. While others will want to focus on concrete problem-solving strategies to get on with their future with little expressed emotion or discussion of the nature of their injury. Either style is effective and attempting to change a person's coping style in the midst of a crisis such as a critical injury is rarely successful. Family members may have a different coping style and it can be distressing to those who need to talk and process the injury to interact with a patient who traditionally does not like to talk or emotionally process their injury and instead wants to focus on the future. The mental health team can provide education to family members whose coping styles differ from that of the patient. Successful processing at this phase can promote post-traumatic growth and resiliency long after discharge. Peer visitors can be especially effective at this phase, as they are usually that one voice who can truly understand what the patient is going through and they have been trained in supportive counseling. Often the patient will seek out those they feel safe with to process some of their feelings. It is necessary to be alert to such crucial conversation opportunities and if you are not prepared or qualified to answer certain questions, ask if you can have someone who can help in that area instead of shutting down a discussion about the future or responding by minimizing the concern.

Managing mood may also be a challenge and low mood or even depression can be a barrier to adhering to treatment. Depression should be assessed and treated with either medication and/or nonpharmacological interventions. Behavioral activation [31] such as getting the patient up, dressed and out of bed, and having one positive activity or event that they can look forward to everyday is particularly effective in the inpatient setting. Proactively asking about concerns they have about eventual discharge from hospital may also open the door to questions about appearance, body image, and social anxiety issues.

Rehabilitation Phase

The success of the transition to the rehabilitation or outpatient phase of care largely depends upon the education and preparation for discharge. The education, interventions, and trust that the burn team has developed from the ICU through the acute phase will set the patient up for success at discharge. The amount of information that needs to be conveyed at discharge regarding wound care, therapies, medications, and outpatient follow-up visits can quickly overwhelm patients. Information will need to be repeated and given in different formats. Having their primary nurse sit down with them and go over the information verbally, as well as providing them with written handouts and even offering a video of range of motion exercises can all be effective multimodal strategies. Patients and their family members should also be reassured that their care does not end at discharge. They will continue to be followed closely by the burn team for as long as they need it and can call or come in often for outpatient appointments and consultations. Outpatient clinic visits should also be multidisciplinary, with each discipline screening, assessing, and intervening on the issues that they managed while in the hospital. Screening for all of the above issues (e.g., mood, anxiety/PTSD, pain) should continue in the outpatient setting and the same screening tools can be used. Common screening tools recommended for use are listed in Table 21.4 [32–38]. Positive responses to the screens should initiate a referral or consultation to a mental health provider.

Emerging needs during the aftercare and reintegration phase (Table 21.5) when survival is no longer an issue includes needs for physical safety and comfort, self-esteem, and acceptance by others. The primary focus is on cosmetic and functional deficits and the emotional impact in personal (body image, self-esteem, sexuality, close family and other relatives), social (casual relationships including encounters with strangers in various social settings), and vocational (productive activity) spheres of life.

Table 21.4 Common screening tools recommended for use in the rehabilitation phase of recovery

Patient stress questionnaire [32]—this is a compilation of the PHQ-9 [28], the GAD-7 [33], the PC-PTSD [34], and the AUDIT [35] and can quickly assess for depression, anxiety, PTSD, and substance abuse in adults
Satisfaction with appearance (SWAP) [36]: can be used to assess body image concerns
Moods and feelings questionnaire (MFQ) [37]: short version can be used to assess for depressive symptoms in children under age 13
PTSD symptom scale (PSS) [38]: can be used to assess PTSD in children

Table 21.5 Emerging needs during the reintegration phase of recovery

Sleep disturbance
Depression
Body image concerns
Pain/itch control
PTSD
Relationship issues
Social discomfort
Work or school issues

Body Image

Oftentimes issues with body image arise in the outpatient setting and need to be addressed. However, just because body image concerns arise in the outpatient setting does not mean that the patient has not been worrying about it earlier. It is very important to address such concerns while preparing the patient and family prior to discharge from hospital. Body image and social anxiety issues can be addressed in the acute phase by taking patient outside the burn unit to practice how to respond to staring, double-takes, and questions. Depression, PTSD, and pain can all be impacted by a person's body image following their burn injury [39]. In one study, body image dissatisfaction at 1 year postdischarge was the most important predictor of overall adjustment [16]. Response to wounds and potential scarring can vary greatly between individuals. Research has shown that those who place more importance on appearance prior to their injury will have more body image dissatisfaction after their injury [16, 40]. Although the Satisfaction With Appearance Scale [36] was developed specifically for burn survivors to assess body image, it is lengthy and primarily used for research purposes and would be a burdensome screening tool in a busy outpatient burn clinic. We recommend screening for body image issues by simply asking if a person is getting out in public, how they are responding to questions or staring, and their confidence level in interacting with the public. These questions can give you clues to their body image and open the door for a more in-depth conversation on the issue. We have also found that asking about sexual desire and function during their review of systems can also lead to a conversation about body image issues. Providing education on the scarring process can be helpful. We stress that their scars will continue to mature over the next year so "acceptance" of their scars is not necessary in the first year as it is not clear what they are being asked to "accept." Peer support visits can be extremely helpful for a patient and family in understanding how the scars mature and what they can reasonably expect. Even after the first year, burn survivors often want to maintain hope for improvement in scars with new technologies such as laser surgery and reconstructive surgical techniques. Burn reconstructive surgeons often struggle with the question of how much surgery is too much and when they should stop. The answer to this dilemma depends upon the burn survivor and a frank discussion with the survivor of the inability for any surgical intervention to erase scars is crucial. The surgeon and survivor will need to decide if the risk of the intervention is worth the potential benefits.

A substantial number of individuals experience significant difficulties with long-term psychosocial adjustment, especially those individuals with changes in appearance [11]. Adjustment difficulties such as coping with staring and teasing when out in public, body image, and relationship issues significantly affect quality of life, and much of the recovery happens not in the safe zone in a hospital but out in the community [11]. Meeting with a Phoenix SOAR peer volunteer can be beneficial for a burn survivor who is deciding how much reconstructive surgery they want to undergo or who is struggling with body image issues. At minimum, preparing a person to face the public with dressings, pressure garments, and pigment changes or scarring needs to be addressed early after discharge. The burn team can at least prepare them for the responses they may get and how to be prepared. It is often overwhelming for the patient to discuss and process these issues prior to discharge. In these circumstances, a conversation with the family about how to assist may be helpful. Helping burn survivors practice specific strategies to use in public and in social situations can assist them in making the successful transformation to a person who thrives after surviving a burn injury [41]. Preparation can be done by offering different social scenarios and helping the survivor to plan responses that are comfortable for them. Guiding them to the Phoenix Society's online resources to access "Beyond Surviving: Tools for Thriving after a Burn Injury" and their online videos is also an excellent resource that also includes the Image Enhancement Program that provides creative make-up techniques for burn survivors. A referral to a mental health provider may also be needed.

Post-traumatic Stress Disorder

As mentioned above, Post-traumatic Stress Disorder (PTSD) can be a major cause of emotional distress following a burn injury. Rates of PTSD over the course of a year vary from 19 to 45 % [2, 4, 42] and can be quite debilitating. PTSD can be a major barrier to returning to work, particularly if the accident occurred on the job. It can also impair sleep and their ability to go out in public. Screening tools are often lengthy and typically need to be administered by a mental health provider. However, one screening tool that may be useful is the Primary Care PTSD Screen (PC-PTSD) [34]. It is a 4-item scale to be used in medical settings and a positive response to any of the 4 items should initiate a referral to a mental health provider for a more thorough assessment. The burn team can ask whether or not a person is getting out in public, if they are having nightmares of the injury or any fears of returning to work. A positive response to these questions should initiate a referral to a mental health provider for more thorough assessment and intervention.

Return to Work

Returning to work is a major step towards reintegration following a burn injury. Research has shown that the sooner a person can return to work, the more likely they are to return to work and the better state of mental health [43]. Returning to work can be an important part of therapy as it forces a person to get up, out of the house, and be active daily. Work can improve mood and improve quality of sleep. The burn team can set a person up for success in this area by encouraging them to contact their employer as soon as possible following the injury and assist with filling out any necessary paperwork. It is rare that a person with a burn injury qualifies for either short- or long-term disability. A gradual return to work plan is recommended that includes consideration of light duty options as soon as possible after discharge; as well as returning to work for a couple of hours for a short time, then progressing to half days, and finally full days. Returning to work in the middle of a typical work week can ease the transition as there are only a couple of days of work until the weekend and then they can rest and start again the following week. Patients should be encouraged to consult their state's employment rules, especially if it is an injury that occurred on the job.

Return to School

Similar to returning to work, the sooner a child can return to school, the better they do emotionally and physically. Public schools are mandated to provide accommodations when needed. This may entail allowing a child to wear splints and pressure garments during the day and getting assistance with range of motion exercises. Accommodations for physical education classes might also be necessary for a short time. It is rare that a child would need home schooling or to change schools as a result of their injury. The Phoenix Society has developed a program entitled, "The Journey Back," for parents, teachers, and hospital staff who are assisting a child with a positive return to school after a burn injury. It is important that the child be prepared for questions and comments from classmates about their injury. Healthcare providers and parents need to discuss different questions and scenarios with the child and rehearse appropriate responses prior to returning to school.

Conclusion

A qualitative analysis [44] examining views of compassionate care within the context of burn care through burn survivors accounts yielded three primary themes: respect the person (by establishing an empathic connection, restoring control through choice, providing individualized care, and going above and beyond); interpersonal and informational communication; and provision of competent care. "Compassion is vital in burn care" [39]. Each step of the recovery from a burn injury is different, just like each burn survivor and family. The journey involves not just healing the body, but also the mind and spirit. Burn care has to support the whole person, while also engaging a survivor's loved ones and support systems. Successful reintegration into society with an acceptable quality of life begins at the initial admission to the burn unit. The multidisciplinary team, in partnership with advocacy organizations, such as the Phoenix Society can work together to help a patient and family not just survive, but thrive following their injury.

References

1. Muangman P, Sullivan SR, Wiechman S, Bauer G, Honari S, Heimbach DM, Engrav LH, Gibran NS. Social support correlates with survival in patients with massive burn injury. J Burn Care Rehabil. 2005;26(4):352–6.
2. Corry NH, Klick B, Fauerbach JA. Posttraumatic stress disorder and pain impact functioning and disability after major burn injury. J Burn Care Res. 2010;31(1):13–25.
3. Smith MT, Klick B, Kozachik S, Edwards RE, Holavanahalli R, Wiechman S, Blakeney P, Lezotte D, Fauerbach JA. Sleep onset insomnia symptoms during hospitalization for major burn injury predict chronic pain. Pain. 2008;138(3):497–506.
4. Wiechman Askay S, Patterson DR. What are the psychiatric sequelae of burn pain? Curr Pain Headache Rep. 2008;12(2):94–7.
5. Edwards RR, Magyar-Russell G, Thombs B, Smith MT, Holavanahalli RK, Patterson DR, Blakeney P, Lezotte DC, Haythornthwaite JA, Fauerbach JA. Acute pain at discharge from hospitalization is a prospective predictor of long-term suicidal ideation after burn injury. Arch Phys Med Rehabil. 2007;88(12 Suppl 2):S36–42.
6. Needham DM, et al. Improving the long-term outcomes after discharge from intensive care unit: report from a stakeholders' conference. Crit Care Med. 2012;40(2):502–9.
7. Inouye SK. Delirium in hospitalized older patients: recognition and risk factors. J Geriatr Psychiatry Neurol. 1998;11:118–25.

8. Fauerbach JA, Pruzinsky T, Saxe GN. Psychological health and function after burn injury: setting research priorities. J Burn Care Res. 2007;28(4):587–92.
9. Kammerer-Quayle B. Behavioral skills and image enhancement training for burn survivors. Essential interventions for improving quality of life and community integration. In: Sood R, editor. Auchauer and Sood's burn surgery, reconstruction, and rehabilitation. Philadelphia: Saunders; 2006.
10. Feller I, Jones CA. Introduction: statement of the problem. In: Fisher SV, Helm PA, editors. Comprehensive rehabilitation of burns. Baltimore/London: Williams & Wilkins; 1984.
11. Acton RA, Mounsey E, Gilyard C. The burn survivor perspective. J Burn Care Res. 2007;28(4):615–20.
12. Blakeney P, Partridge J, Rumsey N. Community integration. J Burn Care Res. 2007;28(4):598–601.
13. Thompson R, Boyle D, Teel C, Wambach K, Cramer A. A qualitative analysis of family member needs and concerns in the population of patients with burns. J Burn Care Rehabil. 1999;20:487–96.
14. Arnoldo BD, Hunt JL, Burris A, Wilkerson L, Purdue GF. Adult burn patients: the role of religion in recovery – should we be doing more? J Burn Care Res. 2006;27(6):923–4.
15. Edwards RR, Smith MT, Klick B, Magyar-Russell G, Haythornthwaite JA, Holavanahalli R, Patterson DR, Blakeney P, Lezotte D, McKibben J, Fauerbach JA. Symptoms of depression and anxiety as unique predictors of pain-related outcomes following burn injury. Ann Behav Med. 2007;34(3):313–22.
16. Thombs BD, Bresnick MG, Magyar-Russell G, Lawrence JW, McCann UD, Fauerbach JA. Symptoms of depression predict change in physical health after burn injury. Burns. 2007;33(3):292–8.
17. McKibben JB, Bresnick MG, WiechmanAskay S, Fauerbach JA. Acute stress disorder and posttraumatic stress disorder: a prospective study of prevalence, course, and predictors in a sample with major burn injuries. J Burn Care Res. 2008;29:22–35.
18. Lawrence JW, Fauerbach JA. Personality, coping, chronic stress, social support and PTSD symptoms among adult burn survivors. J Burn Care Rehabil. 2003;24:63–72.
19. Mahar PD, Wasiak J, et al. Frequency and use of pain assessment tools implemented in randomized controlled trials in the adult burns population: a systematic review. Burns. 2012;38(2):147–52.
20. Wibbenmeyer L, Sevier A, Liao J, Williams I, Latenser B, Lewis II R, Kealey P, Rosenquist R. Evaluation of the usefulness of two established pain assessment tools in a burn population. J Burn Care Res. 2011;32:52–60.
21. Adamis D, Sharma N, Whelan PJ, et al. Delirium scales: a review of current evidence. Aging Ment Health. 2010;14:543–55.
22. Inouye SK, van Dyck CH, Alessi CA, et al. Clarifying confusion: the confusion assessment method. A new method for detection of delirium. Ann Intern Med. 1990;113:941–8.
23. Ely EW, Inouye SK, Bernard GR, et al. Delirium in mechanically ventilated patients: validity and reliability of the confusion assessment method for the intensive care unit (CAM-ICU). JAMA. 2001;286:2703–10.
24. Trzepacz PT, Mittal D, Torres R, et al. Validation of the Delirium Rating Scale-revised-98: comparison with the delirium rating scale and the cognitive test for delirium. J Neuropsychiatry Clin Neurosci. 2001;13:229–42.
25. Patterson DR, Tininenko JR, Schmidt AE, et al. Virtual reality hypnosis: a case report. Int J Clin Exp Hypn. 2004;52(1):27–38.
26. Wiechman AS, Patterson D. A randomized controlled trial of hypnosis for burn wound care. Rehabil Psychol. 2007;52(3):247–53.
27. Wiechman S, Meyer W, Edelman L, Fauerbach J, Gibbons L, Holavanahalli R, et al. Psychological outcomes. Summary article – American Burn Association Consensus Statements. J Burn Care Res. 2013;34(4):363–8.
28. Kroenke K, Spitzer RL, Williams JB. The PHQ-9: validity of a brief depression severity measure. J Gen Intern Med. 2001;16(9):606–13.
29. Jaffe SE, Patterson DR. Treating sleep problems in patients with burn injuries: practical considerations. J Burn Care Rehabil. 2004;25(3):294–305.
30. Ehde DM, Patterson DR, Fordyce WE. The quota system in burn rehabilitation. J Burn Care Rehabil. 1998;19(5):436–40.
31. Martel CR, Dimidjian S, Herman-Dunn R. Behavioral activation for depression. New York, NY: Guilford Press; 2010.
32. Patient Stress Questionnaire – compliments of the Center for Integrated Primary Care, University of Massachusetts Medical School.
33. Spitzer RL, Kroenke K, Williams JBW, Lowe B. A brief measure for assessing generalized anxiety disorder. Arch Intern Med. 2006;166:1092–7.
34. Prins A, Ouimette P, Kimerling R, Cameron RP, Hugelshofer DS, Shaw-Hegwer J, Thrailkill A, Gusman FD, Sheikh JI. The primary care PTSD screen (PC-PTSD): development and operating characteristics. Prim Care Psychiatr. 2003;9:9–14.
35. Saunders JB, Aasland OG, Babor TF, et al. Development of the alcohol use disorders identification test (AUDIT): WHO collaborative project on early detection of persons with harmful alcohol consumption-II. Addiction. 1993;88:791–803.
36. Lawrence JW, Fauerbach JA. Thombs BD A test of the moderating role of importance of appearance in the relationship between perceived scar severity and body-esteem among adult burn survivors. Body Image. 2006;3(2):101–11. Epub 2006 Mar 29.
37. Angold A, Costello EJ, Messer SC, Pickles A, Winder F, Silver D. The development of a short questionnaire for use in epidemiological studies of depression in children and adolescents. Int J Meth Psychiatr Res. 1995;5:237–49.

38. Foa EB, Riggs DS, Dancu CV, Rothbaum BO. Reliability and validity of a brief instrument for assessing posttraumatic stress disorder. J Trauma Stress. 1993;6:459–73.
39. Lawrence JW, Heinberg LJ, Roca R, Munster A, Spence R, Fauerbach JA. Development and validation of the satisfaction with appearance scale: assessing body image among burn-injured patients. Psychol Assess. 1998;10(1):64–70.
40. Thombs BD, Notes LD, Lawrence JW, Magyar-Russell G, Bresnick MG, Fauerbach JA. From survival to socialization: a longitudinal study of body image in survivors of severe burn injury. J Psychosom Res. 2008;64(2):205–12.
41. Acton A. ABC of burns. When we leave hospital: a patient's perspective of burn injury. BMJ. 2004;329: 504–6.
42. Ehde DM, Patterson DR, Wiechman SA, Wilson LG. Post-traumatic stress symptoms and distress following acute burn injury. Burns. 1999;25(7): 587–92.
43. Mason ST, Esselman P, Fraser R, Schomer K, Truitt A, Johnson K. Return to work after burn injury: a systematic review. J Burn Care Res. 2012;33(1): 101–9.
44. Badger K, Royse D. Describing compassionate care: the burn survivor's perspective. J Burn Care Res. 2012;33:772–80.

Burn-Related Child and Adult Abuse

22

David G. Greenhalgh

Introduction

Unfortunately, burns are not always the results of accidents, but on occasion they are the result of intent to injure. Child maltreatment is the *intentional harm or threat of harm to a child by someone acting the role of caregiver, even if for a short time*. While the recipients of most maltreatment are children, intentional injuries also occur to adults. Usually, those people who are vulnerable—children, emotionally and mentally impaired people, and the elderly—are abused. Burns are also a means of assault. There are four types of maltreatment [1]:

1. **Physical abuse**: inflicting bodily injury by force or by forcing physically harmful activity
2. **Sexual abuse**: exposure to sexual acts or materials, passive use for sexual stimuli, actual sexual contact
3. **Emotional abuse**: coercive, demeaning, overly distant behavior by the caregiver that interferes with the child's normal psychosocial development
4. **Neglect**: failure to provide basic shelter, supervision, medical care, or support (most common and life threatening)

This chapter will only cover the physical abuse related to burns but other forms of abuse that are often linked to burns. The goal of this chapter is to teach the caregiver how to recognize intentional maltreatment and then describe the caregiver's role in treating these patients. The responsibilities of the caregiver are also discussed.

The true incidence of burn-related child abuse is not known but studies suggest that burns make up approximately 10 % of all abuse [2–6]. Data are only available for burn admissions and studies state the abuse makes up 4–10 % of pediatric burn admissions [4, 7–12]. No one knows how many children sustain small, intentional burns in the outpatient setting but they certainly do occur [13]. All studies state that intentional burns are more common at the time of toilet training and usually occur in children less than 5 years of age. Stress is usually associated with abuse [4, 11, 14]. These burns are much more common in lower income and broken families. They often occur in single parent families and in those with lower levels of education. Interestingly, these characteristics are not true for sexual abuse, which covers all economic levels. The perpetrator is often not the parent but another person who is caring for the child (such as the boyfriend). Scalds are the most common type of admitted

D.G. Greenhalgh, M.D. (✉)
Shriners Hospitals for Children Northern California, University of California, Davis Medical Center, 2425 Stockton Boulevard, Sacramento, CA 95817, USA
e-mail: dggreenhalgh@ucdavis.edu

D.G. Greenhalgh (ed.), *Burn Care for General Surgeons and General Practitioners*,
DOI 10.1007/978-3-319-29161-1_22

abuse-related burns. Contact burns are usually small and are usually treated as outpatients. Toddlers are at risk since toilet training increases stress and frustration of the caregiver. Finally, child abuse can be considered an "inherited disease" since parents who were abused as a child are more likely to abuse their children.

The physician and all other caregivers have several roles when faced with child abuse. The caregiver must first become suspicious that abuse has occurred and if there is a concern for maltreatment, then that concern needs to be passed on to the authorities—usually child protection services. The responsibility of reporting any concern that abuse has occurred is a legal requirement that is above caregiver/patient confidentiality. In essence, the caregiver must protect the child from any future abuse by letting authorities know about their concern. Failure to report a suspicion of abuse may lead to legal action against them. The caregiver must take care of the child and must document everything and anything that they observe. They are not, however, to be the judge in the case. Typically, the parent or whoever is with the child is told that the burn is suspicious in nature and will require investigation. Otherwise, unless the courts direct the parent that they are not to visit the child, they are treated like any other parent. A parent who has not abused their child will understand the need for such action. Once care is complete, the decision of whom the child is discharged to is up to social services, child protective services, or other legal authorities.

Recognition of Suspected Burn-Related Child Abuse

Recognition of burn-related child abuse is simple in principle—one must match the "story" with the patient's "burn pattern." When the pattern does not match the story the caregiver is obligated to report his or her concern to the authorities. In order to match the story with the burn pattern, the caregiver must know basic principles on how people are burned. *Burn depth* is dependent on four factors:

1. Temperature of the contacting agent
2. Duration of contact
3. Thickness of skin
4. Blood supply to the skin

The first factor, *temperature of the contacting agent* is obvious—hotter agents produce deeper burns. Obviously, molten steel will create a deeper burn than melted wax. In addition, the mechanism of how the heat is transferred is important. Direct contact with hot metal or liquid transfers the heat more efficiently than through convection or radiation of heat. *Duration of contact* is also very important in determining burn depth. The longer the contact the deeper the burn will be. The minimal temperature to cause a burn is around 43.5° Centigrade (C) [15]. At this temperature many hours are required to produce a superficial burn. Moritz and Henriques published their classic papers that described the relationship between temperature of a liquid and depth of injury in the 1940s [16, 17]. At 160° Fahrenheit (F) (71° Centigrade [C]) a full-thickness burn will occur in 1 s. At 120° F (48.9° C), a full-thickness burn will occur in 10 min. This is the basis of one of the most important prevention efforts: to lower household water heater temperatures to 120° F. These efforts have greatly reduced burns in children and probably will lower the incidence of scald-related child abuse. Duration of contact also affects contact burns. As adults, we have learned to quickly withdraw our hands when we touch a hot surface. Young children, however, freeze when they touch a hot surface and thus sustain deeper burns. The *thickness of skin* principle is also simple; thinner skin tends to be a greater risk for full-thickness injury than thicker skin. For instance, when a hand is exposed to extreme heat, the palm with its thicker skin tends to heal spontaneously. The thinner dorsal hand and volar distal forearm often end up to be full-thickness burns because that skin is significantly thinner. The back, being thicker, often heals well because of this fact. Finally, *greater vascularity in the skin* tends to dissipate the heat and thus lessen the depth of injury. The face, being very vascular, is more tolerant of heat than less vascular areas such as the feet.

Since *scald burns* are the most common type of burn in child abuse, one must understand how a liquid burns a person. There are *two principles of scald injury*:

1. Liquids follow the "law of gravity"
   (a) Free liquids fall to the ground
   (b) Liquids in a container have an upper surface that is horizontal
2. The site of burn injury occurs wherever the hot liquid touches the skin

Accidental scald burns typically occur when a hot liquid "spills" onto a child. The liquid contacts the face, shoulder, chest, or back in a wide area and then courses down the body. As the water travels down a standing child, it narrows the contact area to create a classic "V" pattern that also includes drip patterns (Fig. 22.1). If the child is sitting, the hot liquid will often spill between the legs to burn the upper or inner thighs and genitalia. If the child is wearing clothes, the burn pattern may change because the cloth disperses the liquid. In addition, clothing keeps the hot liquid in contact with the skin for a longer period so that area will be deeper than other areas. The classic scenario is hot liquid spilling on to the face, shirt, and pants. The face burn is more superficial because the liquid rapidly falls off the face. The shirt keeps the fluid in contact longer so that the chest is deeper. The pants, being the last to be removed, results in burns to the thighs that are the deepest of all of the injured areas.

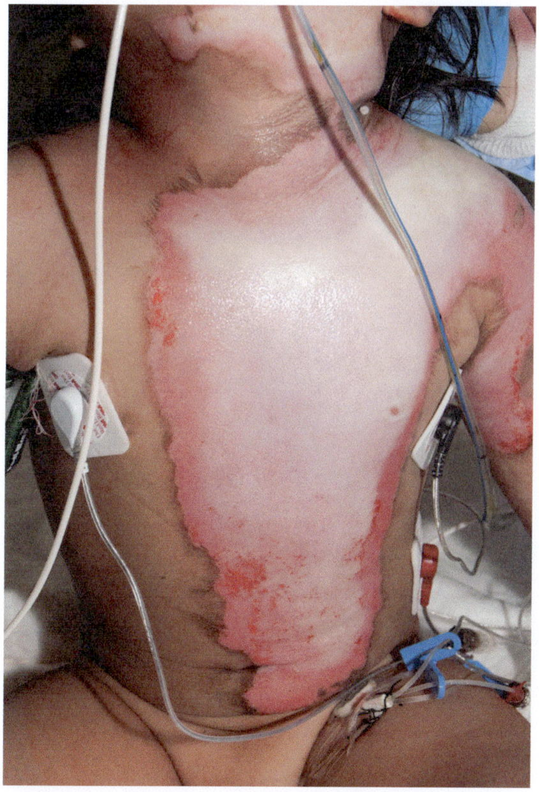

Fig. 22.1 A typical accidental scald injury shows a "V-shaped" pattern as the water runs down the trunk. Typically, there are often "drip" marks. The scald is caused by the hot water falling off the child

Intentional burns often occur by "dipping" a child into a container of hot water—usually a bathtub. These burns may occur accidentally but if the perpetrator describes this injury as a "spill" then one must be concerned about abuse. Since any liquid in a container has a horizontal upper surface, the burn tends to be well demarcated at the top of the injury. The entire burned area is in contact with the hot liquid for the same time so the injury is of uniform depth. Classically, the child is grabbed under the arms and is placed feet and buttocks into the hot bath water. When placed into the tub, they lift their feet, bend their legs, and enter with their feet and buttocks. Therefore, they end up with a demarcated burn that has a line from the lower back, to the lower abdomen and at the lower thighs and upper lower legs—as if the knees are flexed (Figs. 22.2 and 22.3). In several areas, the skin edges are in contact with each other so that no hot water contacts those regions.

The inguinal creases and popliteal regions, which maintain contact, are usually spared (Fig. 22.4). Finally, the buttocks and plantar feet often contact the tub, which is not as hot, so those areas are typically spared or of lesser depth.

Other parts of the body are also subjected to the same principles. Scald burns often occur to the hands when exposed to pouring water. If it is a spill injury, the dorsal hand is injured in an irregular pattern with sparing of the palm as the water falls off the hand (Fig. 22.5). Intentional burns often involve a well-demarcated burn on

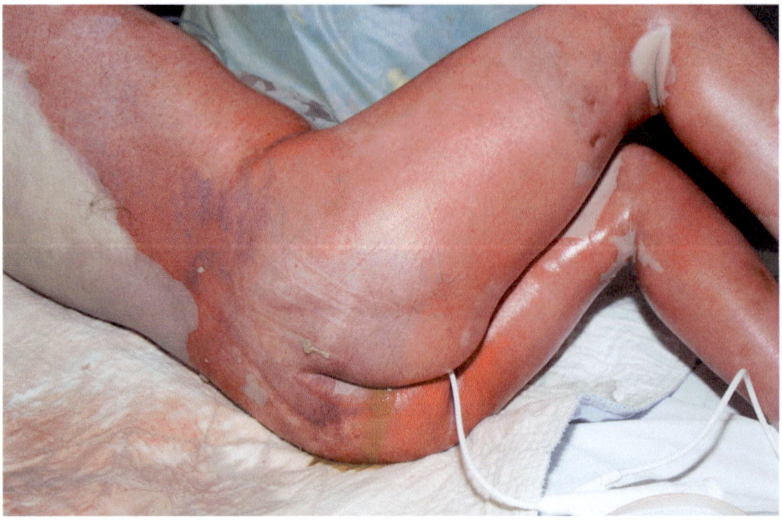

Fig. 22.2 The classic child abuse burn pattern is the "dip" burn. The child is placed feet and buttocks first into hot water. There is a well-demarcated line at the top of where the tub water contacts the skin. This is a severe burn as far as extent of injury

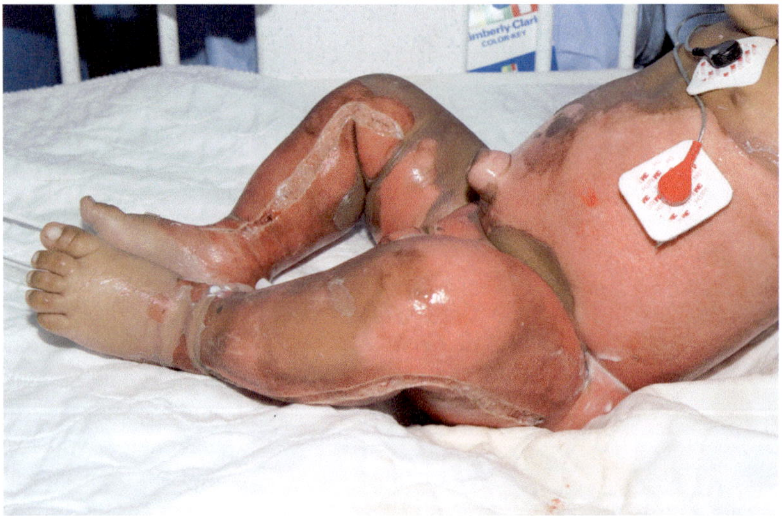

Fig. 22.3 With a "dip" burn there is sparing behind the knees and in the inguinal creases since the skin in that area is in contact with the opposite side (so that water does not touch it)

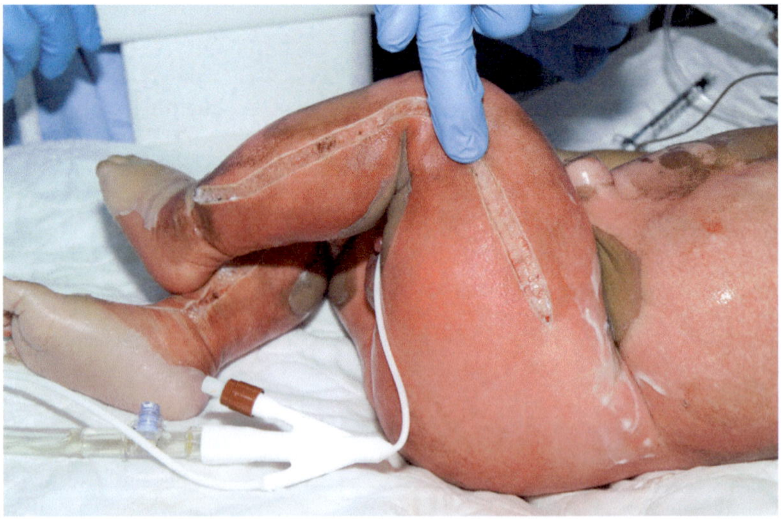

Fig. 22.4 The sparing in the popliteal areas is clearly seen. Since the skin is contacting the opposite side, these areas are spared

the wrist or forearm, and a uniform depth burn throughout the entire hand, as the extremity is forced into the hot liquid (Fig. 22.6). One leg may be placed in hot water to produce a demarcated single lower extremity injury. I have even taken care of a child who had his head dipped into hot water.

There are *characteristics* of the explanation of burn etiology that should raise the suspicion of burn-related child abuse. Just like any patient evaluation, one must consider the *history* provided. Is the story plausible? Could the child really turn on the hot water and get into the tub by him or herself? Does the story change? People who fabricate stories will not provide a consistent explanation of what had happened. On occasion, the perpetrator will try to change the story to fit the burn if the first explanation does not make sense. I had a father who would say "what about this explanation? Does it make the burn make sense?" One should also determine the supervision at the time of burn. Quite often, the perpetrator will state that the baby was left in the care of the young sibling who then is blamed for causing the burn.

When considering the likelihood that the pattern of injury matches the alleged story, one must also understand the *developmental stage of the*

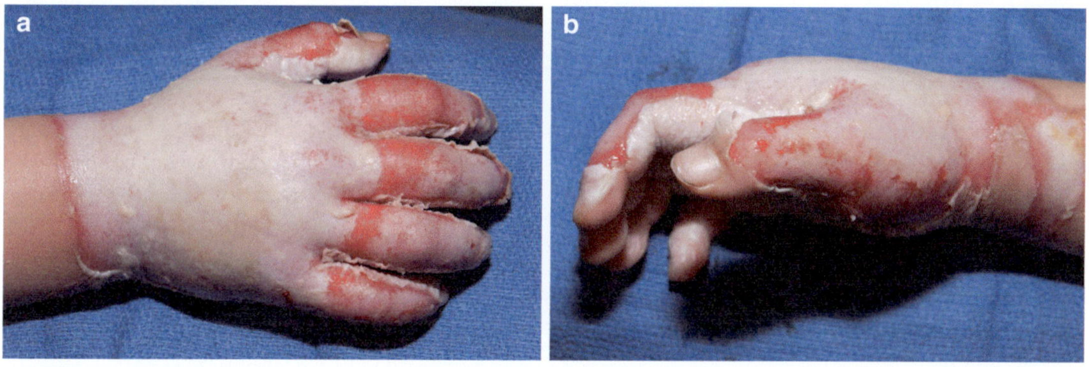

Fig. 22.5 An accidental hand burn usually involves one side of the hand (**a**). By reflex, the fingers usually close to protect the palm (**b**)

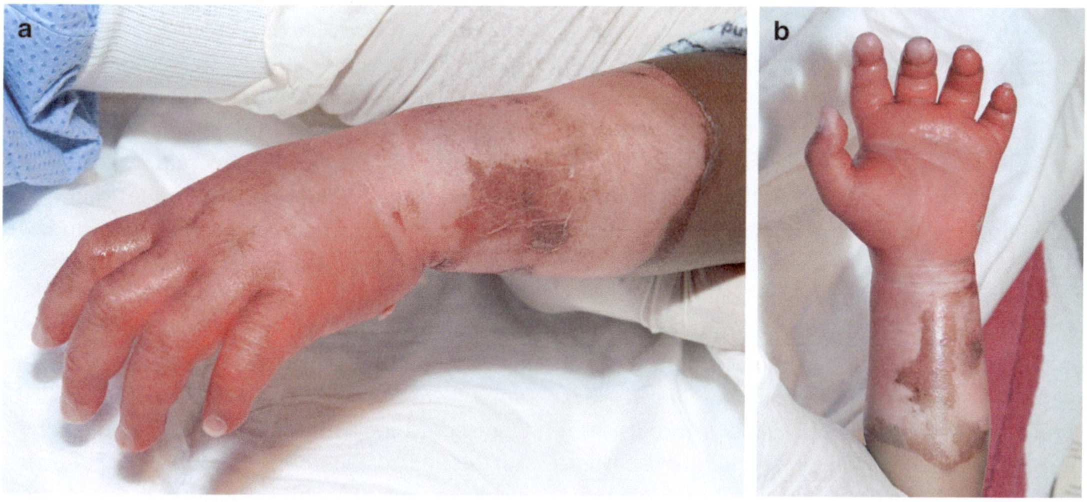

Fig. 22.6 When a hand is forced into hot water the burn usually involves both the dorsal (**a**) and palmar (**b**) aspect of the hand

child. In other words, can the child really do what the perpetrator states he/she did? One must ask what can the child physically do at their current age? Can the child maintain a sitting or standing position? Can the child climb into the tub by himself? Can he climb in the tub without falling or putting hands on the bottom? For instance, I have treated young children with well-demarcated single leg burns with the explanation that they climbed into the tub and stood on one foot. Toddlers are unable to climb into a tub without falling and are unable to stand on one foot and then get out. Very often, the explanation is that the child turned on the hot water but one must ask, can the child grasp the faucet with enough strength or skill to turn it on? Can the child roll over? One child that I treated was 2 months of age when he presented with burns over his posterior legs, buttocks, and back. The story was that the 18-month-old brother placed him in the tub and turned on the hot water. First of all, an 18 month old would not be able to place the child in the tub and create a demarcated burn. Second, a 4 month old is unable to do anything but lie on his back so he would have been unable to maintain a sitting position, or even lift his head off the bottom of the tub.

While it is not the job of the caregiver to be the investigator, the *physical examination* can assist with the investigation. The detective usually determines the maximal temperature of the water and the time required to reach that temperature. Once the depth of injury is determined, one can estimate the duration of contact that occurred at the scene. The distance between the bottom of the buttocks and the top of the burn will also provide the depth of the liquid at the time of injury. This information, along with the size and depth of the tub, will assist with determining how the burn might have occurred. The design of the faucet mechanism will also provide information as to whether a child could turn on the hot water or not. Any information that the child provides should also be documented since, on occasion, the child will say how the injury really occurred. One time I asked a child how she was burned and she stated, "My uncle burned me." This was the only time she stated so but it helped with the investigation. Other findings at the scene are also helpful. If the household is filthy or full of drug paraphernalia one may have more concerns of abuse or neglect.

An *inappropriate response of the child* is also a sign of abuse. If the child fails to cry during painful procedures, such as blood draws or intravenous line placement, then suspicions of abuse should increase. If a child is being chronically physically abused, then crying may lead to more abuse, so he or she learn not to cry when pain is inflicted. The interaction of the child with the parents or caregivers is also important to observe. Most toddlers will not want to leave a mother's side but if they do not care or seem more attached to the caregivers, then one must worry about abuse. One must also watch for signs of fear when exposed to someone such as a boyfriend. Finally, unusual language or age-inappropriate promiscuity may be a sign of sexual abuse.

The child should always have a full physical examination that looks for other signs of injury or abuse. If there are burns of different ages of healing one must be concerned. If the injuries are on unusual sites such as genitalia, eyelids, or buttocks, then suspicions should be raised. There are classic signs of physical abuse such as bruising around the eyes and other areas from punching, and other "grab" marks. Signs of injury from being struck by other objects, such as sticks, whips, and others, should be noted. One should look for more subtle injuries such as retinal hemorrhages and signs of intracranial injuries. One should also perform an examination for fractures, especially in the mid humerus as from the "shaken baby" syndrome. Obtaining total body x-rays is warranted for young children who have significant signs of abuse [18–21]. Finally, checking for sexual abuse is also important.

One must also consider whether there are signs of *neglect*, which is considered one of the worst forms of abuse. Is the child malnourished? One should look for signs of unexpected weight for the age of the child. One should also document whether the child is unusually dirty or is wearing inappropriate clothing. Again, if the house is filthy or used to manufacture illegal drugs raises concerns. Another warning sign is if there are other children with injuries or burns. Clearly, previous reports to child protective services or the law is a warning sign.

There are well-documented warning signs that are often observed in the *parental response*. Most parents are extremely concerned when their child sustains a burn. They will also understand if you tell them that the burn is suspicious and will require some investigation. If, on the other hand, the parents are more concerned with themselves than the child one must worry that something is wrong. The abuser will often be angry or in a hurry instead of being concerned. As stated earlier, the home situation is often one of disarray, with economic and social distress. Parents are often separated or divorced. Physical abuse is more common in the less-educated family than in those with higher levels of education. Drug or alcohol abuse is often more common in the household of the abused child. Frequently, it is not the mother but a boyfriend who really has no interest in the child. On more than one occasion, it appeared as though the mother admitted that she burned the child but it seemed as though she was lying to protect the boyfriend because of fear or love. In addition, other members of the family (such as grandparents) add to the stress by indicating that the mother is doing a poor job or that the boyfriend is a major problem. Finally, child abuse is an "inherited disease" since if a parent was abused as a child, they are more likely to abuse their own children. Many times economic and social stresses are very high and when a child's toileting accident or crying adds to the stress the child is burned.

The *role of the caregiver* is quite simple. They must take care of the child first and foremost. They should tell the parent that the burn is suspicious and will require an investigation. Unless directed to do otherwise by authorities, they should inform the parents of the plan and of the patient's status like they would for any other patient family. All members of the team should document all comments and interactions. They should assist with investigation as described above but no one should judge the family. All caregivers have a *legal obligation* to report any concerns to the authorities. All concerns of potential abuse supersede all claims of professional/client privilege. There are penalties if one fails to report potential abuse.

Burn-Related Adult Abuse

Most burn-related abuse occurs in the young child but one must not forget that adults may also be abused [8, 10, 22–25]. The populations that are most at risk are the elderly, and the physically and mentally disabled. People who depend on others for the majority of their care are at significant risk. Inability to defend oneself is also a risk. Adults are often at risk for being "dipped" in hot water during bathing. They are also at risk for neglect since they are unable to obtain basic needs. Burns are also a means of assault [6, 11, 25–27]. Scalds may occur by throwing hot liquids on to someone. Women are more likely to scald a significant other compared to other forms of assault. Unfortunately, men tend to injure women through flames or chemicals. Men may throw an accelerant onto a woman and ignite it. Chemical burns are often used to intentionally disfigure someone by attacking the face. While the size of the burn may not be large, the chemical tends to lead to severe scarring. This injury seems to be more common in the Middle East and Central Asia.

Summary

Burn-related child and adult abuse is, unfortunately, a form of injury that is not that uncommon. It is the obligation of the caregiver to recognize these injuries and report them to the authorities. The concept is relatively simple; one must match the "story" with the pattern of burn injury. One must also know which families are at greater risk of this type of burn—broken families, socioeconomically depressed, and of lower education levels. Even sadder is the fact that abuse is often transmitted to the next generation since any child who was abused is at higher risk for abusing his or her children. By cooperating with the authorities, the perpetrators can be caught. By improving the social environment in the world, we may reduce the amount of these unfortunate injuries.

References

1. Wissow LS. Child abuse and neglect. N Engl J Med. 1995;332(21):1425–31.
2. Dubowitz H, Bennett S. Physical abuse and neglect of children. Lancet. 2007;369(9576):1891–9.
3. Scalzo A. Burns and child maltreatment. St. Louis, MO: GW Medical Publishing Inc.; 1994.
4. Hummel III RP, Greenhalgh DG, Barthel PP, et al. Outcome and socioeconomic aspects of suspected child abuse scald burns. J Burn Care Rehabil. 1993;14(1):121–6.
5. Lane W, Bair-Merritt MH, Dubowitz H. Child abuse and neglect. Scand J Surg. 2011;100(4):264–72.
6. Reiland A, Hovater M, McGwin Jr G, Rue III LW, Cross JM. The epidemiology of intentional burns. J Burn Care Res. 2006;27(3):276–80.
7. Peck MD, Priolo-Kapel D. Child abuse by burning: a review of the literature and an algorithm for medical investigations. J Trauma. 2002;53(5):1013–22.
8. Greenbaum AR, Donne J, Wilson D, Dunn KW. Intentional burn injury: an evidence-based, clinical and forensic review. Burns. 2004;30(7):628–42.
9. Andronicus M, Oates RK, Peat J, Spalding S, Martin H. Non-accidental burns in children. Burns. 1998;24(6):552–8.
10. Gravante G, Esposito G, Delogu D, Montone A. Intentional burn injuries. Burns. 2006;32(4):526–7.
11. Kumar S, Singh US, Verma AK, Ali W, Krishna A. Intentional and non-intentional burn related deaths: a comparative study of socio-demographic profile. Burns. 2015;41(2):265–70.
12. Thombs BD. Patient and injury characteristics, mortality risk, and length of stay related to child abuse by burning: evidence from a national sample of 15,802 pediatric admissions. Ann Surg. 2008;247(3):519–23.
13. Shavit I, Knaani-Levinz H. Images in emergency medicine. Child abuse caused by cigarette burns. Ann Emerg Med. 2008;51(5):579. 82.
14. Wibbenmeyer L, Liao J, Heard J, Kealey L, Kealey G, Oral R. Factors related to child maltreatment in children presenting with burn injuries. J Burn Care Res. 2014;35(5):374–81.
15. Greenhalgh DG, Lawless MB, Chew BB, Crone WA, Fein ME, Palmieri TL. Temperature threshold for burn injury: an oximeter safety study. J Burn Care Rehabil. 2004;25(5):411–5.
16. Moritz AR, Henriques FC. Studies of thermal injury: II. The relative importance of time and surface temperature in the causation of cutaneous burns. Am J Pathol. 1947;23(5):695–720.
17. Moritz AR, Henriques Jr FC. The reciprocal relationship of surface temperature and time in the production of hyperthermic cutaneous injury. Am J Pathol. 1947;23(5):897.
18. Maguire S, Moynihan S, Mann M, Potokar T, Kemp AM. A systematic review of the features that indicate intentional scalds in children. Burns. 2008;34(8): 1072–81.
19. Degraw M, Hicks RA, Lindberg D. Incidence of fractures among children with burns with concern regarding abuse. Pediatrics. 2010;125(2):e295–9.
20. Fagen KE, Shalaby-Rana E, Jackson AM. Frequency of skeletal injuries in children with inflicted burns. Pediatr Radiol. 2015;45(3):396–401.
21. Hicks RA, Stolfi A. Skeletal surveys in children with burns caused by child abuse. Pediatr Emerg Care. 2007;23(5):308–13.
22. Peck MD. Epidemiology of burns throughout the World. Part II: intentional burns in adults. Burns. 2012;38(5):630–7.
23. Greenbaum AR, Horton JB, Williams CJ, Shah M, Dunn KW. Burn injuries inflicted on children or the elderly: a framework for clinical and forensic assessment. Plast Reconstr Surg. 2006;118(2):46e–58e.
24. Modjarrad K, McGwin Jr G, Cross JM, Rue III LW. The descriptive epidemiology of intentional burns in the United States: an analysis of the National Burn Repository. Burns. 2007;33(7):828–32.
25. Natarajan M. Differences between intentional and non-intentional burns in India: implications for prevention. Burns. 2014;40(5):1033–9.
26. Kaufman MS, Graham CC, Lezotte D, et al. Burns as a result of assault: associated risk factors, injury characteristics, and outcomes. J Burn Care Res. 2007; 28(1):21–8. discussion 9.
27. Das KK, Khondokar MS, Quamruzzaman M, Ahmed SS, Peck M. Assault by burning in Dhaka, Bangladesh. Burns. 2013;39(1):177–83.

Burn Prevention for the Surgeon

23

Ernest J. Grant

The surgeon is in a unique position to promote fire and burn prevention efforts by regularly participating in national, state, and local programs that encourage fire and burn safety education. Additionally, they should also use their influence as head of the health care team to actively endorse legislative agendas that create and maintain a safe environment for all. Finally, whether conducting an initial interview or discharge teaching, as physicians, they are in a unique position to discover potential unsafe activities that may be occurring in the home and should take the appropriate steps to help their patients and families maintain a safer home environment, while continuing to remain culturally sensitive. The surgeon should remember that the best way to treat a burn is to prevent it from occurring in the first place. This chapter presents a historical review of burn prevention efforts, identifies and discusses high-risk populations, and outlines some specific measures that can help reduce the incidence of specific burn injuries.

E.J. Grant, Ph.D., R.N., F.A.A.N. (✉)
North Carolina Jaycee Burn Center, UNC Hospitals, 5th Fl. P.S.T., 101 Manning Dr., Chapel Hill, NC 27514, USA
e-mail: Ernest.Grant@unchealth.unc.edu

Historical Perspective

On a yearly basis, approximately 45,000 Americans are burned significantly enough to require hospitalized treatment. This number also includes the approximately 25,000 individuals whose burns are so significant that they required treatment at one of the 132 designated burn care facilities in the United States and Canada [1, 2]. The National Fire Protection Association (NFPA) reports that fires accounted for 3240 civilian deaths in 2013, the latest date in which figures are available [3]. Although these numbers represents significant improvement over the decades in which data related to fire and burn injuries have been collected, such injuries still rank fourth as the leading cause of unintentional injury deaths in the United States [4]. The publication of the report "America Burning" in 1973 and "America Burning Re-commissioned" in 2000 [5, 6] started a revolution in fire and burn safety awareness that would continue for decades into the future. This publication laid the foundation that identified among other things: (1) the need for the establishment of codes and standards; (2) fire protection planning programs and most importantly; (3) fire and life safety education programs. During the four decades after the initial report, more American homes (96–97 %) have been documented as having at least one *working* smoke alarm [7]. Additionally, adoption of local, state, and national regulations that enforce safer building

D.G. Greenhalgh (ed.), *Burn Care for General Surgeons and General Practitioners*,
DOI 10.1007/978-3-319-29161-1_23

codes and standards such as clearly defined exits and building egress procedures, sprinklers, and fire notification procedures has also led to a reduction in fire and burn injuries. However, the continued high number of fire- and burn-related injuries drives home the need for continued public education. The next section will provide an in-depth historical overview of prevention efforts.

Past Prevention Efforts

One of the most widely known and publicized fires occurred in the United States in 1942. It is known as the Boston Coconut Grove nightclub fire that claimed the lives of 491 individuals. An investigation of the fire revealed that a number of code violations existed such as blocked or locked exits, overcrowding, flammable materials within the building(s), and a lack of sprinklers and smoke alarms [8–10]. As a result of this fire, remarkable advances were made in burn treatment [comprehension of inhalation injuries, fluid resuscitation, and the use of antibiotics] and public safety [revolving doors must also have swing doors, disaster planning, and no combustible materials in places of assembly] [10–13]. It was thought that the enactment of these public safety endeavors would keep the public safe should another fire of this magnitude were to occur again. The likelihood of such safety endeavors being enacted on their own, before such a horrific event, probably would never have occurred.

Shortly after the Cocoanut Grove Fire, another devastating fire occurred that would also awaken the public's conscious regarding fire and burn safety. On July 6, 1944, the big tent of the Ringling Brothers Circus suddenly became inflamed while nearly 7000 people were watching the show. The entire tent was completely demolished within 6 min. One hundred sixty-eight individuals died (two-thirds of them children) and hundreds were severely injured [14, 15]. Following this disaster, flame-retardant compounds were used on circus tents to minimize any future fire spread [14–16]. A review of the fire investigator's reports for both of these fires noted that when the fire occurred, individuals panicked and attempted to head towards the exits in which they had entered out of habit, or because of blocked exits, thus causing congestion and confusion as others attempted to escape as well as the large amount of recorded injuries and deaths.

Over the next 25 or so years following the circus fire, scant progress was made in the effort to promote fire and burn safety. Examples of such progress may include the passage of the 1953 Flammable Fabrics Act. This act was designed to regulate the manufacture or sale of highly flammable clothing [17]. The introduction of the home smoke alarm in the mid-1960s also made a major impact towards the promotion of fire and burn safety. In the early 1970s, the Department of Housing and Urban Development (HUD) project "Operation Breakthrough" stated that smoke detectors should be required in all the homes participating in this project [18]. Additional safety modification included a few attempts at behavioral change (closing the matchbox cover before striking, locking away matches and lighters) or product usage warnings (flammability labeling on fuel cans, safe use of space heaters). Such efforts garnered little success.

Members of the health care team that provided burn care services recognized the need for fire and burn safety education. For example, Dr. Carl Moyer published an article in 1954 entitled "The Treatment of Severe Thermal Injury" in which he stated "The real solution lies not in treatment of burns, but in the prevention, not in the therapeutic but in sociologic medicine. We are not going to stop using fires, warming our houses, cooking our food, bathing in warm water" [14, 19]. Dr. Moyer had the foresight to recognize that behavioral modification alone was not the answer to a prevention-focused initiative.

Present-Day Efforts

Over the last four decades (1960s to 2010s), efforts at promoting fire and burn prevention have made great strides at the local, state, and national levels. During this time period, national campaigns such as Fire Prevention Week©, Burn Awareness Week, and the National Scald Prevention Campaign® that promoted widespread safety initiatives such as the use of smoke alarms, reduction of hot water heater temperatures, and home escape planning may have contributed to the public's awareness of prevention safety [20–22]. In addition, the adoption of formal safety programs promoted by professional organizations such as the NFPA's "Learn-not-to-Burn®" curriculum; public safety programs such as Safe Kids Worldwide; governmental organizations such as the CDC's "National Action Plan for Child Injury Prevention"; and the Consumer Products Safety Commission (CPSC) provide fire and life safety educators with the necessary tools to promote consistent unified safety messages and practice guidelines. Nationally, many public school systems adopted mandatory fire and burn safety education as a component of their health and safety curriculums. The surgeon must realize the importance of ensuring the fire and life safety messages are accurate, adhered to, and remain up-to-date. It is very easy for the public to become complacent with fire and life safety messages since they do not encounter such tragedies on a daily basis. Members of the public may be easily lured into a false sense of security because of all the initiatives taken to maintain a safe environment such as a fully sprinklered building, clearly defined exits, and safety inspections and safety messages. However, as recently as 2003, a major fire occurred at the Station nightclub in Warwick, RI. One hundred people died and over 200 individuals were injured by the band's pyrotechnic display. Egress from the nightclub, (which was not equipped with sprinklers) was hampered by the crowd rushing the main entrance to the building in an attempt to escape; an overcrowded venue with blocked on not obvious exits; combustible interior finishes and incorrect exit doors …a similar problem that had occurred in other similar major US fires [23].

The Five-Step Process

As the population of fire and life safety advocates began to increase, two main strategies have been employed to address fire and life safety programs. The use of the "Five-step Process" and the "Three Es" influenced the approach safety advocates utilized to help tackle and address the fire and burn safety problems. The "Five-Step Process" created by the U. S. Fire Administration was specifically designed to assist with public fire education planning. This process describes a systematic approach to designing, implementing, and evaluating community safety education programs (see Table 23.1). The manual is designed to assist individuals that may be new to community safety education understand some of the basic concepts about how to get started with an organization's community safety education programs. It was also designed to provide some hints and techniques on a variety of topics, such as methods for locating partners to assist with community education or techniques for locating resources for your safety programs [24]. The five steps identified in this process consist of the following:

Step 1: Conduction of a community risk analysis.
Step 2: Development of community partnerships.
Step 3: Create an intervention strategy.
Step 4: Implement the strategy.
Step 5: Evaluate the results.

A description of the components and application of the "Five-Step Process" is detailed in Table 23.1.

Table 23.1 Five essential steps in promoting an injury prevention program

Essential steps	Resources/prevention programs
1. Conduct a community assessment	American Burn Association (ABA) www.ameriburn.org
2. Define the injury problem	American Association of Retired persons (AARP)
3. Set goals and objectives	Nat'l Center for Injury Prevention and Control (NCIPC/CDC)
4. Plan and test interventions	National Fire Protection Association (NFPA) www.nfpa.org
5. Implement and evaluate interventions	US Fire Administration (USFA) www.usfa.fema.org
	American Council of the Blind
	National Center for Health Statistics (NCHS)
	National Fire Incident Reporting System (NFRIS)
	The National Institute on Deafness and Other Communication Disorders (NIDOCD)

Reprinted from Ref. [14] with permission from Elsevier

The Five Es

Initially known as the "Three Es" concept (Table 23.2) was another approach fire and life safety advocates have used to identify risk factors and subsequently develop a strategic plan to alleviate potential injuries. The components of the "three Es" are *Education, Environment, and Enforcement.* In 2000, the National Fire Academy (NFA) added the components of "*economic incentive*" and "*emergency response*" because of their importance to community risk reduction [25]. This concept is known and referred to as the "Five Es" of prevention. Each of these concepts may be utilized in primary, secondary, and tertiary prevention initiatives. The "*Education*" component promotes the dissemination of information to at-risk individuals or targeted groups. The information disseminated usually includes a detailed description of the injury or risk at hand and the necessary steps the target audience (or individual) could (or should) take to avoid them; it also promotes an attitude or behavior change. This component is useful when: (1) there is new information about a risk that the target audience may already be familiar, but are unfamiliar with the new information; (2) No other approach to promote or demonstrate safety behavior may exist; (3) advocates may be seeking to influence policy makers and design engineers, and (4) there is a recognized need to teach a specific behavior or skill [25, 26]. This method is only effective if individuals recognize their vulnerability and take the initiative to do what will keep them safe.

Table 23.2 The five "Es" of prevention

"E"	Explanation
Education	Education is used to inform the target group about potential hazards or risks based upon their current behavior. Education may not cause the individual to change their behavior, but does increase injury awareness. An educational example would be informing about the need to change their smoke alarm every 10 years
Environment	Environment refers to the use of passive interventions that promote fire and burn safety behaviors. There is no direct action required by the consumer. The use of and installation of a long-life or ten year smoke alarm is a good example of environmental change
Enforcement	Attempts to reduce unsafe behavior through the use legislative codes, standards, or regulations. Regulations may govern the actions of manufacturers, consumers, or local government. A law requiring landlords to have a working smoke alarm installed in all rental property is an example of regulations that may reduce the possibility of loss of life in the event of a fire.
Economic incentive	Incentives that may be used to influence or persuade individual behaviors either positively or negatively. Positive incentives may be used as a reward (monetary, gifts, etc.) for individuals behaving in a certain manner. Negative incentives may be the issuance of tickets, fines, or punishment for not behaving in a certain manner. An example of a positive incentive may be a discount on homeowner's insurance if a smoke alarm is present.
Emergency response	Emergency response initiatives are used by EMS personnel to reduce the potential of a risk. Recognizing potential community dangers or planning for community disasters are example of how emergency response may be used as part of the five "Es" of prevention For example, after practicing for a local disaster (chemical spill, tornado drill or hurricane evacuation) an evaluation of the event may assist community planners in determing available resources or needs.

The environmental approach is the second component of the three E concept. This technique embraces the concept that environmental changes could reduce injury risks. Changes may include the physical surroundings such as changes to a pathway or exit route; products such as safety equipment utilized in vehicles, and the social environment such as attitudes towards fire play. The unique concept surrounding the use of the environmental approach is that it does not depend upon the actions of others, but are usually passive, automatic, or constant in their protective effects [26]. The installation of the home smoke alarm is a good example of the environmental approach. It provides the three protective concepts (passive, automatic, and constant) with little effort by the consumer other than a battery chance or alarm replacement every 10 years.

The third "E" refers to the concept of enforcement. The enforcement approach seeks to effect a behavioral change through the process of legislative initiatives, such as laws/policy, codes, and standards. This process may require or prohibit actions thought necessary to keep the public safe. A good example of this process is the recent enactment of Reduced Ignition Propensity Cigarette Legislation (also known as fire-safe or self-extinguishing cigarettes) in all 50 states. According to the NFPA, 2012 was the first year such laws became effective in all 50 states. A projection linking the percentage decline in fire deaths to the percentage of smokers covered suggests that when smoking material fire death numbers are analyzed for the year 2012, the reduction in civilian deaths will reach roughly 30 % [27]. Other examples of how such laws may require or prohibit specific actions to promote safety are listed in Box 23.1.

As previously mentioned, the NFA added two additional "Es" in 2000. The notion of "economic incentive" implies measures that may be undertaken to influence behaviors in a positive or negative manner. For example, a positive incentive may be a discount on a homeowner's insurance coverage if proof is provided that the home has a working smoke alarm. In addition to discounts, other positive incentives may include such things as offering monetary rewards, sales or coupons for the purchase of safety equipment. An example of a negative economic incentive may be issuance of fines or citation for failing to enact certain safety behaviors such as proper storage of flammables [25].

The "emergency response" premise refers to interventions that may be taken by emergency responders to mitigate risks [25]. This is achieved by responders having a thorough knowledge of the available community resources and capabilities when formulating a community risk assessment plan. Having a working knowledge of resources may necessitate the need to enhance identified areas of weakness. For example, if it is discovered that a particular manufacturer within the community used extremely hazardous chemicals as a part of their manufacturing process, having that knowledge will allow emergency responders to better plan for and practice a response in the event of a spill. As a part of the planned response, it may be discovered that a lack of capabilities for a specific response dictates further training and specific knowledge, equipment or tools to help mitigate this deficiency before emergency services are overwhelmed by demands.

The application of consistent messaging follows a long period of safety messages being taught in a variety of ways and is a relatively new concept that has been embraced by present-day fire and life safety advocates. The application of consistent messages and guidelines reduces the potential of recipients receiving mixed messages. An example of a mixed message would be teaching the concept of the "Stop, drop, and roll" (SDR) procedure should an individual's clothing catch afire. Should the safety technique be taught as "stop," "drop," and "roll," or "stop," "drop," "*cover your eyes*," and then "roll," or "Stop," "drop," and "*roll all the way over [or side-to-side]*" to extinguish the flame. According to the NFPA, the correct technique is to stop, drop to the ground, and cover your face with your hands. Roll over and over or back and forth until the fire is out [28]. A good slogan has three characteristics: it is easily understood, easily remembered, and effectively incorporates the essential aspects required to protect the intended audience. The current Stop, Drop, and Roll (SDR) slogan has the characteristics of being a good slogan, having only four terms ("stop," "drop," and "roll") that members of the general public are able to understand and remember easily. Another important aspect of the SDR message is that the public is able to associate the technique with a specific situation and the message is simple [28].

Future Implications

The future of fire and burn prevention initiatives is looking brighter. The surgeon must recognize that such initiatives should incorporate new educational approaches such as the use of technology (communication, digital, data analysis, and robotics/interactive play) and other resources such as product redesign, marketing, and legislative initiatives to achieve a successful prevention-focused program. It is imperative that the surgeon recognize that the future of burn prevention lies in the team approach [14]. Examples of how to use such programs, initiatives, and endeavors may consist of the following:

Enhanced Organizational Awareness on Prevention

As the head of the Burn Team, the surgeon should recognize the influence they may have with hospital administration to get them to support burn prevention initiatives. By blending a combination of marketing skills and public education, the surgeon should be able to achieve the full support of hospital administrators to back prevention-focused initiatives. From a marketing perspective, these initiatives create a branding opportunity and name recognition for both the burn center and the hospital within the community. It also creates an opportunity to collaborate with the local fire service and other safety-oriented organizations within the community. Having the surgeon (or his/her team representative) champion such causes reinforces the notion that prevention is an important, cost-effective risk reduction tool [24]. Additionally, achieving verification by such organizations as the American Burn Association, the American Trauma Society, etc., may well depend upon how successful burn center sponsored prevention programs are supported by the facility in which it is located.

Greater Comprehension of Data Collection and Analysis

We are living in a society that collects data about everything. However, there are some areas in which available data is lacking or unattainable. The National Fire Incident Reporting System (NFIRS) and the ABA Burn Registry collect data on most fires and burns that occur in the United States and Canada respectively [24, 29]. Be that as it may, data obtained only represents a nominal portion of potential information regarding fires and burns as many fire departments and burn centers do not contribute to these databases. The surgeon should start an initiative within their community to collaborate and team with other agencies such as law enforcement, fire departments, health department, and fire marshal's offices that may collect fire and burn data. Gathering and analyzing data is an essential part of planning and developing an effective program. The success of a burn prevention strategy depends on the availability of demographic data and reliable burn statistics, including mortality rates and, more importantly, morbidity rates [14]. Before a strategy can be designed, developed, implemented, and evaluated, the problem must be identified and analyzed. By collecting data, injury prevention personnel are able to (1) identify the magnitude of the type of injury, (2) monitor trends and specific areas of burn injury, (3) identify problems that may occur, and (4) evaluate burn prevention or intervention efforts [14, 30]. Using such tools as GPS mapping, the surgeon could use data obtained to design a specific injury prevention campaign for a specific neighborhood or zip code. GPS mapping may also help design culturally sensitive programs for a targeted area that may reflect a growing ethnicity. Other team members could ensure the success of such program by providing on-going monitoring to evaluate the success of such programs and make adjustments accordingly.

Integrated Use of Prevention Interventions

The "five Es" concept as described earlier provides an opportunity for the surgeon to choose the best approach when planning a prevention strategy. However, the surgeon should remember that the most effective strategies incorporate all five concepts (education, engineering enforcement, economic incentive, and EMS) to ensure the most successful outcome. The five interventions working together tackle the problem from all sides so the ability to reduce death and injuries is improved dramatically [25].

Enhanced Application of Technology

There is no doubt that technological advancements made within the past few years have greatly contributed to the reduction of deaths and injuries associated with fires and burns. Appliances with automatic shut-off switches, exterior oven doors that remain cool when the interior is hot, residential sprinklers, and improvement in advanced warning systems are just a few examples of risk reduction technology. The surgeon should embrace computer technology as a tool and incorporate its use to assist with prevention strategies. Various apps are available that monitors the efficiency of early warning devices (smoke and Co alarms) and reminds the consumer when critical values have been reached or the need to replace such devices. Computer simulations that allow the consumer to draw a blueprint of their home could assist the homeowner in planning and determining the best escape routes to take in the event of a fire or when practicing home escape planning. Preloaded safety programs and messages may be downloaded onto computers that would allow the consumer the opportunity to watch and learn safety information at their convenience and in their native language. Such programs would allow the consumer to replay information they may not have understood. Interactive programs would allow the consumer to direct specific questions and concerns to program officials, thus creating a tailor-made personalized safety program. As technology continues to advance, surgeons and prevention specialist need to work with engineers and manufacturers to assist with designing products that will continue to promote a safe environment.

The Role of the Surgeon in Promoting Burn Prevention

As previously mentioned, the surgeon is in a unique position to help promote burn prevention. When promoting such efforts, the surgeon's role is that of remembering the importance of considering such aspects as cultural, socioeconomic, and community resources. For example, depending upon their culture, location, and economic condition, individuals may use portable heating equipment such as a kerosene heater as an alternative heating and cooking source to save money. Poorer households may be less likely to have a safe heating system, code compliance electrical services, smoke alarms, or other fire-safe security measures. Their financial difficulties may present a potential challenge for the surgeon when assessing their prevention needs [14]. However, if the surgeon has a working knowledge of community resources he/she may be able to connect the individuals with available resources to alleviate a potential injury.

Though their main role is health promotion, the surgeon should also seize every opportunity to emphasize prevention as well. The surgeon should see their role as taking a proactive stance in promoting fire and burn prevention strategies. This may be performed on many fronts. For example, conducting a TV or radio interview concerning a fire in which one or several individuals may have sustained a burn injury creates the perfect teaching moment. Simply stating that an early warning device such as a *working* smoke alarm and prevention education could have prevented the incidence or given the injured an opportunity to escape sends a message to others in the community of the need to check their smoke alarm.

The surgeon must also recognize the importance and benefits of building a coalition of similar minded agencies and organizations (local, state, and national) when deciding whether to address legislative initiatives that may or may not promote a safe environment for the community. For example, if the local or state government is considering permitting the sale of pyrotechnics within the community or across the state, the lone voice of the surgeon voicing concern that permitting such sales may result in an increase in burn and traumatic injuries may not be enough to deter the enactment of such legislation. However, the formation of a coalition with similar local, state, and national life safety organizations, such as the National Fire Protection Association®, SafeKids Worldwide®, local fire safety educators, Emergency Nurses Association, Pediatric Society, American Trauma Society, Academy of Family Physicians to site a few, could be enough to deter such legislative actions. Additionally, the coalition could compile resources such as data (incidents frequency, body parts injuries, estimated costs, time lost from work or school, suppression costs, property damage), money, technology, and content expertise. The formation of a coalition also ensures that everyone involved has the same message, data, and concerns. A legislative initiative that enforce or enrich current and new regulations may help to reduce fire and burn injuries. Government officials are more likely to respond to groups that present as a united front with a consolidated initiative and concern than the lone voice of one individual.

Age-Related Burn Prevention

A burn injury may occur to anyone at any time; however certain individuals are more vulnerable than others. Individuals who are at an increased risk may include infants, young children, older adults, and persons with disabilities. These individuals may lack the ability to escape a fire or life-threatening situation or the ability to tolerate the physical stress a burn injury may impose on the body. Suggested prevention strategies and coalition partners associated with each of the identified groups are addressed.

Infants and Preschool-Aged Children

Because they have little control over their environment, this very vulnerable group depends upon their parents or caregivers for safety and protection. Burns and fires are the fifth most common cause of accidental death in children and adults and account for an estimated 3500 adult and child deaths per year [31]. Scald burns (caused by hot liquids or steam) and contact burns (caused by touching a hot object) are the most common types of burn-related injuries among young children [14]. Therefore, any fire and burn prevention initiative and strategies should be focused on educating parents and caregivers to create a safe environment such as reducing hot water heater temperatures to 120 °F/48 °C or just below the medium setting. An example of the time and temperature necessary to produce a scald burn in the older and infants is outlined in Table 23.3. The installation of anti-scald valves in the shower or tub could also prevent the possibility of a bathroom-related scald injury. Kitchen safety for this special group includes instructing parents and caregivers to turn pot handles away from the edge of the stove and cook on the back burners of the stove. Creating a "no kid zone" around the stove, ovens, or hot items is another kitchen safety burn prevention tip [32]. Additional ways to reduce scald injuries is outlined in Box 23.1. Enlisting the assistance of infant and preschool-aged childhood organizations such as a local social services

Table 23.3 Relationship between the temperature of tap water and time elapse before a scald injury occurs in the adult and infant

Temperature		Degree burn			
		Adult		Infant	
Degrees centigrade	Degrees Fahrenheit	2nd	3rd	2nd	3rd
70	158	Instant	Instant	Instant	Instant
65	149	Instant	1 s	Instant	Instant
60	140	2 s	5 s	Instant	1 s
55	131	11 s	20 s	2 s	5 s
50	122	2 min	7 min	11 s	20 s
45	113	1 h 46 min	2 h 7 min	2 min	7 min
40	104	–	–	1 h 46 min	2 h 7 min

Reprinted from Ref. [14] with permission from Elsevier and Courtesy of the N. C. Jaycee Burn Center, UNC School of Medicine, Chapel Hill, NC

Box 23.1. Suggested Ways to Reduce Scald Injuries Caused by Hot Liquids

- Ensure that the hot water heater is set at a temperature of 90°–120°F (32.2–48.9 °C).
- Install tempering valves (anti-scald devices) in all faucets and shower heads.
- When preparing a bath, always turn on the cold water first, then, gradually add hot water to the desired temperature.
- Always test the water temperature with your hands before putting children into or stepping into the tub.
- If uncertain about the water temperature, use a commercial thermostat or bath thermometer to check the temperature.
- When using the microwave, always read and follow directions and warnings on microwaveable foods. Open microwave heated containers away from your body as contents may be hot.
- Never cuddle or hold children (or pets) when drinking hot drinks.
- Do not cook with children or pets in the kitchen or cooking area. Create a "No Kids/Pet" zone three feet in front of the stove.
- Always turn pot handles in when cooking on the stove.
- When possible, only cook on back burners.
- Keep small appliances (crock pots, toaster ovens) at the back of the counter, with their cords out of the way of children.

organization, daycare association, children's advocacy group, and pediatrician group may also help the surgeon promote safety initiatives. Such organization may be able to provide age appropriate learning characteristics that may enhance the program's design.

School-Aged Children

Elementary and junior high school students are more prone to sustaining a burn injury when their clothing ignites. This usually is associated with curiosity or fascination while playing with matches or lighters or spilling gasoline on their clothing while attempting to refuel the lawnmower [33]. Other burn-related injuries may be the result of unsupervised cooking or horseplay in kitchen. Modern fashion trends call for children to wear very loose-fitting clothing which if ignited would support combustion due to the air between the garment and the skin [34]. Once their clothing has ignited, children may instinctively run, providing oxygen and increasing flame propagation, and resulting in more severe burns. Educational strategies that promote the "Stop, Drop, and Roll" technique is an important lifesaving behavior for this group to know. This behavior gives them a means to protect themselves and minimize fire spread by limiting thc supply of air, thus smothering the flames. Kitchen safety for this age group centers on adult supervision. Performing simple tasks such as using the microwave to heat soups and popcorn could result in a burn injury. Providing clear safety instructions such as opening microwaved products away from the face may reduce the potential of a burn injury. Collaborating with organizations such as the fire service, boy and girl scouts and the local clubs or organizations within the schools may prove beneficial for such safety initiatives.

Older Adults

Current projections estimate close to 17 % of the total US population will be older than 65 by the year 2020. This percentage will continue to rise annually until it peaks at more than 20 % in 2050 [2, 35–38]. The older adult population is susceptible to fire- or burn-related injuries for a number of reasons such as changes in physical and mental abilities, comorbidities such as diabetes, aging/frailty, malnutrition, and impaired senses. A study [39] conducted in 2008 noted inadequate safety equipment in the homes of 50 % of the older adults and 30 % had tap water temperatures in excess of 60 °C (140 °F). Older adults, like young children, have thinner skin, so exposures to burning substances such as hot liquids can cause a deeper burn with even brief exposure. Marketing and other research studies have shown repeatedly that one of the most major concerns of older Americans is their health and safety [14]. The above data make apparent the message of fire and burn prevention should be carried to the older adult population in such a manner that they will be motivated to take action on their own behalf. To be effective educators, surgeons need to be able to assess and remedy knowledge deficits and beliefs about fire and burn safety in older adults. However, having knowledge is insufficient, persons who learn the risks and dangers of burns would be expected to assess their environment and make changes that would decrease their risk for injury from fire and burn.

However, this population may not have the means to make the necessary changes. A few key elements for the surgeon to consider when preparing to present fire and burn safety education to older adults are:

- Encourage their participation during discussion topic.
- Keep the message short and simple.
- Repeat key messages.
- Provide local examples.
- Emphasize positive behaviors.
- Host mid-morning classes.

The surgeon should consider collaborating with organizations that focus on the health and safety of the older adults such as the local council on aging, fire department, and social services. Additional agencies to form a partnership with may include the local meals-on-wheels program and home health agencies. When contemplating a senior-specific fire and burn safety program, the surgeon must also be aware that some program participants may have low literacy skills. Appy (2005) pointed out that adults with low literacy skills put themselves in danger of failing to receive and understand basic fire prevention and protection messages and to utilize essential fire safety devices [40]. Therefore safety programs should include a variety of communicative means such as simple words, pictures, and simple pictorial diagrams and videos to ensure that the intended message is received without creating an embarrassing situation for the learner or the instructor.

Burn Prevention for Individuals with Disabilities

There are wide variations in the definition of a disability. According to the Americans with Disabilities Act (ADA), a disability is defined as (1) a physical or mental impairment that substantially limits one or more of the major life activities of an individual, (2) a record of such an impairment, or (3) being regarded as having such an impairment. Major life activities are functions such as thinking and caring for oneself, performing manual tasks, walking, seeing, hearing, speaking, breathing, learning, and working [41]. Individuals with disabilities face unique challenges if they are unprepared in the event of an emergency. Even if steps have been taken to be prepared for emergencies, individuals may still be at risk if their safety depends upon caregivers that may be absent or otherwise distracted. The surgeon should remember that safety education should be based around the abilities of the individual and should include them and their caretakers to help reinforce the lessons. Partnering with local and national organizations that provide specific disability services (deaf and hard of hearing, blind services, brain trauma, etc.) may prove to be very beneficial when designing programs specifically designed for this very high-risk population. To be more effective at reaching individuals with disabilities or their caregivers, programs must consider providing (1) materials in alternative formats such as large print, braille, audiotapes, or disk, (2) sensitivity training for instructors, and (3) means of communications between emergency service providers and people with disabilities or their caregivers. Table 23.4 identifies burn prevention strategies and educational topics for individuals with disabilities.

Table 23.4 Burn prevention strategies and educational campaigns for individuals with disabilities

Prevention strategies	Educational topics
Identify the nearest emergency exits	Plan and practice escape around abilities
Install and maintain smoke alarms	Never leave stove unattended while cooking
Have a fire extinguisher available and learn how to use it	Never leave smoking materials unattended
Live near an exit	Educational materials in alternate format
Plan and practice an escape plan	Fire sprinkler protection
Involve the fire department	

Reprinted from Ref. [14] with permission from Elsevier

Vision-Hearing and Mobility Impaired Persons

Individuals with vision, hearing, and mobility impairments must take extra precautions when it comes to their health and well-being, especially in regard to fire and burn safety. Interactions with an environment in which they cannot see, hear, or maneuver around may create potential health and safety hazards. As a result of their disabilities, these individuals may be at an increased risk of injury or death in the event of a fire or burn injury. When designing fire and burn safety programs related to individuals with special needs, the surgeon should seek assistance from local and national organizations that provide assistive services to these high-risk groups. The surgeon should also keep in mind that safety programs should be based around the individual's disability and capabilities. For example, a home escape plan for an individual with partial vision lost may include the use of an exit sign that flashes when the fire alarm is activated. Individuals with total blindness may need to have a visual/light alarm signals in the areas in which they dwell as well as known area of refuge to shelter in place [42]. A safety program designed for individuals that may be deaf or hard or hearing should include the installations of a visual and tactile smoke alarm. These alarms are designed as an assistive device rather than compensate for the inability to hear [14]. Individuals with mobility and thought impairments may be restricted from swift actions when faced with a challenging situation such as the need to escape in the event of a fire. Safety programs for this particular group should first focus on the individuals and their caregivers recognizing their vulnerability due to their limitations. The next step should center on educating these individuals to practice techniques that decrease their chances of accidentally sustaining a burn injury in the event of fire or while cooking or other activities of daily living such as bathing. Discussion should center on the installation of anti-scald devices in the kitchen and bathroom. Educational programs should focus on the use of assistive devices that are designed to meet the specific disability needs of the individual, thus making a potential challenging situation no longer insurmountable.

Summary

The surgeon is in a unique position to lead fire and burn prevention programs. Their intimate interactions with individuals that have sustained a burn injury due to a lack of sufficient education, failure to practice safety maneuvers, or installation of safety equipment or early warning devices in the home should serve as a catalyst for the surgeon to promote fire and burn safety. During initial interviews or upon discharge, the surgeon should rely on their assessment skills (or members of the Burn Team) to determine whether their patients may be returning to an unsafe environment. If such a situation is discovered, appropriate social contacts and referrals should be made to ensure that culturally sensitive needs of the patient and their family are met. Finally, the surgeon should lead by example and pledge to practice fire and burn safety in their personal lives at all times.

References

1. American Burn Association. Burn incidence and treatment in the United States: (2015) fact sheet. 2015. http://www.ameriburn.org/resources_factsheet.php.
2. Grant EJ. Preventing burns in the elderly. Home Healthc Nurse. 2014;31(10):561–73. doi:10.1097/01.NHH.0000436217.56972.58.
3. National Fire Protection Association. An overview of the U. S. Fire problem: fire analysis and research. 2015. http://www.nfpa.org/research/reports-and-statistics/printable-fact-sheets.
4. Peck MD. Epidemiology of burns throughout the world. Part I: distribution and risk factors. Burns. 2011; 37(7):1087–100. doi:10.1016/j.burns.2011.06.005.
5. National Commission on Fire and Control and the United States Fire Administration. America Burning: The Report of the National Commission on Fire Prevention and Control. (Library of Congress Card Number 73–600022). 1973. http://www.usfa.fema.gov/downloads/pdf/publications/fa-264.pdf.
6. United States Fire Administration. America Burning Recommissioned (USFA Publication No. HQ-00-144). Washington, DC. 2000. https://www.fema.gov/news-release/2000/12/13/america-burning-recommissioned-issues-final-report.
7. Aherns M. Smoke alarms in U.S. home fires. Quincy, MA: National Fire Protection Association; 2014.
8. Reilly WA. Report concerning the Cocoanut Grove Fire, November 28, 1942. Boston: City of Boston Printing Dept; 1944.
9. Grant CC. Last dance at the Cocoanut Grove. Nati Fire Protect Assoc J. 1991;85(3):74–76.
10. Esposito JC. Fire in the grove. Cambridge, MA: Da Capo Press; 2005.
11. Moulton RS. The Cocoanut Grove night club fire, Boston, November 28, 1942. Natl Fire Protect Assoc J. 1943;11:1–19.
12. Saffle JR. The 1942 Fire at Boston's Cocoanut Grove Night Club. Am J Surg. 1993;166(6):581–91.
13. Hall Jr JR, Cote AE. An overview of the fire problem and fire protection. In: Cote AE, Grant CC, Hall Jr JR, Solomon RE, editors. Fire protection handbook, vol. 1. Quincy, MA: National Fire Protection Association; 2008. Sec. 3.25.
14. Grant EJ. Burn prevention. In Flynn MB, editor. Crit Care Nurs Clin North Am 16(1):127–38. Philadelphia: Elsevier Saunders; 2004.
15. Brown RJ. The day the clowns cried. 2015. http://www.historybuff.com/library/reffire.html.
16. Goldberg K. The Hartford circus fire of 1944. The concord review. 1990. http://www.tcr.org/tcr/essays/Web_Hartford.pdf.
17. U.S. Consumer Products Safety Commission. Flammable Fabrics Act: Public Law 88, Chapter 164; 83d Congress, 1st Session, H.R.5069. U.S. Government Printing Office. 1953. https://books.google.com/books/about/Flammable_Fabrics_Act.html?id=4vI9AAAAYAAJ.
18. Milke J. The history of smoke detection: a profile of how the technology and role of smoke detection has changed. 2011. www.nfpa.org/~/media/files/…/sup-det11milkeabstract.pdf?la=en.
19. Moyer CA. The treatment of severe thermal injury. West J Surg Gynecol. 1954;62:107–20.
20. National Fire Protection Association. About fire prevention week. 2015. http://www.nfpa.org/safety-information/fire-prevention-week.
21. American Burn Association Burn Awareness Week. 2015. http://ameriburn.org/preventionBurnAwareness.php.
22. National Scald Prevention Campaign. 2012. http://ffburn.org/wp-content/uploads/2012/06/NationalScaldPrevention.pdf.
23. Grosshandler WL, Bryner NP, Madrzykowski D, Kuntz K. Report of the technical investigation of the station nightclub fire, vol 1. 2005. National Institute of Standards and Technology. (21521 K).
24. U.S. Fire Administration. Public fire education planning a five step process (FA-219). 2008. https://www.usfa.fema.gov/downloads/pdf/publications/fa-219.pdf.
25. U.S. Department of Homeland Security, Federal Emergency Management Agency. Executive analysis of community risk reduction course. 2012. https://www.usfa.fema.gov/downloads/pdf/coffee-break/fm/fm_2013_13.pdf.
26. Christoffel T, Gallagher SS. Injury prevention and public health. 2nd ed. Burlington, MA: Jones & Bartlett publishers; 2005.
27. Coalition for Fire-Safe Cigarettes. Fire-safe cigarette legislation. 2015. http://www.nfpa.org/safety-information/for-consumers/causes/smoking/coalition-for-fire-safe-cigarettes.
28. National Fire Protection Association. Educational messages desk reference. Quincy, MA: National Fire Protection Press; 2015. http://www.nfpa.org/safety-information/for-public-educators/educational-messaging/educational-messages-advisory-committee.
29. The American Burn Association. National Burn Registry, burn repository data. 2015. http://www.ameriburn.org/NBR.php.
30. Hunt JL. The presidential address: back to the future: the ABA and burn prevention. J Burn Care Rehabil. 2000;21(6):474–83.
31. Johns Hopkins Medicine. Burns in Children factsheet. 2015. http://www.hopkinsmedicine.org/healthlibrary/printv.aspx?d=90, P01887.
32. American Burn Association. Pediatric scalds: a burning issue factsheet. 2015. http://www.ameriburn.org/Preven/PediatricScalds_2-27-15.pdf.
33. Nationwide Children's Hospital. Burn prevention: pre-school and school age. 2105. Accessed from: http://www.nationwidechildrens.org/burn-prevention-preschool-and-school-age.
34. Rodgers GB, Adair PK. Exemption to the children's sleepwear flammability standards: a description of policy consideration and an evaluation of the effect on burn injuries to children. J Consum Pol 2009;32(1): 59–71. http://link.springer.com/article/10.1007%2Fs10603-009-9092-y. doi 10.1007/s10603-009-9092-y.

35. Miller AM, Iris M. Health promotion attitudes and strategies in older adults. Health Educ Behav. 2002;29(2):249–67.
36. Ortman JM, Velkoff VA, Hogan H. An Aging Nation: the older population in the United States. U.S. Department of Commerce Economics and Statistics Administration. U.S. Census Bureau. 2014. http://www.census.gov/prod/2014pubs/p25-1140.pdf.
37. Transgenerational.org. The demographics of aging. 2009. http://transgenerational.org/aging/demographics.htm.
38. U.S. Census Bureau. The next four decades, the older population in the United States: 2010 to 2050. 2010. http://www.census.gov/prod/2010pubs/p25-1138.pdf.
39. Davidge K, Fish J. Older adults and burns. Geriatr Aging. 2008;11(5):270–5.
40. Appy M. The Home Safety Council and its challenge. Am J Prev Med. 2005;28(1):70–1. doi:10.1016/j.amepre.2004.09.022.
41. U.S. Department of Commerce. Americans with disabilities: 1994–95. Economic and Statistic Administration, U. S. Bureau of Census, Household Economic Studies, 1997; Washington, DC: Current Population Reports # p70–61.
42. United States Fire Administration. Fire risks for the blind or visually impaired. Emmitsburg, MD: TriData Corp; 1999.

Index

D.G. Greenhalgh (ed.), *Burn Care for General Surgeons and General Practitioners*,
DOI 10.1007/978-3-319-29161-1

MIX
Papier aus verantwortungsvollen Quellen
Paper from responsible sources
FSC® C105338
FSC
www.fsc.org

If you have any concerns about our products,
you can contact us on
ProductSafety@springernature.com

In case Publisher is established outside the EU,
the EU authorized representative is:
Springer Nature Customer Service Center GmbH
Europaplatz 3, 69115 Heidelberg, Germany

Printed by Libri Plureos GmbH
in Hamburg, Germany